MASTER
MEDICINE

Systematic
Pathology

For Paulina, Aaron, David and Abraham.
Thanks for all the encouragement
PB

and

For Mark
CW

Commissioning Editor: Timothy Horne
Project Development Manager: Barbara Simmons
Project Manager: Frances Affleck
Designer: George Ajayi

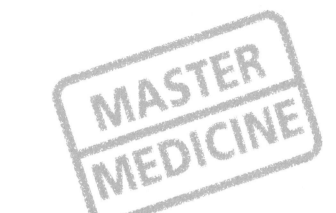

Systematic Pathology

A clinically-orientated core text with self-assessment

PAUL BASS BSc MD FRCPath

Consultant Histopathologist and Honorary Clinical Senior Lecturer
Southampton University Hospitals NHS Trust
Southampton

SUSAN BURROUGHS BSc BM MRCPath

Consultant Histopathologist
Salisbury Health Care NHS Trust
Salisbury

CLAIRE WAY BSc MBChB MRCPath

Specialist Registrar in Histopathology
Southampton University Hospitals NHS Trust
Southampton

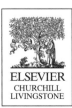

ELSEVIER
CHURCHILL
LIVINGSTONE

EDINBURGH   LONDON   NEW YORK   OXFORD   PHILADELPHIA   ST LOUIS   SYDNEY   TORONTO   2005

ELSEVIER
CHURCHILL LIVINGSTONE

An imprint of Elsevier Limited

First published 2005

ISBN 0443 070075

British Library Cataloguing in Publication Data
A catalogue record for this book is available from the British Library

Library of Congress Cataloging in Publication Data
A catalog record for this book is available from the Library of Congress

Notice
Medical knowledge is constantly changing. Standard safety precautions must be followed, but as new research and clinical experience broaden our knowledge, changes in treatment and drug therapy may become necessary or appropriate. Readers are advised to check the most current product information provided by the manufacturer of each drug to be administered to verify the recommended dose, the method and duration of administration, and contraindications. It is the responsibility of the practitioner, relying on experience and knowledge of the patient, to determine dosages and the best treatment for each individual patient. Neither the Publisher nor the authors assumes any liability for any injury and/or damage to persons or property arising from this publication.

The Publisher

 ELSEVIER your source for books, journals and multimedia in the health sciences

www.elsevierhealth.com

Working together to grow libraries in developing countries
www.elsevier.com | www.bookaid.org | www.sabre.org

ELSEVIER   BOOK AID International   Sabre Foundation

The publisher's policy is to use **paper manufactured from sustainable forests**

Printed in Spain

Contents

Using this book

Learning about systemic pathology provides the building blocks for understanding disease processes, which is something that all doctors require in order to practise effectively.

Over the last five years, there have been radical changes to many undergraduate medical courses, with increasing emphasis on communication and clinical skills, ethics, special study modules and interprofessional learning. These are delivered within different curriculum models, such as integrated, graduate entry or problem-based learning. In some curricula, pathology is not taught as an identifiable 'course' and it can be difficult for students to identify the important subject matter that must be learnt.

All the material in this book is core pathology. It is the basis of clinical medicine and is essential for good clinical practice. Much of the detail found in larger textbooks has been eliminated, so if you know and understand the information in this book, you will have an adequate basis for your ward-based and postgraduate studies. Larger textbooks can be used for reference if you wish to study topics in more depth, but it is not necessary to read them from cover to cover. Revision 'crammers' consisting largely of lists are favoured by some, but they encourage simple retention of facts rather than understanding, and they are unlikely to be of use unless you already understand the material.

It is important that you develop the skills of deep learning that will underpin a lifetime of learning. Qualified doctors learn until they retire. Systemic pathology has immediate relevance and importance to clinical medicine and as such is easier to learn than some basic science subjects. The ability to apply pathology knowledge to clinical situations is fundamental to the diagnostic process. The use of clinical examples and case histories in this book is designed to make the subject more interesting, memorable and understandable.

General principles of assessment

Most medical school assessments or exams are of summative type; they are designed to pass or fail and to enable you to move on to the next stage of the course. Formative assessment is a different kind of assessment where the results are used to give feedback to the students about their strengths and weaknesses and about their progress. In this book the self-assessment questions are intended to give you some idea of where there are gaps in your knowledge.

Assessment methods

Multiple choice questions

The multiple choice question (MCQ) is a popular form of assessment in many medical courses because the questions are relatively easy to set and can be marked quickly and efficiently in large numbers by mechanical means. MCQs mainly test knowledge, understanding and reasoning skills. The most valid and useful MCQs are those that use the 'best-matched answer' format.

Some MCQs use negative marking, where points are deducted for wrong answers. This system is designed to prevent guessing. Nevertheless, studies have shown that you are, on average, more likely to be right than wrong if you have a hunch about the right answer, even if you are not sure. An over-cautious approach can result in answering too few questions to pass, so it is probably best to 'play your hunches' if you have to. If there is no negative marking, you should attempt all questions as you have nothing to lose.

Short answer questions

Short answer questions are used to test knowledge, reasoning and understanding and sometimes problem solving. The examiners usually devise a prototype answer and marks are simply awarded for every item or cluster of items required. Start your answer with some kind of definition and go on from there. It is a good idea to use simple diagrams wherever possible. You can then refer to them in your explanation.

No extra points will be given for information that is not strictly relevant, therefore read the question and answer the question that is set. Unless the instructions for the paper indicate that different questions have different weights of marks, spend roughly the same amount of time on each question. There is sometimes a temptation to spend longer on questions that you believe you can answer particularly well, but this is unlikely to compensate fully for a question that is answered badly or not at all because of lack of time. It may be a good idea to start with the questions about which you feel less confident; as the pressure increases towards the end of the exam you can concentrate on your areas of strength.

Essay

The essay gives you a chance to show how much you understand and your ability to relate one area of knowledge to another. It also tests your ability to organise and present information logically and clearly. Some essays also allow you to develop an argument rather than simply set down facts. It is a communication exercise; marks may be given not just for factual content but for use of English, presentation (including handwriting) and structure of the essay and how the points and arguments are expounded. Use side headings (underlined if necessary) and diagrams. These help to make things clear and will often enable you to communicate your knowledge to the examiner.

It is vital that you read the question carefully and answer only the question that is set. Examiners will not award marks for irrelevant material, so don't waste your time presenting it. Do not spend too long on an essay on a favourite topic, or you will have insufficient time for other questions.

Essays are time consuming to mark and may be subject to marker bias and for this reason are often denigrated. Nevertheless, a well-set and properly marked essay can test a variety of skills, and essay papers are still encountered in many medical schools.

Viva

The viva voce or oral examination is an integral part of many examinations in medicine, both undergraduate and postgraduate. It can be an alarming experience, but it is your opportunity to show the examiners not just how much you can recall but your breadth and depth of understanding.

All students find vivas stressful. Sometimes you will feel as though your mind has gone blank when the examiner asks a question. Don't panic; take a deep breath and think for a second or two before jumping in with the first thing that comes into your head. Try to imagine how you would start the answer if you were writing it down. A simple definition is often a good start. If you do not understand the question then say so and ask for it to be repeated. The viva is a two-way communication process and examiners cannot expect you to give your best if they do not express themselves clearly.

If the question requires an answer listing the causes of a disease, assemble your causes in order of importance. Do not put the most rare one at the top of the list. Common things occur commonly. For example, haemorrhoids or rectal polyps are common causes of rectal bleeding, whereas amoebiasis would be a very rare cause in the UK. It may help to assemble topics in a logical way that demonstrates your understanding of basic principles and also acts as an aide-mémoire so that you don't forget important areas. For example, you can divide causes of intestinal obstruction into factors within the lumen, within the wall and outside the wall. Likewise, an intestinal polyp can be inflammatory, hamartomatous or neoplastic. Neoplasms can be benign or malignant, primary or metastatic.

If you mention a rare disease, the examiner may ask you more about it. This is fine if you know the subject, but not if you don't, so try to keep the conversation to areas in which you are confident. Most examiners try to be empathic and sympathetic. Nevertheless, they are usually trying to determine the limits of your knowledge and understanding, so you will probably be asked some questions that you cannot answer. If you haven't a clue, it is perfectly acceptable to say you don't know so the examiner can move on to a different area.

Spotter

The spotter exam consists of a series of 'stations' at which there will be a specimen, test result or diagram about which you have to answer questions. You are allowed a certain time at each station and then you move on to the next one, usually when a bell rings. More sophisticated versions of the spotter may include a clinical case in which you move through a series of stations which all relate to the one case. For example, a pathology image showing myocardial infarction may be followed by stations with chest X-rays, ECGs or cardiac enzyme results.

Students often feel pressurised during spotter exams and it is a good idea to jot down a précis of the question at a station if you cannot respond, so that if there are a few spare minutes at another easier station, you can go back to the one that you had trouble with.

OSCEs

Pathology is the link between basic science and clinical medicine, and so you may be required to demonstrate pathological knowledge in a wide variety of OSCEs (objective structured clinical examinations). Ensure you are up to date with the regulations for death certification and asking for autopsy consent, since these may be the focus of an OSCE station.

Using the self-assessment sections in this book

A mixture of assessment methods for you to use have been included in this book. The answers provided will give you some idea of where your knowledge gaps are and will also help you to organise your answers effectively.

There are factual answers to all the MCQs and answers with discussion points for the case histories.

The answers for the OSCE, short answer and viva questions are not comprehensive. Where appropriate, an outline answer has been suggested and a way of approaching the answer to show that you can organise, prioritise and apply your knowledge to different situations.

Dr Clair du Boulay
Director of Medical Education,
Southampton University Hospitals

1 Cardiovascular system

Overview

Pathology of the cardiovascular system, the heart and blood vessels, is responsible for a large proportion of deaths in the UK each year, and also causes considerable morbidity through heart failure, stroke and peripheral vascular disease. The major underlying disease processes responsible include atherosclerosis, hypertension and diabetes mellitus. Lifestyle modification can play a significant role in reducing disease risk, particularly in relation to smoking, exercise, body weight and fat consumption. This chapter covers atherosclerosis and its complications, ischaemic heart disease, hypertension, valvular heart disease, cardiomyopathies and congenital heart disease. Many cardiac pathologies result in heart failure, which may initially primarily involve either the left or right ventricle. The basic pathology of vasculitis and vascular tumours is also reviewed.

1.1 Atherosclerosis, aneurysms and ischaemic heart disease

Learning objectives

You should:

- Understand the pathogenesis and clinical consequences of atherosclerosis
- Be able to discuss pathology and complications of myocardial infarction
- Know how lifestyle modifications can reduce the risk of ischaemic heart disease

Atherosclerosis

Atherosclerosis (also called atheroma) is an inflammatory, degenerative disease of large and medium sized arterial vessels. It is characterised by the development of fibrolipid plaques within the intima of the vessel wall. In smaller arteries, including the coronary vessels that supply the myocardium, these plaques can cause severe narrowing (stenosis) of the lumen, with significant impairment of blood flow. The clinical consequences depend on the speed of development of the stenosis, and on whether the affected tissue has any additional source of blood supply (known as collateral supply). In large arteries, such as the abdominal aorta, the inflammatory atherosclerotic process damages the muscular wall causing weakness and dilatation. This is known as aneurysm formation (see Box 1). As the aneurysm enlarges there is an increasing risk of rupture, with resultant catastrophic haemorrhage.

Four major *risk factors* are recognised for atherosclerosis.

1. Smoking
2. Hypercholesterolaemia (raised low density lipoproteins)
3. Hypertension
4. Diabetes mellitus

Minor risk factors include increasing age, male gender, obesity, family history and stress.

Pathogenesis of the fibrolipid atherosclerotic plaque

Atheromatous plaques are probably initiated by injury to the endothelial cells of the arterial intima. An inflammatory response is evoked to the damage, which results in an infiltrate of macrophages, and proliferation of smooth muscle cells from the media of the vessel wall. These smooth muscle cells migrate into the intima and begin to produce collagen. Both the macrophages and the smooth muscle cells may accumulate lipid within their cytoplasm, giving a vacuolated appearance on light microscopy ('foam cells'). Free cholesterol and necrotic inflammatory debris also become incorporated within the plaque lesion.

Figure 1 shows a normal muscular artery and a typical atheromatous plaque with a fibrous tissue cap and a lipid-rich, necrotic centre. It is important to realise that the actual composition of individual plaques varies, and can change over time. Plaques that are particularly rich in lipids may be more unstable and susceptible to rupture or haemorrhage (see later section on ischaemic heart disease). Older plaques can become heavily calcified. The plaque surface is prone to develop superimposed thrombosis, which can rapidly increase the severity of the obstruction to blood flow. At autopsy, it is common to find a recent thrombus complicating an atheromatous coronary artery plaque in patients who died after acute myocardial infarction.

Clinical complications of atherosclerosis

- **Coronary arteries:** angina, myocardial infarction, heart failure, sudden death (cardiac arrhythmia).
- **Cerebral arteries:** transient ischaemic attacks, stroke.
- **Aorta:** abdominal aneurysm formation (risk of rupture and death) (see Box 1).
- **Mesenteric arteries:** intestinal ischaemia and infarction.
- **Renal arteries:** renal artery stenosis (hypertension, ischaemic kidney).
- **Lower limbs:** intermittent claudication, gangrene.

Aortic dissection

Also called dissecting aneurysm, although this is an inaccurate term as the aorta is not significantly dilated. In aortic dissection, blood tracks into the muscular wall of the blood vessel. The entry point of blood into the aortic media is through an intimal tear, usually within the proximal 10 cm of the ascending aorta. Occasionally, there is a second distal luminal tear, through which blood re-enters the circulation, producing a 'double-barrelled' aorta. More commonly, however, the haemorrhage extends outwards with vessel rupture and catastrophic extamural haemorrhage into:

- the pericardium, causing cardiac tamponade
- the mediastinum, causing haemothorax
- the abdominal cavity (haematoperitoneum).

The dissection can also involve the great vessels of the neck, compromising cerebral blood flow. Dissection of the coronary arteries is a rare cause of acute myocardial ischaemia.

There is a strong association with systemic hypertension and with Marfan's syndrome.

Ischaemic heart disease

Ischaemia is due to lack of oxygen, and in the overwhelming majority of ischaemic heart disease (IHD) cases this is due to reduced blood flow through coronary arteries narrowed or occluded by atherosclerosis. However, the left ventricular myocardium is also at risk

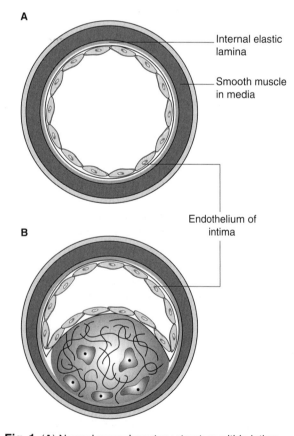

A

Internal elastic lamina

Smooth muscle in media

Endothelium of intima

B

Fig. 1 (**A**) Normal muscular artery structure within intima (endothelium), internal elastic lamina and media. (**B**) An atherosclerotic plaque composed of lipid and fibrous tissue is present in the intima causing internal narrowing (stenosis) of the vessel lumen and thinning of the underlying muscular media.

Box 1 Aneurysms

Definition
Abnormal dilatation of a vessel wall, which communicates with the lumen—almost always arterial

Pathogenesis

Inflammation
- Atherosclerotic aneurysm (abdominal aorta, iliac arteries, popliteal arteries)
- Polyarteritis nodosa
- Kawasaki disease (coronary arteries)

Infection (mycotic aneurysm)
- Syphilis
- Direct spread from adjacent infection

Congenital defect
- Berry aneurysm (Circle of Willis, see Chapter 14 Nervous System)

Metabolic
- Diabetes mellitus (retinal capillary microaneurysms)

Hypertension
- Charcot–Bouchard aneurysms (deep white matter of cerebral hemispheres)

Trauma

Complications
- Rupture with haemorrhage (often fatal if aorta or cerebral vessels involved)
- Compression of adjacent structures
- Thrombus formation (vessel occlusion and distal thromboembolism)
- Secondary infection
- Sclerosing periaortitis (dense fibrosis surrounding abdominal aortic aneurysm which can entrap ureters)

of ischaemia when there is pathological hypertrophy, for example in systemic hypertension or aortic valve stenosis. Under these conditions, cardiac perfusion may be insufficient to meet the metabolic needs of the increased muscle mass. Rarely, cardiac ischaemia can result from decreased oxygen-carrying capacity of the blood in severe anaemia (even though the coronary arteries may be normal).

Myocardial infarction

Cell death (necrosis) caused by ischaemia is known as infarction. Cardiac muscle cells cease to function within 30–60 seconds of loss of blood supply. Irreversible cell injury requires at least 20 minutes of anoxia (no oxygen). Cardiac muscle cells do not divide in post-natal life (i.e. they are 'permanent' cells) and infarcted myocardium is eventually replaced by fibrous scar tissue.

Regional (transmural) infarction—is caused by occlusion of a single coronary artery. The arterial block-

age results from atherosclerosis complicated by thrombosis or by intraplaque haemorrhage, which rapidly expands the atheromatous plaque (see Fig. 2). The commonest sites for clinically significant coronary atherosclerosis are:

- proximal left anterior descending artery (up to 50%)
- right coronary artery (30%)
- left circumflex artery (up to 20%)
- left main coronary artery.

Regional infarction most frequently affects part of the anterior wall of the left ventricle, or part of the interventricular septum, with extension into the right ventricle in a small proportion of cases. Isolated right ventricular infarction is very uncommon.

The subendocardial region of the myocardium is the muscle area most vulnerable to hypoxia.

Subendocardial infarction—can occur when there is a global decrease in cardiac blood flow due to systemic hypotension ('shock'). Myocardial necrosis is usually limited to the inner third of the muscle but can involve the territory of more than one coronary artery.

Unusual causes of myocardial infarction include coronary artery dissection, arteritis or spasm.

Macroscopic and microscopic changes in myocardial infarction
- Less than 24 hours—microscopic changes only (increased eosinophilic staining of cardiac muscle cells, loss of nuclei, muscle cells become buckled).
- From 24 to 72 hours—infarct becomes apparent macroscopically at autopsy as an area of pallor or yellow discolouration, with a peripheral rim of haemorrhage. Microscopically the dead muscle fibres provoke an inflammatory response, initially consisting of neutrophil polymorphs, followed by macrophages. The infarct becomes soft.
- Up to 2–3 weeks—the dead tissue is removed and replaced by blood vessel proliferation and myofibroblasts (granulation tissue).
- Weeks to months—collagen is produced and the scar becomes progressively less cellular, less vascular and more fibrotic.

Biochemical markers of myocardial infarction
Necrotic cardiac muscle releases enzymes, which can be measured in the serum and are helpful in confirmation of the diagnosis.

- **Heart-specific troponins**—released 2–4 hours after cell death, remaining elevated for up to one week. Troponin T and I are highly specific for myocardial damage.
- **Creatine kinase (CK)**—starts to rise after a few hours of infarction, and falls again within 48 hours. CK is

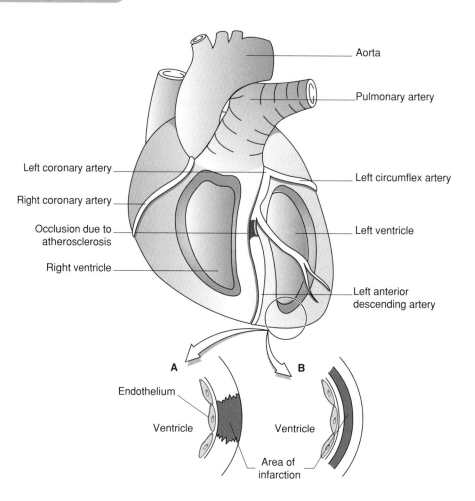

Fig. 2 Major coronary arteries and types of myocardial infarction: (**A**) regional and (**B**) subendocardial.

Aorta

Pulmonary artery

Left coronary artery

Right coronary artery

Occlusion due to atherosclerosis

Right ventricle

Left circumflex artery

Left ventricle

Left anterior descending artery

A

B

Endothelium

Ventricle

Ventricle

Area of infarction

also released from injured skeletal muscle cells; measurement of the specific cardiac isoenzyme is therefore more diagnostically helpful.

- **Aspartate aminotransferase (AST)**—also non-specific as it is released by damaged liver cells.
- **Lactate dehydrogenase (LDH)**—peaks at 3–6 days and may remain elevated for two weeks. May be useful in patients presenting late after suspicious chest pain.

Complications of myocardial infarction
Immediate
- Arrhythmias
- Acute cardiac failure
- Cardiogenic shock
- Sudden death.

Early
- Infarct rupture (3–7 days).

Later
- Mural thrombosis
- Cardiac aneurysm.

Dressler's syndrome (pericarditis associated with circulating antibodies to heart muscle) occurs from two weeks to two years post infarction.

Reinfarction can occur at any time. Cardiac failure and arrhythmias may also be late complications. The presence of myocardial scarring increases the risk of sudden death from ventricular arrhythmia.

1.2 Hypertension, cardiomyopathies and myocarditis

Learning objectives

You should:

- Know the aetiology, risk factors and complications of hypertension, so as to be able to identify patient risk factors amenable to treatment by lifestyle modification, and to investigate patients appropriately for causes of secondary hypertension

- Understand the term cardiomyopathy, its classification, major causes and complications

Hypertension

Chronically raised systemic blood pressure is a major cause of morbidity and mortality. Hypertension can cause, or significantly contribute to:

- atherosclerosis
- hypertensive heart disease (left ventricular hypertrophy)
- chronic renal failure
- cerebrovascular disease (intracerebral haemorrhage, ruptured Berry aneurysm)
- retinopathy.

'Normal' blood pressure varies within a population and with age, but evidence suggests that a sustained pressure of 140/90 mmHg or greater is associated with increased risk of disease. Persistent diastolic blood pressure in excess of 100 mmHg requires treatment. Very high elevation (e.g. 240/120 mmHg) can result in accelerated disease—'malignant hypertension'.

In approximately 10% of cases, systemic hypertension is secondary to another disease (Box 2). The mechanism of primary hypertension is unclear but the following defects have been found in patients:

- abnormal renal excretion of sodium
- abnormal sodium and calcium metabolism in vascular smooth muscle
- abnormalities of renin–angiotensin mechanism, probably in part related to polymorphisms in key genes.

Family history, obesity and excessive alcohol intake are further associated factors. The aetiology of essential hypertension is complex and clearly involves a combination of genetic and environmental factors. Modest, but clinically significant, reductions in blood pressure may be achieved by weight loss, regular physical exercise, moderation of alcohol intake and possibly by reduction of salt in the diet.

Blood-vessel changes are similar in both primary and secondary hypertension, with homogenous thickening of arteriolar walls and narrowing of the vascular lumen ('hyaline arteriosclerosis'). Marked cellular proliferation ('onion skinning') and blood-vessel necrosis may occur in malignant hypertension. Hypertensive heart disease is characterised by concentric hypertrophy of the left ventricle.

Cardiomyopathy

Cardiomyopathy is defined as heart-muscle disease not caused by ischaemic, hypertensive, valvular or congenital heart disease. Although uncommon, cardiomyopathies are an important cause of cardiac failure and sudden death in young adults. The aetiology of specific cardiomyopathies is shown in Box 3. Ninety per cent are of the dilated type.

Hypertrophic cardiomyopathy (HOCM)—is characterised by asymmetrical left ventricular hypertrophy (as opposed to the concentric hypertrophy seen in hypertensive heart disease and aortic valve stenosis). The interventricular septum is particularly thickened. Microscopically, the cardiac muscle cells are enlarged and haphazardly organised (myocyte disarray). There is often fibrosis between muscle cells. Many cases show autosomal dominant inheritance. Genetic defects include cardiac myosin genes on chromosome 14. Complications of hypertrophic cardiomyopathy include:

- atrial fibrillation
- atrial thrombus and systemic embolism
- infective endocarditis of the mitral valve
- cardiac failure
- sudden death.

Box 2 Secondary hypertension

Renal disease
- Glomerulonephritis
- Polycystic kidney disease
- Renal artery stenosis
- Chronic pyelonephritis
- Renal cell carcinoma

Endocrine disease
- Adrenal cortical tumours
- Cushing's disease
- Phaeochromocytoma
- Diabetes mellitus
- Acromegaly

Coarctation of the aorta

Iatrogenic
- Steroid therapy

Note that hypertension can be either a cause or a consequence of chronic renal impairment

---

Box 3 Cardiomyopathy

Genetic
- Hypertrophic cardiomyopathy (HOCM)
- Haemochromatosis

Post-infectious
- Dilated cardiomyopathy (many cases are probably caused by viral infection)

Toxic
- Alcoholic cardiomyopathy
- Drug induced (chemotherapy agents—adriamycin commonest)

Metabolic
- Amyloid heart disease

Idiopathic

Dilated cardiomyopathy—is characterised by dilatation of all four cardiac chambers with progressive cardiac failure. The heart is typically enlarged (2–3 times normal weight) and flabby at autopsy. Mural thrombi may be present. The microscopic findings are not specific, but there is often patchy ventricular fibrosis. Cardiomyopathy caused by alcohol, chemotherapy agents and haemochromatosis is of the dilated type.

Restrictive cardiomyopathy—describes a condition of 'stiff' ventricles, which fail to relax, impeding diastolic filling. The ventricles are of normal size but the atria are dilated. Microscopically there is non-specific myocardial scarring. Causes include radiation fibrosis and cardiac involvement by amyloid (see Box 4).

Myocarditis

Myocarditis is inflammation of the heart muscle. It may be asymptomatic, or cause:

- acute cardiac failure
- sudden death
- chronic cardiac failure (usually due to dilated cardiomyopathy).

Acute myocarditis may be suggested at autopsy by a pale, flabby heart, but histological examination is necessary for diagnosis. Microscopically there is multifocal

---

Box 4 Amyloid

Definition
An abnormal extracellular accumulation of protein with specific physical and chemical properties (including β-pleated sheet conformation on X-ray crystallography).

Demonstration
On light microscopy, amyloid appears pink in tissue sections stained with Congo Red. When sections are viewed with polarised light, the amyloid changes colour to bright green. Amyloid fibrils can also be recognised on electron microscopy.
    All forms of amyloid contain a glycoprotein (P component) as a minor constituent. The major amyloid protein varies and is reflected in the disease classification.

Classification
- AL amyloid (light chains of immunoglobulins—multiple myeloma)
- AA amyloid (serum amyloid A protein—long-standing chronic inflammation)
- Haemodialysis associated amyloid (β_2-microglobulin)
- Hereditary amyloidosis (serum amyloid A protein or transthyretin)
- Localised cardiac amyloid (transthyretin)
- Isolated atrial amyloid (atrial natriuretic factor)
- Endocrine-associated amyloid (calcitonin in medullary carcinoma of thyroid)

Box 5 Causes of myocarditis

Infection
- Viral (Coxsackie, ECHO)
- Bacterial (meningococcus)
- Fungal (Candida)
- Parasitic (Chagas' disease, toxoplasmosis)

Immune-mediated
- Post-infective (including rheumatic fever)
- Systemic lupus erythematosus
- Transplant rejection

Idiopathic
- Sarcoidosis

---

myocardial chronic inflammation associated with cardiac muscle-cell death. The aetiology of myocarditis is shown in Box 5.

1.3 Congenital heart disease

Learning objectives

You should:

- Know the commonest types of congenital heart disease and the aetiological factors that may cause congenital cardiac defects

- Understand what is meant by cyanotic congenital heart defects

---

Congenital heart disease—describes abnormalities of the heart and major vessels present at birth. The incidence in live-born infants is approximately 1 in 200. The common lesions include:

- isolated defects in cardiac chamber walls—atrial septal defect, ventricular septal defect
- persistence of embryonic structures—patent foramen ovale, patent ductus arteriosus
- stenosing lesions ('narrowings')—aortic valve stenosis, pulmonary stenosis, coarctation of the aorta
- transposition of the great arteries
- complex anomalies—Fallot's tetralogy.

The aetiology is unknown in many cases but there is evidence of genetic predisposition. A small percentage of cases are associated with chromosome abnormalities, particularly Turner's syndrome (45XO syndrome), with coarctation of the aorta, and Down's syndrome (trisomy 21), with atrial and ventricular septal defects. Intrauterine infection with rubella may cause multiple congenital cardiac defects. Atrial septal defects are a feature of fetal alcohol syndrome.

Some congenital heart defects, such as small atrial septal defects, may be clinically inconsequential or present only in later adult life.

Abnormal connections between the cardiac chambers permit shunting of blood from one side of the circulation to the other. In post-natal life, atrial and ventricular septal defects usually cause shunting of blood from the left side of the heart (high pressure) to the right side (low pressure). This increases the work of the right ventricle (pressure and volume overload) and can lead to right ventricular hypertrophy and pulmonary hypertension. Structural narrowing of pulmonary arteries occurs in response to chronically raised pulmonary vascular pressure, and the flow of blood through the shunt may be reversed (i.e. it becomes a right-to-left shunt, known as Eisenmenger's syndrome).

Some congenital cardiac defects cause right-to-left blood shunts from their onset. Deoxygenated blood bypasses the lungs and passes directly from the right heart into the systemic circulation. If the shunt is large enough, cyanosis will be clinically apparent as blue discolouration of the skin and nail beds.

Cyanotic congenital heart defects include:

Fallot's tetralogy
- Ventricular septal defect.
- Outflow obstruction to the right ventricle.
- Aorta overriding the ventricular septal defect.
- Right ventricular hypertrophy.

Transposition of the great vessels
- The aorta emerges from the right ventricle and the pulmonary artery arises from the left ventricle. To be compatible with post-natal life, there must also be either an atrial or ventricular septal defect.

1.4 Valvular heart disease

Learning objectives

You should:

- Understand the pathological causes and pathophysiological consequences of stenosis and incompetence of all the cardiac valves, but particularly the mitral and aortic valves

- Understand the pathology of infective endocarditis, so as to be able to identify patients at risk and, when appropriate, ensure prophylactic treatment is given

Valvular stenosis and incompetence

Damage to the cardiac valves can result in stenosis (narrowing of the valve orifice with obstruction to blood flow) or incompetence (regurgitation of blood back through a leaking valve). Valve disease can be congenital (see Section 1.3) or acquired. In non-congenital cases the clinically significant lesions almost always affect the mitral or aortic valves.

Abnormal movement of deformed valves and abnormal blood flow causes characteristic murmurs and added sounds on cardiac auscultation.

Rheumatic heart disease

Rheumatic heart disease (RHD) is a major cause of acquired mitral valve disease. The incidence has dramatically decreased in the UK over recent decades but is still relatively common in Third World countries. The initiating event is usually a pharyngeal infection by Group A β-haemolytic streptococci, followed several weeks later by rheumatic fever (RF), an immunologically mediated multisystem disorder. RF results from the cross-reaction of antistreptococcal antibodies with normal host tissues—direct bacterial infection does not occur. During acute RF there is often a pancarditis with inflammation of pericardium, myocardium and endocardium. Myocarditis can occasionally cause acute heart failure, arrhythmias and death. However, it is recurrent attacks of RF that produce the most significant cardiac lesions. Repeated acute inflammation of the endocardium covering heart valves leads to fibrosis and deformity. Valve leaflets become thickened and fused, resulting in 'fishmouth' or 'buttonhole' mitral valve stenosis. The aortic valve may also be affected. Complications include:

- atrial fibrillation
- valvular and atrial thrombus formation with systemic embolism
- cardiac failure
- infective endocarditis.

Mitral valve prolapse

Mitral valve prolapse, also known as 'floppy mitral valve', is a common condition involving approximately 5% of adults. Young females and Marfan's syndrome patients are particularly affected. One or both mitral valve leaflets are enlarged and prolapse into the left atrium during systole. The condition is usually incidental but occasionally can cause mitral regurgitation, infective endocarditis, valvular thrombosis or arrhythmias.

Infective endocarditis (IE)

Infection of the endocardium or vascular endothelium can occur in:

Table 1 Causes and consequences of valvular heart disease

Valve lesion	Causes	Consequences
Mitral stenosis	Rheumatic heart disease	Increased left atrial pressure; left atrial dilatation, atrial fibrillation Increased pulmonary venous pressure, leading to pulmonary hypertension and right ventricular hypertrophy
Mitral incompetence	Rheumatic heart disease Infective endocarditis Left ventricular dilatation Papillary muscle ischaemia, fibrosis or rupture Mitral valve prolapse Leaking prosthetic valve	Left atrial dilatation Left ventricular hypertrophy, due to volume overload (Acute mitral incompetence caused by rupture of necrotic papillary muscle in myocardial infarction can result in acute cardiac failure)
Aortic stenosis	Senile calcification of normal valve Calcification of congenitally bicuspid valve Rheumatic heart disease	Left ventricular hypertrophy, due to pressure overload (increased gradient across stenotic valve); ischaemia of hypertrophic ventricular myocardium (angina, arrhythmias, cardiac failure, sudden death)
Aortic incompetence	Rheumatic heart disease Infective endocarditis Leaking prosthetic valve Aortic root dilatation (aortic dissection, arthritis, Marfan's syndrome, syphilis)	Left ventricular hypertrophy, due to volume overload; left ventricular failure

- previously damaged heart valves (e.g. RHD, calcific aortic stenosis)
- congenital heart disease
- prosthetic heart valves or vascular tissue
- normal heart valves (uncommon causes, acute severe endocarditis).

IE is usually a chronic/subacute illness caused by low-virulence organisms colonising abnormal tissue. Normal heart valves can be infected by high virulence bacteria or fungi, especially in IV drug abusers or the immunosuppressed (AIDS, diabetes, alcoholics, transplant recipients).

Common pathogenetic bacteria in IE include:

- *Streptococcus viridans*—normal flora of upper respiratory tract; low virulence.
- *Streptococcus faecalis*—normal flora of perineum and gut; low virulence.
- *Staphylococcus aureus*—can be member of normal mucocutaneous flora; high virulence.
- *Staphylococcus epidermidis*—normal skin flora; low virulence.

Other organisms include *Coxiella, E. coli, Chlamydia* and *Candida*.

Colonisation occurs following transient bacteraemia (bacteria floating in the bloodstream, distinct from septicaemia, which is clinical illness caused by bacteria multiplying in the blood). Such bacteraemia may result from dental work, endoscopy, surgery or established infection elsewhere in the body. Organisms may be introduced in prosthetic material or by intravascular catheters such as central venous pressure (CVP) lines. Patients known to have damaged or prosthetic heart valves are at risk of

developing IE after episodes of transient bacteraemia with low virulence organisms, and so require prophyiactic antibiotic therapy prior to undergoing any procedure that might seed organisms into the bloodstream.

Layers of microorganisms and fibrinous inflammatory debris build up at the site of colonisation, forming

---

Box 6 Infective endocarditis: clinical notes

Acute endocarditis

Typically presents with fever and acute valvular incompetence. In IV drug abusers the tricuspid valve is often affected (organisms are injected directly into arm or leg veins). Blood cultures will often be positive for the causative virulent organism. Early antibiotic treatment is necessary and emergency valve replacement may be indicated if valve destruction has caused cardiac failure.

Subacute endocarditis

May give rise to non-specific chronic symptoms of malaise, fatigue, weight loss and anorexia. There is often a fluctuating pyrexia and a heart murmur (particularly a regurgitant or changing murmur). Extracardiac clinical features frequently reflect embolisation of cardiac vegetations, immune complex deposition or sepsis, and include:

- Splinter haemorrhages in the nails
- Petechial haemorrhages in the skin and conjunctivae
- Glomerulonephritis
- Cerebral infarction (or history of transient ischaemic attacks)
- Finger clubbing
- Splenomegaly
- Disseminated abscesses or infarcts

'vegetations', which can be seen on an echocardiogram. Complications include:

- valve perforation with acute incompetence
- valve thrombosis
- perivalvular abscess
- dehiscence of prosthetic valves
- septic embolisation of the vegetations with distant infarction and abscess formation in the brain, kidney, spleen, bone, and elsewhere.

1.5 Heart failure

Learning objectives

You should:

- Understand the pathological causes of heart failure in order to appropriately investigate patients with this condition

- Be able to describe the typical changes seen at autopsy in the organs of a patient that has died from cardiac failure

- Understand the clinical features of left and right heart failure and be able to relate these to the underlying pathological changes

Heart failure—occurs when one or both cardiac ventricles are unable to maintain an output sufficient for the body's metabolic needs. Although the left or right ventricle may fail individually at first (depending on the underlying pathology) eventually both ventricles will fail together, producing congestive cardiac failure and generalised enlargement of the heart (cardiomegaly). However, it is helpful to consider the aetiology and clinical effects of left and right heart failure separately.

Left ventricular failure

Left ventricular failure (LVF) results from a loss of myocardial contractility, due to the sudden or gradual dysfunction, or death, of cardiac muscle cells. Less frequently, there may be significant impairment of ventricular filling during diastole. The latter situation occurs when the left ventricular wall is abnormally 'stiff' and unable to distend adequately.

Loss of myocardial contractility
- Ischaemic heart disease
- Hypertensive heart disease
- Valvular heart disease
- Dilated cardiomyopathy.

Inability to fill ventricle adequately
- Massive ventricular hypertrophy (hypertension, hypertrophic cardiomyopathy, aortic stenosis)
- Amyloidosis (restrictive cardiomyopathy).

Other causes
- Pericardial disease that impedes cardiac filling (pericardial effusion or constrictive pericarditis)
- High-output cardiac failure (anaemia or thyrotoxicosis).

Markedly increased blood volume due to iatrogenic fluid overload or renal failure can precipitate or exacerbate cardiac failure.

Right ventricular failure

Right ventricular failure (RVF) is most often encountered as a consequence of left ventricular dysfunction. Myocardial infarction only infrequently involves the right side of the heart, and then this is usually as an extension of a predominantly left ventricular infarct. Primary right ventricular failure can occur as a result of chronic lung disease. The right ventricle is spared the effects of systemic hypertension. However, raised pressure in the pulmonary circulation will affect the right ventricle, causing hypertrophy. This is recognised by the pathologist at post mortem by an increase in the thickness of the right ventricular wall, which is normally less than 5 mm, and an increase in isolated right ventricular weight (normally less than 50–60 g; total heart weight depends on sex and body weight, but is usually 250–350 g in the absence of any cardiac disease). Lung diseases causing pulmonary hypertension include:

- chronic bronchitis
- emphysema
- recurrent pulmonary emboli
- pulmonary fibrosis.

Clinical features of heart failure

Ventricular failure causes back-damming of blood in the supplying veins, venules and capillaries. This raises the hydrostatic pressure, in capillaries and venules, to the point where the hydrostatic pressure exceeds the plasma oncotic pressure throughout the course of the vessel. The result is that tissue fluid is not reabsorbed into the circulation and accumulates extravascularly, causing oedema. Dilated congested capillaries and venules may also rupture, causing microscopic tissue haemorrhages.

In left ventricular failure, these changes first appear in the pulmonary circulation. Back-pressure is transmitted through pulmonary veins into the alveolar capillaries of the lungs. Thus, oedema develops first in the pulmonary air spaces, causing shortness of breath. Patients dying with pulmonary oedema have dark-red, 'wet' lungs at post mortem, due to the accumulation of blood and oedema. Lung weights (normally 250–300 g) are often doubled or trebled by the fluid, which is easily demonstrated when the lung surfaces are cut with a knife and the fluid squeezed out, like water from a sponge. Microscopically, 'heart failure cells' are often prominent—these are alveolar macrophages containing haemosiderin pigment, a marker of previous capillary haemorrhage. Fluid accumulation within the pleural cavities may produce bilateral serous effusions.

In right ventricular failure, the inferior and superior vena cavae and their feeding veins become congested. Clinically this is evident as raised jugular venous pressure in the neck. Congestion may extend into many organs, especially the liver, which becomes enlarged and shows a characteristic patchy, pale and reddish cut surface at post mortem (which pathologists like to describe as 'nutmeg liver'). Splenomegaly is also common. Oedema develops in the dependent areas of the body, affecting the legs of seated and ambulant patients, and the sacral area in patients confined to bed. Ascites (pale straw fluid) may develop in the peritoneal cavity.

In severe left ventricular failure, symptoms and signs will also result from failure to adequately perfuse the systemic organs. The systemic blood pressure is decreased, the skin appears pale and cold as circulation is diverted to conserve vital organs, especially the brain. Intestinal ischaemia can result in haemorrhage or infarction. Renal ischaemia stimulates the renin–angiotensin system, causing fluid retention that may exacerbate oedema. Severe kidney ischaemia causes acute tubular necrosis and acute renal failure. In advanced heart failure, even the cerebral circulation may be compromised sufficiently to cause symptoms of confusion and diminished consciousness. The effects of low cardiac output are confounded by the fact that many patients with cardiac failure also have significant atherosclerotic disease in their major visceral arteries, which further limits blood flow to the organs.

1.6 Thrombosis, embolism and vasculitis

Learning objectives

You should:

- Understand the basic pathology of thrombogenesis, and the risk factors for development of deep vein thrombosis

- Know the types of embolus that can occur, and the pathology of pulmonary embolism

- Know the common causes of vasculitis

Thrombosis and embolism

Thrombus formation is covered in the *Pathology* volume of the *Master Medicine* series, but is briefly reviewed here.

Three factors are involved in thrombogenesis
- Vessel-wall abnormality (endothelial dysfunction)
- Vascular stasis or turbulent flow
- Increased blood coaguability.

Thrombosis can occur in the arterial system, as a complication of atherosclerosis or aneurysms. It can also arise within the heart, for example left ventricular mural thrombus following myocardial infarction, left atrial thrombus in atrial fibrillation, and valvular thrombus in rheumatic heart disease. In the venous system, thrombus can occur in superficial varicose veins of the legs and in deep veins of the legs and pelvis. The latter is potentially more dangerous as it can embolise to the lungs causing dyspnoea, haemoptysis, pulmonary infarction, acute right heart failure or sudden death. The consequences depend on the size of the embolus and the site at which it occludes pulmonary arterial blood flow. Fatal cases of pulmonary embolism at autopsy often show a large, coiled thrombus filling the main pulmonary arterial trunk—'saddle embolus' (see Fig. 3). Smaller emboli that lodge more peripherally in the lung may be asymptomatic or cause transient discomfort. Recurrent embolisation can cause pulmonary hypertension and right ventricular hypertrophy.

Predisposing factors for deep vein thrombosis are:

Venous stasis
- Immobility
- Post-surgery
- Late pregnancy (pelvic vein compression).

Vessel damage
- Trauma
- Surgical manipulation.

Increased coagulability
- Neoplasia
- Oral contraceptives
- Inherited anticoagulant protein deficiency
- Smoking
- Old age.

Other forms of emboli include (see also p. 30)
- Fat embolism—following trauma with bone fractures
- Air embolism—following chest trauma
- Atherosclerotic plaque embolism
- Amniotic fluid embolism—during delivery of a baby
- Nitrogen embolism—decompression sickness
- Infective endocarditis—septic embolism, which can cause infection as well as infarction at the site of impaction.

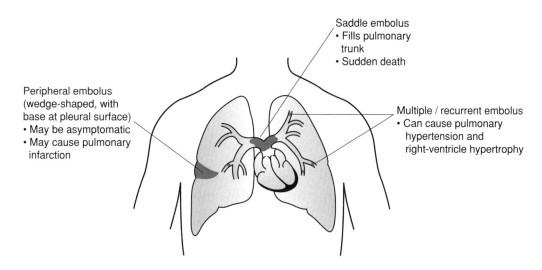

Fig. 3 Pulmonary embolism.

Vasculitis

Inflammation of blood vessels can affect arteries, veins and capillaries. The aetiology most frequently appears to be immunological, with deposition of immune complexes in vessel walls. Some vasculitides are associated with antineutrophil cytoplasmic antibodies (ANCA). These antibodies show two distinct patterns on direct immunofluorescence examination—perinuclear (p-ANCA) and cytoplasmic (c-ANCA). Over 80% of patients with Wegener's granulomatosis have circulat-ing c-ANCA at some stage of their disease. The pathogenetic role of ANCA is uncertain, but the antibodies are useful in diagnosis and in monitoring disease activity and the effects of treatment.

The more commonly encountered and important vasculitides are shown in Table 2. Vasculitis can also occur in connective tissue disease such as rheumatoid arthritis. Infectious vasculitis occurs when microorganisms invade blood vessels from an adjacent source of sepsis, or via haematogenous spread from distant sites of infection.

Table 2 Vasculitis

Disease	Vessel type	Clinico-pathological features	Mechanism of disease
Giant cell arteritis	Temporal arteries, also aorta	Segmental granulomatous inflammation, headache, visual impairment	Unknown
Polyarteritis nodosa	Medium-sized (muscular) arteries	Focal vessel-wall necrosis, aneurysm formation, multiple organ involvement with ulceration, infarcts and haemorrhage	Unknown (possibly immune complex related)
Wegener's granulomatosis	Arteries, arterioles, capillaries, venules	Necrotising vasculitis, granulomatous inflammation of the respiratory tract, glomerulonephritis (often severe)	Immunologically mediated, c-ANCA elevated in active disease
Kawasaki disease	Coronary arteries	Acute illness—necrotising vasculitis, cervical lymphadenopathy, skin rash and erythema, coronary artery aneurysm is a late complication	Unknown (possibly infection, possibly immune system dysfunction)
Henoch–Schönlein purpura	Arterioles, capillaries, venules	Haemorrhagic rash on buttocks and legs due to acute necrotising vasculitis, 30% have glomerulonephritis	Immunological (IgA immune complexes)
Cutaneous hypersensitivity vasculitis	Arterioles, capillaries, venules	Skin rash, vessel necrosis with acute inflammation (neutrophil polymorphs)	Immunological reaction to drugs, microorganisms or other antigens

1.7 Pericardial disease

Learning objective

You should:

- Know the causes of pericardial fluid accumulation and pericarditis

Pericardial serous effusions occur in congestive cardiac failure. Haemopericardium is seen in ruptured myocardial infarction, aortic dissection and trauma. Rapid accumulation of greater than about 200 ml of blood into the pericardium prevents ventricular filling and causes cardiac arrest.

Pericardial inflammation (*pericarditis*) has various causes:

Infections
- Bacteria
- Viruses
- TB
- Fungi

Immunological
- Rheumatic fever
- Systemic lupus erythematosus
- Post-myocardial infarction (Dressler's syndrome).

Other causes
- Uraemia
- Post-surgery
- Neoplasia
- Trauma.

1.8 Vascular and cardiac neoplasms

Learning objective

You should:

- Know the common benign and malignant tumours that arise in blood vessels

Haemangiomas—are common benign neoplasms of blood vessels, usually of capillary type. Haemangiomas occur in the skin and in many solid organs.

Kaposi's sarcoma—is a low-grade vascular proliferation usually classified as a neoplasm, but recently linked to human herpes virus 8 infection. Kaposi's sarcoma occurs in elderly East European males as an indolent disease, and also arises in African children (more aggressive). Kaposi's sarcoma frequently develops in AIDS patients.

Angiosarcoma—is an uncommon malignant tumour of endothelial cells, usually arising on the head and neck of elderly patients. It can also arise in solid organs. Hepatic angiosarcoma is associated with industrial exposure to polyvinyl chloride.

Cardiac myxoma—is the commonest tumour of the heart, arising in the atria. Although benign, cardiac myxomas can cause valvular obstruction.

The heart and pericardium can become secondarily involved by malignant tumours, particularly by direct spread of bronchial carcinoma or malignant pleural mesothelioma.

Self-assessment: questions

Multiple choice questions

1. The following investigations may be indicated in a young adult with hypertension:
   a. Urinary tract ultrasound
   b. Urinary catecholamine measurement
   c. Urinary oestrogen measurement
   d. Renal artery angiography
   e. Plasma glucose measurement.

2. The following are correctly paired:
   a. Patent ductus arteriosus—infective endocarditis
   b. Fallot's tetralogy—tricuspid stenosis
   c. Atrial septal defect—early cyanotic heart disease
   d. Turner's syndrome—coarctation of the aorta
   e. Ventricular septal defect—pulmonary hypertension.

3. Early complications of myocardial infarction include:
   a. Papillary muscle rupture
   b. Complete heart block
   c. Cardiogenic shock
   d. Ventricular aneurysm
   e. Dressler's syndrome.

4. The following conditions can cause a dilated cardiomyopathy:
   a. Haemochromatosis
   b. Amyloidosis
   c. Viral myocarditis
   d. Alcohol abuse
   e. Chemotherapeutic agents.

5. The following are normal constituents of atherosclerotic plaques:
   a. Cholesterol
   b. Smooth muscle cells
   c. Collagen
   d. Neutrophil polymorphs
   e. Foamy macrophages.

6. Isolated left ventricular failure causes:
   a. Pulmonary oedema
   b. Haemosiderin-laden alveolar macrophages
   c. Ascites
   d. 'Nutmeg' liver
   e. Raised jugular venous pressure.

7. The following are risk factors for coronary heart disease
   a. Alcohol consumption of 1 unit per day
   b. Raised HDL cholesterol

c. Post-menopausal state
d. Modest hypertension
e. Diabetes mellitus.

8. The following are correctly paired:
   a. Giant cell arteritis—temporal artery involvement
   b. Atherosclerosis—granulomatous inflammation
   c. Wegener's granulomatosis—respiratory-tract disease
   d. Polyarteritis nodosa—c-ANCA
   e. Henoch–Schonlein purpura—IgA nephropathy.

9. Aortic dissection:
   a. Is a complication of atherosclerosis
   b. Often commences distal to the aortic arch
   c. Is associated with systemic hypertension
   d. Can occur in patients with inherited connective tissue disorders
   e. Is inevitably fatal.

10. Regarding myocardial infarction:
    a. Macroscopic changes will be evident in the myocardium after 10 hours
    b. The right ventricle alone is affected in 10% of cases
    c. The underlying pathology always involves coronary artery atherosclerosis
    d. Irreversible myocardial cell injury requires at least 20 minutes of anoxia
    e. The subepicardial region of the heart muscle is the most susceptible to hypoxia.

11. Regarding vascular tumours:
    a. Kaposi's sarcoma occurs only in HIV-positive patients
    b. Kaposi's sarcoma is associated with cytomegalo-virus infection
    c. Angiosarcoma often arises in the skin
    d. Angiosarcoma can be an industrial disease
    e. Capillary haemangiomas have potential for malignant behaviour.

12. The following are correctly paired:
    a. Mitral stenosis—left ventricular hypertrophy
    b. Rheumatic fever—staphylococcus aureus
    c. Mitral incompetence—myocardial infarction
    d. Aortic stenosis—sudden cardiac death
    e. Mitral valve disease—cerebrovascular accident.

13. The following are risk factors for infective endocarditis:
    a. Rheumatic heart disease

b. Prosthetic heart valves
c. Immunosuppression
d. Endoscopy
e. Myocardial infarction.

Case histories

Case history 1

> A 67-year-old female presents with angina. ECG shows changes of left ventricular hypertrophy. An echocardiagram shows left ventricular thickening and an abnormal bicuspid aortic valve.

1. What are the pathological causes of left ventricular hypertrophy?
2. What is the significance of a bicuspid aortic valve?
3. What other cardiovascular complications might occur in this patient?

Case history 2

> A 58-year-old man presents complaining of chest pain. He has a history of hypertension. The blood pressure in his left arm is 180/100, while that measured in his right arm is 140/90. Chest X-ray shows minor widening of the mediastinal structures, which may be related to the aorta. ECG shows no evidence of acute ischaemia. He collapses and dies suddenly and a coroner's autopsy is performed to ascertain the cause of death. On opening the chest, a haemopericardium is apparent.

1. What are the possible causes of haemopericardium?
2. What is the clinical significance of hypertension and of the blood pressure difference between the arms?
3. What inflammatory conditions can affect the aorta?

Case history 3

> A 27-year-old drug addict is seen in Accident and Emergency having overdosed on heroin. Clinical examination and investigations during admission show swinging pyrexia, splinter haemorrhages and a cardiac murmur.

1. Which other investigations are indicated?
2. Of what further cardiovascular complications is the patient at risk?

Case history 4

> A 48-year-old female consults her GP for advice on coronary heart disease prevention. Her mother and paternal grandfather both died of 'heart attacks' before their seventieth birthdays. She has no history of cardiac symptoms herself, and is reluctant to take any regular medications.

1. What lifestyle advice would you give to this patient?
2. In view of her family history, what investigations might be considered?

Viva questions

1. What changes would you expect to see in the organs at the post mortem examination of a patient with congestive cardiac failure?
2. Discuss the risk factors for pulmonary embolism.

Self-assessment: answers

Multiple choice answers

1. a. **True.** If there are indications from urinalysis (proteinuria, haematuria) or from serum urea, creatinine and electrolyte measurements, that renal disease is present. Renal ultrasound can demonstrate kidney size, scarring and the presence of tumour masses or polycystic renal disease.
   b. **True.** If phaeochromocytoma is suspected (See Ch. 6).
   c. **False.**
   d. **True.** If renal artery stenosis is suspected.
   e. **True.** Fasting hyperglycaemia would suggest an underlying endocrine pathology—diabetes, acromegaly or Cushing's disease—with secondary hypertension.

2. a. **True.**
   b. **False.** There is pulmonary outflow tract stenosis; the tricuspid valve is unaffected.
   c. **False.**
   d. **True.**
   e. **True.** With larger defects, there is a significant left-to-right shunt, increasing pressure in the pulmonary circulation.

3. a. **True.** Infarct rupture is most common in the first 3–7 days.
   b. **True.**
   c. **True.**
   d. **False.** Ventricular aneurysm develops within the scar that forms as the infarcted muscle is replaced by fibrous tissue; it is a late complication, arising weeks or months after the infarct.
   e. **False.** This is an immunological reaction that develops at least 2 weeks after infarction.

4. a. **True.**
   b. **False.** Amyloid produces a restrictive cardiomyopathy.
   c. **True.**
   d. **True.**
   e. **True.**

5. a. **True.**
   b. **True.**
   c. **True.**
   d. **False.**
   e. **True.**

6. a. **True.**
   b. **True.**
   c. **False.**
   d. **False.**
   e. **False.**

7. a. **False.** This level of alcohol consumption is associated with a lower risk of coronary heart disease than abstinence. However, high alcohol intake is associated with greater cardiovascular morbidity.
   b. **False.**
   c. **True.** Women are relatively protected against ischaemic heart disease during reproductive years.
   d. **True.**
   e. **True.** Diabetes is associated with a two-fold increase in ischaemic heart disease.

8. a. **True.**
   b. **False.**
   c. **True.**
   d. **False.**
   e. **True.**

9. a. **False.**
   b. **False.** The dissection usually commences in the proximal 10 cm of the aorta.
   c. **True.**
   d. **True.** There is an increased incidence in patients with Marfan's syndrome.
   e. **False.**

10. a. **False.** Naked-eye changes are unlikely to be evident until at least 24 hours post-infarction
    b. **False.** Isolated right ventricular infarction accounts for only 3% of all infarcts, but the frequency of partial right ventricular involvement in inferior left ventricular infarcts is approximately 40%.
    c. **False.** Beware the 'always' and 'never' questions! The rare causes of myocardial infarction (with little or no coronary artery atheroma) include coronary artery aneurysm, dissection, arteritis and embolism.
    d. **True.**
    e. **False.** The most sensitive region to hypoxia is the subendocardium.

11. a. **False.**
    b. **False.** Herpes virus 8.
    c. **True.** Especially the head and neck of elderly patients.

d. **True.** Vinyl chloride exposure has been associated with angiosarcoma in the liver.

e. **False.** They are entirely benign neoplasms.

12. a. **False.** The left atrium is usually hypertrophic.

b. **False.** Rheumatic fever follows Group A β-haemolytic streptococcal infection.

c. **True.** If the infarct involves the papillary muscle.

d. **True.**

e. **True.** Both mitral stenosis and regurgitation can cause atrial enlargement and fibrillation, with a high risk of atrial thromboembolism to the brain.

13. a. **True.**

b. **True.**

c. **True.**

d. **True.** In patients with previously damaged or prosthetic valves, or certain types of congenital heart disease (e.g. patent ductus arteriosus).

e. **False.**

Case history answers

Case history 1

Pathological causes of left ventricular hypertrophy include:

- hypertension
- aortic stenosis
- mitral valve incompetence
- hypertrophic cardiomyopathy.

The first two are the commonest.

Congenitally bicuspid aortic valves occur in 1–2% of the UK population, and are more susceptible to becoming pathologically narrowed due to valve calcification. This occurs at an earlier age than calcific stenosis developing on a previously normal three-cusped aortic valve.

A congenitally abnormal valve is a risk factor for infective endocarditis, with its multiple complications. Bicuspid aortic valves can become incompetent as well as stenotic. Left ventricular hypertrophy can cause angina, sudden cardiac death (through a fatal cardiac arrhythmia), or gradual left ventricular failure.

Case history 2

Causes of haemopericardium include:

- ruptured myocardial infarction (commonest)
- aortic dissection
- trauma.

Hypertension and differing arm blood pressures may be features of aortic dissection. If the dissection involves the aortic arch, blood tracking in the aortic media can partly obstruct the major arterial vessels (carotid and left subclavian arteries), and therefore reduce blood flow and pressure in the upper limbs. Of course hypertension is very common in the UK population, and very few patients presenting with raised blood pressure and chest pain will have aortic dissection. Remember that hypertension is a major risk factor for ischaemic heart disease.

Aortic inflammation (vasculitis/aortitis) can occur in giant cell arteritis and in Takayasu's disease (a histologically similar but clinically distinct granulomatous vasculitis). In previous decades, tertiary syphilis was a common cause of aortitis with thoracic aortic aneurysm, but this condition is now extremely rare in the UK. Atherosclerosis is, of course, an inflammatory condition that commonly results in distal abdominal aneurysms. Rarely, infective aortitis results in mycotic aneurysm formation.

Case history 3

The features are highly suggestive of infective endocarditis. Blood cultures are required for identification of the organism(s) responsible—these are more likely to be positive in acute endocarditis than in subacute cases, where multiple culture specimens can be negative, especially if antibiotic therapy has been commenced. An echocardiogram will demonstrate valvular vegetations. Complications are discussed in Section 1.4, but include:

- valve incompetence, +/− acute cardiac failure
- septic embolisation and infarction
- glomerulonephritis
- distant organ abscess formation.

Case history 4

Remember that the four main risk factors for atherosclerosis, and therefore for coronary heart disease, are: smoking; hypertension; diabetes; and hypercholesterolaemia. Giving up cigarettes, maintaining a normal body weight, taking regular physical exercise, moderating excess alcohol intake and reducing cholesterol and saturated fats in the diet can all help reduce the risk of ischaemic heart disease.

Heart disease is very common, so it may be mere coincidence that this patient reports a family history. However, hypercholesterolaemia and Type II diabetes certainly can show familial clustering, so fasting cholesterol and dipstick urine testing or fasting blood glucose might be appropriate. A strong history of multiple young cardiac deaths in the family raises the possibility of a more unusual inherited cause, such as an uncommon form of hyperlipidaemia, hypertrophic cardiomyopathy or an unusual conduction defect.

Viva answers

1. Changes in the heart will reflect the underlying cause of the cardiac failure—there may be fibrosis of the left ventricle in ischaemic heart disease, with hypertrophy in hypertension, aortic stenosis or mitral incompetence. There is often generalised cardiac chamber enlargement (cardiomegaly) in biventricular failure. Other features can include valvular heart disease (vegetations, valve thickening, distortion or calcification), and right ventricular hypertrophy in patients with pulmonary hypertension. Ventricle hypertrophy is confirmed by measuring the isolated ventricular weight but may be suggested by increased muscle thickness.

The lungs frequently show marked vascular congestion and pulmonary oedema. The pleural cavities may contain straw-coloured effusions (transudates). The liver has a 'nutmeg' appearance on its cut surface, due to venous congestion, which is most severe in the perivenular (centrilobular) part of the liver lobules. The liver may show mild enlargement. Vascular congestion is also seen in the spleen and kidneys. Pitting subcutaneous oedema can be demonstrated in the dependent areas (usually lower legs).

2. You need to know what pulmonary embolism is, its clinical consequences, and the risk factors for deep vein thrombosis. Be prepared to discuss the basic pathophysiology of thrombogenesis. This is all covered in Section 1.6.

2 Respiratory system

Overview

The respiratory system extends from the nasal orifices to the periphery of the lungs and the pleura, and includes the nasal passages, paranasal sinuses, larynx and lungs. The pathology of these structures will be discussed in this chapter. Respiratory diseases are so commonplace that they will inevitably be encountered in whichever branch of medicine you decide to follow. Many bed-ridden patients develop some degree of bronchopneumonia. Pneumonia is also a frequent cause of hospital admission, and is often fatal in the elderly and infirm. Obstructive and restrictive (interstitial) lung diseases are common, causing significant morbidity among the general population. Last but not least, lung cancer is not only the most common malignancy in men, with dramatically increasing frequency in women, but it is also the most frequently fatal malignancy. Lung disease in general is a major cause of morbidity and mortality across the globe, and its importance in clinical practice cannot be overemphasised.

2.1 Nasal passages and paranasal sinuses

Learning objective

You should:

- Know the major inflammatory conditions and tumours that can affect the nasal passages and paranasal sinuses

Structure and function

The nasal passages and sinuses lie in continuity and are lined by respiratory-type epithelium. The function of the nasal sinuses is to warm, humidify and clean inspired air.

Inflammatory disorders

Inflammatory diseases are the commonest disorders to affect the nasal passages and paranasal sinuses.

Rhinitis

Inflammation of the nasal passages has two main causes:

1. **The common cold** (infective rhinitis). This is almost invariably initiated by a virus.
2. **Hay fever** (allergic rhinitis). This is initiated by allergens, the inflammatory reaction being mediated via Type I and Type III hypersensitivity reactions.

Nasal polyps

These inflammatory swellings are common and result from recurrent inflammation of the nasal passages. They are often bilateral (in contrast to nasal tumours which are usually unilateral).

Sinusitis

Inflammation of the sinuses is frequently a complication of acute rhinitis. Swelling of the nasal mucosa obstructs the drainage orifices of the sinuses. This leads to stasis of the secretions within the sinuses, with consequent infection and inflammation.

Tumours

Tumours of the nasal passages and sinuses are uncommon.

Benign

The most frequent benign tumours are:

- squamous papilloma
- inverted papilloma (transitional cell papilloma)
- haemangioma
- angiofibroma.

Malignant

The malignant tumours include:

- squamous cell carcinoma
- transitional cell carcinoma
- adenocarcinoma
- plasmacytoma
- olfactory neuroblastoma.

2.2 The larynx

Learning objectives

You should:

- Know the major inflammatory conditions and tumours which can affect the larynx
- Know the aetiology and behaviour of laryngeal carcinoma

Structure and function

The larynx connects the trachea to the pharynx. It is a complex organ with numerous connective tissue elements. The lining epithelium varies from non-keratinising stratified squamous to respiratory-type. The function of the larynx is to allow air into the trachea and to produce sound for speaking. The epiglottis prevents food from entering the trachea.

Inflammatory disorders

Laryngitis

Inflammation of the larynx can be the result of infection, overuse of the voice, mechanical irritation or exposure to tobacco, other chemical agents, or allergens. Infective laryngitis can be caused by a number of viruses and bacteria. The laryngeal inflammation is usually mild, but if it is severe, such as in diphtheria, the resultant oedema and exudate can cause laryngeal obstruction, particularly in children.

Epiglottitis

The most commonly implicated organism in epiglottitis is the bacteria *Haemophilus influenzae*. Infection results in marked oedema and enlargement of the epiglottis, which can cause life-threatening airway obstruction in children.

Tumours

Benign

The commonest benign tumours are:

- laryngeal polyps ('singers' nodes'). These are most often found in smokers or people who overuse their larynx
- squamous papilloma.

Malignant

The most frequent malignant tumour of the larynx is squamous cell carcinoma, which typically affects males over 40 years of age. This tumour is associated with cigarette smoking, and there may be an increased risk in those exposed to asbestos. Arising most often on the vocal cords, the carcinoma invades locally and can later cause widespread distant metastases.

2.3 The lungs

Learning objectives

You should:

- Understand the structure and function of the lungs
- Know the major groups of lung disorders
- Know the various types of infective, obstructive, restrictive, vascular and neoplastic lung conditions
- Understand the aetiology and pathogenesis of important respiratory diseases

Structure and function of the lungs

The function of the lungs is to exchange gases between the inspired air and the blood. Inspired air passes from the trachea into the main left and right bronchi. Each bronchus then branches dichotomously giving rise to progressively smaller airways, hence the term 'respiratory tree' (Fig. 4). Progressive branching of the bronchi forms bronchioles. Bronchioles branch until they form terminal bronchioles. The part of the lung distal to each terminal bronchiole is called the *acinus*, or *terminal respiratory unit*. Branching of the terminal bronchioles gives rise to respiratory bronchioles, which in turn branch into alveolar ducts. Each alveolar duct branches and empties into blind-ended alveolar sacs, where gas exchange occurs. A group of 3–5 acini is referred to as a *lobule*.

The trachea, bronchi and bronchioles are lined by respiratory-type epithelium. The alveoli are lined by Type I and Type II pneumocytes beneath which lies a connec-

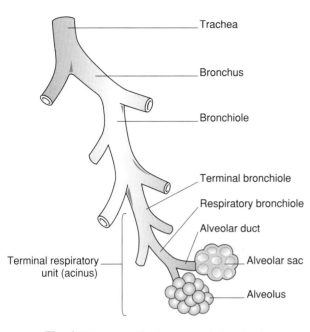

Trachea

Bronchus

Bronchiole

Terminal bronchiole

Respiratory bronchiole

Alveolar duct

Alveolar sac

Alveolus

Terminal respiratory unit (acinus)

Fig. 4 Structure of the lower respiratory tract.

tive tissue membrane. This membrane separates the alveoli from the pulmonary capillaries, but allows rapid and efficient diffusion of gases.

Disorders of the lungs can be divided into five major groups:

1. Inflammatory
2. Obstructive
3. Restrictive (interstitial)
4. Vascular
5. Neoplastic.

Inflammatory disorders

Bronchitis

Acute bronchitis can be caused by infection or exposure to irritant chemical agents such as tobacco smoke, sulphur dioxide, and chlorine. Infective inflammation of the bronchi is usually accompanied by inflammation of the trachea and larynx (acute laryngotracheobronchitis or 'croup'), which is clinically more severe in children. Acute infective bronchitis is most commonly initiated by viruses such as respiratory syncytial virus (RSV), although bacteria can also be a cause. Episodes of acute bronchitis are often seen in people with chronic bronchitis, causing an exacerbation of the established disease.

Bronchiolitis

There are three main types of bronchiolitis:

Primary bronchiolitis is most commonly seen in infants, in whom it can cause symptoms of acute respi-

ratory distress. The inflammation is usually caused by viruses, especially RSV. Resolution is usual, but a minority of patients develop bronchopneumonia.

Follicular bronchiolitis is seen in patients with rheumatoid arthritis. Lymphoid aggregates with germinal centres compress the airways.

Bronchiolitis obliterans can occur from a number of diseases and disease states, and is characterised by the obliteration of bronchiolar lumina by masses of organising inflammatory exudate.

Bacterial pneumonia

Pneumonia is defined as an inflammatory condition of the lung characterised by consolidation (solidification) of the pulmonary tissue. In infective pneumonia, the causative organism infects the lung parenchyma, causing the formation of an inflammatory exudate within the alveolar spaces with consequent consolidation.

Pathogenesis
The respiratory system employs a number of defence mechanisms to clear or destroy any inhaled microorganisms. These include:

- nasal secretions
- the mucociliary apparatus
- alveolar clearance by macrophages
- coughing, and sneezing.

Pneumonia can result whenever these defence mechanisms are impaired (see Table 3)

Classification
Classically, pneumonia is classified according to the main anatomical pattern of consolidation into either bronchopneumonia or lobar pneumonia (Fig. 5).

Bronchopneumonia is characterised by patchy consolidation of the lung. Those individuals most at risk are the elderly, infants, and people with debilitating illnesses. Typical aetiological organisms include streptococci, staphylococci, pneumococci, *Haemophilus influenzae*, *Pseudomonas aeruginosa*, and coliform bacteria. The consolidation is multilobular and frequently bilateral and basal. Histologically, a neutrophil-rich exudate fills the bronchi, bronchioles and adjacent alveolar spaces.

Lobar pneumonia is characterised by consolidation of a large portion of a lobe or an entire lobe, and it typically affects otherwise healthy adults aged between 20 and 50 years. The most common pathogenic organism is *Streptococcus pneumoniae*. Less common causal organisms are *Klebsiella pneumoniae*, staphylococci, streptococci, and *Haemophilus influenzae*.

Table 3 Defects in lung defence mechanisms predisposing to infection

Defect in defence mechanism	Causes
Loss or suppression of the cough reflex	Coma, sedation, neuromuscular disorders, drugs
Impairment of ciliary function	Immotile cilia syndrome (Kartagener's syndrome)
Injury to the mucociliary apparatus	Cigarette smoking
Accumulation of secretions	Cystic fibrosis, bronchiectasis
Interference with alveolar macrophage function	Cigarette smoking, hypoxia
Flooding of the alveoli	Pulmonary congestion and oedema
Reduction in immune response	Immunosuppression

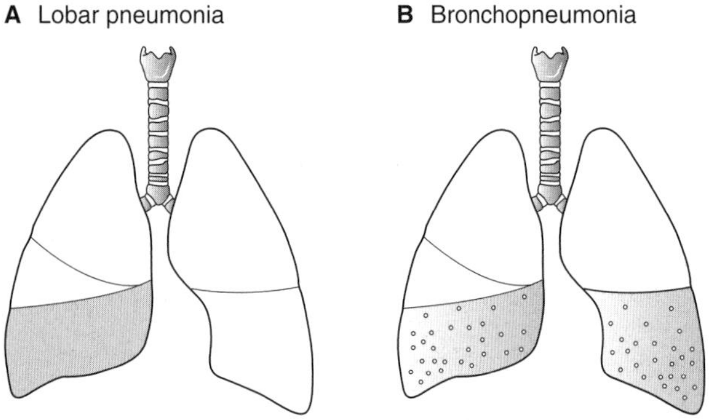

A Lobar pneumonia   **B** Bronchopneumonia

Fig. 5 The distribution of disease in (**A**) lobar pneumonia and (**B**) bronchopneumonia.

There are four stages in the pathological progress of untreated lobar pneumonia:

1. **Congestion**—This stage lasts for about 24 hours. It is characterised by vascular engorgement and the passage of exudate into the alveolar spaces. The affected lung is heavy and red.
2. **Red hepatisation**—This stage lasts for a few days. The exudate in the alveolar spaces now contains inflammatory cells, red blood cells and fibrin. A pleural fibrinous exudate forms (pleuritis/pleurisy). The lung is airless, red and solid.
3. **Grey hepatisation**—This stage also lasts for a few days. The inflammatory cells and red cells are destroyed while the fibrin continues to accumulate. The lung is firm and has a grey-brown, dry surface.
4. **Resolution**—This occurs on about the 8th day. The exudate undergoes enzymic digestion and is then resorbed or coughed up. The lung parenchyma returns to normal. The pleural exudate is either resorbed or undergoes organisation.

Atypical pneumonia

The term 'atypical' in the context of pneumonia is used when the inflammatory changes in the lungs are confined to the alveolar septa and interstitium, without a signifi-cant alveolar exudate. Characteristically, patients have few localising symptoms even with severe atypical pneumonia. As such, atypical pneumonia should be suspected when the chest X-ray is much worse than the symptoms.

Immunocompromised patients are particularly at risk.

Aetiology

In immunocompetent individuals the causes of atypical pneumonia are:

- Viruses, e.g. influenza, RSV, adenovirus
- Bacteria, e.g. *Legionella pneumophila* (Legionnaire's disease)
- Mycoplasma
- *Coxiella burnetii* (Q fever).

In immunocompromised individuals the causes of atypical pneumonia are:

- Viruses, e.g. CMV, measles, varicella
- Bacteria, e.g. *Pneumocystis carinii*, *Chlamydia*
- Fungi, e.g. *Candida*, *Aspergillus*.

Aspiration pneumonia

When food or liquid is aspirated into the lung, there is resultant irritation of the pulmonary tissue by the acidic gastric contents and introduction of organisms from the oropharynx. Inflammation and consolidation of the affected part of the lung may ensue. At risk clinical situations include sedation, coma, anaesthesia, and acute alcoholism.

Lung abscess

A lung abscess is a local suppurative process within the lungs (often walled off), accompanied by necrosis of the lung tissue.

Aetiology and pathogenesis

Under the right conditions, almost any pathogen can cause a lung abscess. An abscess may form as a result of:

- Aspiration or bacterial pneumonia
- Entrapment of septic emboli in the lungs (e.g. embolisation of vegetations in infective endocarditis)

- Infection of a pulmonary infarct
- Airway obstruction. An abscess may form beyond the obstruction, which may be a tumour or a foreign body
- Miscellaneous situations, such as following penetrating trauma to the lung or the spread of infection from neighbouring organs.

Complications

With antibiotic therapy, many resolve and heal completely leaving a fibrous scar. A persistent abscess may require surgical treatment. Possible complications of a lung abscess include an empyema, pyopneumothorax, haemorrhage, and spread of infection to distant sites to cause, for example, brain abscesses or meningitis.

Tuberculosis

The term 'tuberculosis' refers to the disease caused by *Mycobacterium tuberculosis* (found within infected respiratory secretions and air droplets) and less commonly *Mycobacterium bovis* (found in the milk of diseased cows). Tuberculosis (TB) is the single most important infectious cause of death in the world. Up until the mid-

1980s, western countries had seen a decline in the number of clinical cases because of:

- improved hygiene and social conditions
- the introduction of effective antibiotics against the bacilli
- the introduction of immunisation with bacille Calmette–Guérin (BCG).

At present the incidence of TB is rising in the USA, Europe, and Africa, most probably due to the increasing incidence of HIV infection. Furthermore, antibiotic-resistant strains are now being isolated. The lung is the commonest site for infection. TB is classically divided into two phases, primary and post-primary (secondary) TB (Fig. 6).

Primary tuberculosis

Inhaled *M. tuberculosis* passes into the lungs and initiates a non-specific inflammatory response. Alveolar macrophages phagocytose the organism and transport it to the hilar lymph nodes. These naive macrophages are unable to kill the organism, and so more macrophages are recruited. Meanwhile, the bacilli multiply, lyse the host cell and then infect more macrophages. At this

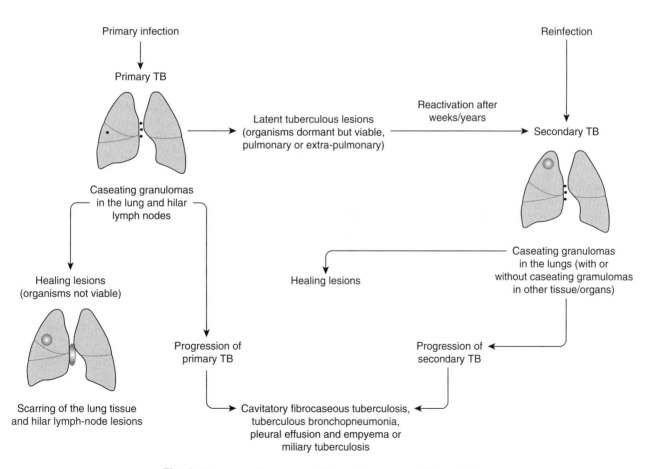

Fig. 6 Diagrammatic representations of the course of tuberculosis.

point, the organisms can potentially disseminate via the bloodstream to other parts of the lung and more distant sites. In immunocompetent hosts, the mycobacteria activate T-cells, which can cause lysis of infected macrophages and stimulate macrophages to mature into epithelioid cells, which are effective killers of *M. tuberculosis*. Some epithelioid cells fuse to become multinucleate giant cells. Consequently, a granuloma forms consisting of epithelioid cells, giant cells and a central area of caseous necrosis corresponding to lysed infected macrophages. The bacilli are unable to survive in such acidic and oxygen-poor conditions, and so infection is controlled. A calcified scar forms in both the affected lung parenchyma (Ghon focus) and the hilar lymph nodes, which together are referred to as a primary Ghon complex. Importantly, bacilli may still survive in these scarred foci for many years. Primary TB is asymptomatic in most cases. Rarely, particularly with infants, children or immunocompromised adults, the primary lesion may progress, resulting in cavitation, tuberculous bronchopneumonia, pleural effusion and empyema, or miliary TB.

Post-primary (secondary) tuberculosis
Most post-primary TB represents reactivation of previous primary TB. During primary infection, the bacilli may attempt to disseminate and establish themselves at sites of high oxygen tension and low blood flow, such as the lung apices. Development of post-primary TB may occur if the host is susceptible, with the formation of typical caseating granulomas. These lesions either heal spontaneously, or with treatment, resulting in a fibrocalcific scar. Alternatively, post-primary TB may progress resulting in cavitatory fibrocaseous TB, tuberculous pneumonia, pleural effusion and empyema, or miliary TB.

Miliary tuberculosis
If the tuberculous bacteraemia becomes heavy during primary or post-primary TB, miliary TB may result. Miliary TB is characterised by numerous granulomas in many organs, and may be fatal if left untreated.

Obstructive airways disease

This group of disorders is characterised by an increase in resistance to airflow, owing to partial or complete obstruction at any level of the respiratory tree. The major obstructive disorders are chronic bronchitis, emphysema, asthma, and bronchiectasis. The symptom common to all these disorders is 'dyspnoea' (difficulty breathing), but each have their own clinical and anatomical characteristics.

Chronic bronchitis and emphysema almost always coexist, and the term chronic obstructive pulmonary disease (COPD) is often used to refer to them.

Chronic bronchitis

Chronic bronchitis is defined clinically as cough with sputum production for at least three months in at least two consecutive years. The condition tends to affect middle-aged men who are smokers. Typically, patients with severe disease are cyanotic (blue), and are then referred to as 'blue bloaters'.

Aetiology
Undoubtedly, the single most important cause is cigarette smoking.

Pathogenesis
Irritants, such as tobacco smoke, cause two main abnormalities, which lead to airway obstruction:

1. Increase in size (hypertrophy) of submucosal glands and a marked increase in the number (hyperplasia) of goblet cells. There is consequent hypersecretion of mucus, mainly in the large airways, which results in mucus plugging and overproduction of sputum.
2. A respiratory bronchiolitis affecting the smaller airways of less than 2 mm in diameter.

Infection does not appear to play a role in the initiation of chronic bronchitis, but is an important cause of exacerbations.

Emphysema

Emphysema is characterised by abnormal permanent dilatation of the air spaces distal to the terminal bronchioles, accompanied by destruction of their walls without obvious fibrosis. The clinical symptoms of emphysema do not appear until at least one-third of the lung parenchyma is destroyed. Typically, patients overventilate to remain well oxygenated, and are then referred to as 'pink puffers'.

Classification
Emphysema is classified into four main types according to the anatomical distribution of the lesions and based on the appearance of the lungs with the naked eye or hand lens (Fig. 7).

A. Centrilobular (centriacinar) emphysema—in this type there is involvement of the central or proximal parts of the acinus with sparing of the distal alveoli. The lesions are closely associated with cigarette smoking and are more common in the upper lobes.

B. Panlobular (panacinar) emphysema—in this type all airways distal to the terminal bronchioles (i.e. the entire acinus) are involved. The lower lobes are more commonly affected, particularly the bases. Panacinar emphysema is associated with α_1-antitrypsin deficiency.

because they are unable to inhibit elastase secreted by inflammatory cells. Airway-wall destruction ensues. The process is further compounded by smoking, mainly because smokers have more inflammatory cells in their lungs.

Irregular emphysema is thought to be due to air-trapping caused by fibrotic scarring. The scars are the result of a previous inflammatory process.

Pathology

In the advanced stages of the disease, the lungs may appear voluminous and bullae may be seen. Microscopically, there are abnormal fenestrations in the walls of the alveoli with complete destruction of the septal walls.

Asthma

Asthma is a chronic relapsing disorder characterised by hyperreactive airways leading to episodic, reversible bronchoconstriction, owing to increased responsiveness of the tracheobronchial tree to various stimuli. These sudden episodes of bronchoconstriction are manifested by sudden attacks of dyspnoea, coughing and wheezing. Between attacks, patients are often asymptomatic. Rarely, symptoms may be severe and prolonged (status asthmaticus). Severe asthma and status asthmaticus are both medical emergencies and can prove fatal.

Asthma is divided into two basic types:

1. Extrinsic asthma
2. Intrinsic asthma.

Extrinsic asthma

This type of asthma is induced by exposure to an extrinsic allergen, and is mediated by a Type-I hypersensitivity reaction.

Atopic allergic asthma—this is the most common type of asthma. It usually begins in childhood and patients may also suffer from other atopic disorders such as hay fever or eczema. There is often a family history of asthma, hay fever, or eczema. The asthma is triggered by environmental allergens such as dust, pollen, food and animal dander. Inhalation of such allergens triggers a Type-I IgE-mediated hypersensitivity reaction, which is characterised by an immediate response and a late phase reaction caused by the local release of inflammatory mediators from a variety of cell types (Fig. 8). The precise pathogenesis of asthma involves interactions between many cell types and mediators, and these interactions are not fully understood. A number of chemical mediators are implicated in the asthma response. Histamine, prostaglandin D2, leukotrienes, platelet-activating factor, tumour-necrosis factor (TNF), chemokines and various interleukins are among those substances thought to be important.

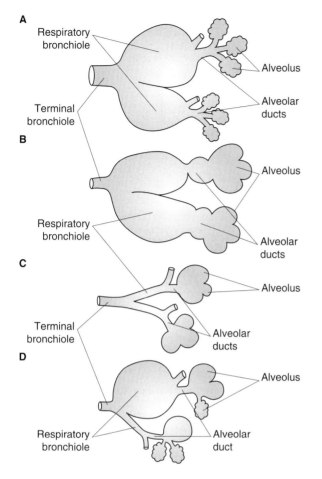

Fig. 7 The classification of emphysema. (**A**) Centrilobular, (**B**) panacinar, (**C**) paraseptal, (**D**) irregular emphysema.

C. Paraseptal emphysema—in this type the distal (peripheral) part of the acinus is involved, with sparing of the proximal part. It is usually more severe in the upper lobes. The affected airways can become very dilated forming cyst-like structures which are termed 'bullous' if they reach over 10 mm in diameter. These bullae may rupture resulting in a spontaneous pneumothorax.

D. Irregular emphysema—in this type the acinus is irregularly involved. Irregular emphysema is almost invariably associated with scarring.

Pathogenesis

Current evidence indicates that emphysema is due to an imbalance between protease and antiprotease activity in the lung. Support for this theory is based on the association between α_1-antitrypsin deficiency and the development of emphysema. α_1-Antitrypsin inhibits the actions of proteases, particularly elastase, which is secreted by neutrophils. α_1-Antitrypsin deficiency is a genetic disorder showing an autosomal recessive pattern of inheritance. Homozygous patients have reduced levels of the enzyme and have a tendency to develop emphysema

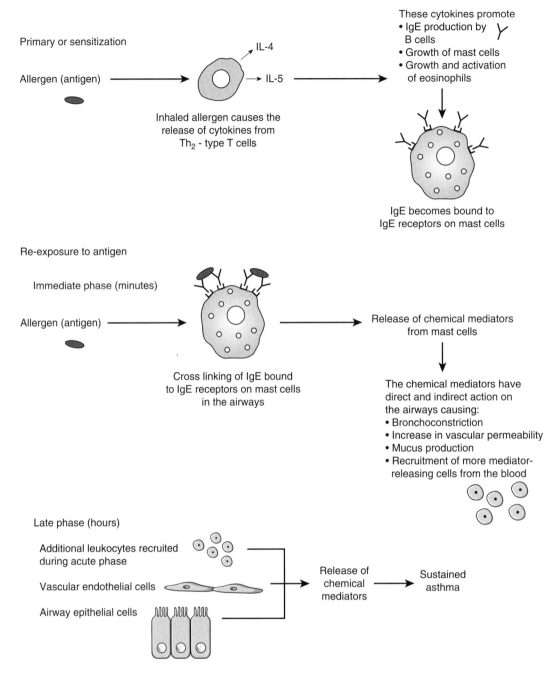

Primary or sensitization

Allergen (antigen) →

IL-4

IL-5

Inhaled allergen causes the release of cytokines from Th₂ - type T cells

These cytokines promote
• IgE production by B cells
• Growth of mast cells
• Growth and activation of eosinophils

IgE becomes bound to IgE receptors on mast cells

Re-exposure to antigen

Immediate phase (minutes)

Allergen (antigen) →

Cross linking of IgE bound to IgE receptors on mast cells in the airways

Release of chemical mediators from mast cells

The chemical mediators have direct and indirect action on the airways causing:
• Bronchoconstriction
• Increase in vascular permeability
• Mucus production
• Recruitment of more mediator-releasing cells from the blood

Late phase (hours)

Additional leukocytes recruited during acute phase

Vascular endothelial cells

Airway epithelial cells

Release of chemical mediators →

Sustained asthma

Fig. 8 A model of mechanisms in the pathogenesis of asthma.

The following morphological changes are seen in the lungs in cases of severe asthma:

1. Mucous plugging of bronchi. These plugs may contain whorls of shed epithelium (Curschmann's spirals).
2. Oedema and inflammation of the bronchial walls. Histologically, there is prominence of eosinophils. Eosinophil membrane protein can be seen as crystals, called Charcot–Leyden crystals.
3. Over inflation of the lungs distal to the obstruction.
4. Mucous gland hypertrophy.
5. Bronchial wall smooth muscle hypertrophy.
6. Thickening of the bronchial basement membrane.

Occupational asthma—this form of asthma is triggered by agents inhaled at work, e.g. fumes, dusts, gases and other chemicals. The airway reaction is thought to be mediated by Type-I and Type-III hypersensitivity.

Allergic bronchopulmonary aspergillosis—this type of asthma is induced by the inhalation of spores of the fungus *Aspergillus fumigatus*. The inhaled spores induce Type-I and Type-III hypersensitivity reactions.

Intrinsic asthma

Intrinsic asthma can be induced by pulmonary infection (usually viral), ingestion of aspirin, cold, exercise, and stress. The mechanism leading to the bronchoconstriction appears to be non-immunological. The pathogenesis remains uncertain.

Bronchiectasis

Bronchiectasis is characterised by permanent dilatation of bronchi and bronchioles. Affected patients suffer from cough with the production of copious amounts of foul-smelling sputum.

Pathogenesis

Both obstruction and infection are usually necessary for development of bronchiectasis. Obstruction of the bronchial lumen results in secondary inflammation and fibrosis. The damaged bronchial walls weaken and eventually become irreversibly dilated. The obstruction can be due to a foreign body, tumour, inspissated mucus, or external compression. Persistent infection results in inflammation and leads to extensive weakening and destruction of the airway walls. Either infection or obstruction may be the initiating factors in the development of bronchiectasis. Persistent infection may lead to obstruction of airways, and obstruction may lead to secondary infection.

It therefore follows that bronchiectasis may be associated with congenital or hereditary disorders such as cystic fibrosis, Kartagener's syndrome, or immunodeficiency states.

Complications

Complications such as empyema formation, brain abscess and amyloidosis are now rare.

Interstitial (restrictive) lung diseases

The interstitium of the lung consists of the basement membrane of the endothelial and epithelial cells, collagen fibres, elastic tissue, fibroblasts and occasional inflammatory cells. In this group of disorders, there is diffuse infiltration of the interstitium, leading to increased amounts of tissue in the lung and causing reduced lung compliance and lung volume, and reduced oxygen diffusing capacity. The functional changes are restrictive rather than obstructive, and affected patients develop symptoms of progressive breathlessness and cough.

Many conditions belong to this group of disorders and, although each begins as a distinct entity, they all ultimately cause scarring and destruction of the lung, referred to as 'honeycomb lung'.

Pathogenesis

Regardless of the type of interstitial lung disease, the earliest change seen in the lungs is the influx of inflammatory cells into the alveoli and alveolar walls. This distorts the normal structure of the alveoli and results in the release of chemical mediators, which injure parenchymal cells and promote fibrosis. Ultimately, with remodelling, the alveoli are replaced by cystic spaces separated by fibrous connective tissue (honeycomb lung).

Classification

There are many ways in which the interstitial lung diseases can be classified, and these are shown in Table 4.

Pneumoconiosis

This term is used to refer to a group of lung diseases resulting from the inhalation of dusts, fumes and vapours.

Coalworkers' pneumoconiosis (CWP)—this condition is caused by inhalation of coal dust. Because coal dust particles are less than 2–3 µm in size, they travel all

Table 4 Classification of interstitial lung diseases

Classification according to aetiology		Classification according to speed of onset of damage	
Known aetiology	**Unknown aetiology**	**Acute interstitial diseases**	**Chronic interstitial diseases**
Environmental agents	Idiopathic pulmonary fibrosis	ARDS	Idiopathic pulmonary fibrosis
Radiation		Drugs and toxins	Pneumoconiosis
Hypersensitivity pneumonitis	Sarcoid	Acute radiation pneumonitis	Sarcoid
Following adult repiratory distress syndrome (ARDS)	Goodpasture's syndrome	Diffuse pulmonary haemorrhage syndromes	Collagen vascular diseases
	Idiopathic pulmonary haemosiderosis		
Drugs and toxins	Collagen vascular diseases		

the way to the alveoli. The coal dust is ingested by alveolar macrophages, which then aggregate around the airways and lymphatics. During their attempts to degrade the particles, macrophages release inflammatory chemical mediators, which cause parenchymal injury and induce fibrosis. The effect of coal dust on the lungs progresses through three stages. Progression through the stages, with continued exposure to coal dust, varies significantly from person to person.

1. **Anthracosis** refers to the presence of coal-dust pigment within the lung, and is asymptomatic.
2. **Simple CWP** refers to focal accumulations of dust-laden macrophages within the lung. This stage can be further subdivided into macular and nodular CWP. Coal macules are lesions measuring 1–2 mm in diameter; while coal nodules are larger and contain collagen fibres. The effect of simple CWP on lung function is minimal.
3. **Complicated CWP/progressive massive fibrosis (PMF)** refers to the presence of large, blackened nodules (> 10 mm) within the lung with extensive scarring. The condition generally takes several years to develop, but ultimately the progressive fibrosis results in severely compromised lung function.

Silicosis—silicates are inorganic minerals found in stone and sand. Silica particles are particularly fibrogenic and, after inhalation, enter the terminal respiratory units, where they stimulate the release of chemical mediators from macrophages. They also have toxic effects on macrophages and epithelial cells, denaturing their cell membranes. Grossly, affected lungs contain multiple fibrous nodules, which may coalesce to form large scars. Fibrotic lesions may also occur in the hilar lymph nodes and their characteristic appearance on radiography is referred to as 'eggshell calcification'. With progression of the disease there is severe impairment of lung function.

Asbestosis—asbestos is a family of silicates that form fibres. Two distinct geometric forms of asbestos exist:

1. Serpentine: curly flexible fibres. Includes the chrysotile form.
2. Amphibole: straight stiff fibres. Includes the crocidolite and amosite forms.

Amphiboles are more pathogenic than serpentines. The long, thin fibres have a small enough diameter (0.25–0.5 μm) to reach all the way to the alveoli and become impacted there. Alveolar macrophages attempt to ingest and degrade the fibres but, in so doing, release chemical mediators that cause tissue injury and fibrosis resulting in asbestosis. The fibrosis tends to be diffuse rather than nodular. During the attempts at engulfment and digestion, asbestos fibres become coated by mucopolysaccharides and haemosiderin, producing a beaded appearance under microscopy (asbestos bodies). As well as asbestosis, exposure to asbestos can cause other pathological changes in the lungs:

- pleural plaques—the commonest manifestation of asbestos exposure (they are asymptomatic)
- bronchogenic carcinoma
- mesothelioma
- other extrapulmonary neoplasms, e.g. laryngeal, gastrointestinal.

Berylliosis—results from prolonged exposure to beryllium. Workers in the nuclear and aerospace industries are at risk, but new cases of chronic berylliosis are now rare. Beryllium induces the formation of pulmonary and systemic granulomatous lesions. The pulmonary granulomas eventually become fibrotic.

Caplan's syndrome—this refers to the coexistence of rheumatoid nodules with a pneumoconiosis.

Idiopathic pulmonary fibrosis

In this condition there is diffuse pulmonary fibrosis of unknown aetiology. The disorder typically affects individuals between 45 and 65. With progression of the disease, respiratory failure with or without cor pulmonale ensues. Although some patients benefit from treatment with corticosteroids, the median survival is less than five years.

Hypersensitivity pneumonitis (extrinsic allergic alveolitis)

This is caused by intense prolonged exposure to antigens which evoke Type-III and Type-IV hypersensitivity responses. Conditions such as farmer's lung, pigeon breeder's lung, and humidifier lung are included in this type of interstitial lung disease.

Drugs and toxins

After they are absorbed into the body, some drugs (e.g. bleomycin, nitrofurantoin, gold, penicillamine and amiodarone) and some other toxic substances (e.g. paraquat) can cause fibrosis within the lungs.

Ionising radiation

The toxic effects of radiation on the lungs is dose dependent, with increased exposure to radiation increasing the risk of diffuse alveolar damage (acute radiation pneumonitis). The condition is most commonly seen in those undergoing radiation therapy for pulmonary or other thoracic tumours. Some cases of acute radiation pneumonitis respond to corticosteroid treatment, but others progress leading to interstitial fibrosis in the affected area (chronic radiation pneumonitis).

Sarcoidosis

This condition is characterised by non-caseating granulomas within many tissues and organs. There is lung and lymph node involvement in the vast majority of cases. The chest X-ray of affected individuals typically shows bilateral hilar lymphadenopathy.

Pulmonary involvement in collagen vascular disorders

Systemic sclerosis (scleroderma)
Systemic lupus erythematosus (SLE)
Rheumatoid arthritis, pulmonary involvement occurs in one of four forms:

- chronic pleuritis
- diffuse interstitial fibrosis
- intrapulmonary rheumatoid nodules
- rheumatoid nodules with pneumoconiosis (Caplan's syndrome).

Diffuse pulmonary haemorrhage syndromes

Goodpasture's syndrome—in this condition, circulating anti-glomerular basement membrane (anti-GBM) antibodies cross-react with pulmonary alveolar basement membrane, resulting in intrapulmonary haemorrhage.

Idiopathic pulmonary haemosiderosis—typically affects children and is manifest by recurrent episodes of intra-alveolar haemorrhage.

Vasculitides causing intra-pulmonary haemorrhage—involvement of the lung by vasculitides such as hypersensitivity angiitis, Wegener's granulomatosis, and SLE can cause intrapulmonary haemorrhage.

Adult respiratory distress syndrome

Adult respiratory distress syndrome (ARDS) is characterised by rapid onset of respiratory distress, initiated by the delivery of a massive insult to the alveolar capillary walls. Endothelial damage allows leakage of proteins and fibrin into the alveoli with the formation of hyaline membranes, which act as barriers to gas exchange. The insult can occur in a number of clinical settings, but infection and physical injuries such as burns and head injuries are the most common causes. The condition is fatal within a few days in 50% of cases despite intensive therapy. For the majority of survivors, there is permanent lung damage with fibro-

sis. Resolution of the inflammation and complete recovery is unusual.

Bronchiolitis obliterans organising pneumonia

The major pathological finding in bronchiolitis obliterans organising pneumonia (BOOP) is polypoid plugs of loose fibrous tissue (Masson's bodies) filling the bronchioles. Aetiologies include infections, inhaled toxins, drugs, collagen vascular diseases and bronchial obstruction.

Miscellaneous

Other less-common causes of interstitial lung disease include condition such as histiocytosis X, pulmonary eosinophilia, and pulmonary alveolar proteinosis.

Vascular diseases of the lungs

Pulmonary oedema and congestion

Pulmonary oedema signifies increased fluid in the lung interstitium, causing breathlessness and cough productive of frothy, pink sputum. There are several causes of pulmonary oedema:

Common causes
- Increased venous hydrostatic pressure.

Uncommon causes
- Injury to the alveolar capillary bed, e.g. ARDS
- Blockage of lymphatic drainage
- Lowered plasma oncotic pressure.

The commonest cause of pulmonary oedema is increased venous hydrostatic pressure, most often resulting from left ventricular failure. When the increasing hydrostatic pressure exceeds the oncotic pressure within the pulmonary capillaries, fluid is forced out of the vessels and into the lung interstitium, with resultant pulmonary oedema. Oedematous lungs are heavy, congested and wet. Histologically, the alveolar capillaries are engorged, and frothy, pink precipitate can be seen within the alveoli. Alveolar microhaemorrhages may be seen with associated haemosiderin-laden macrophages ('heart failure cells').

Pulmonary embolism

An embolus is a detached intravascular solid, liquid or gaseous mass, which is carried by the blood to a site distant from its point of origin. Pulmonary embolism refers to the occlusion of some part of the pulmonary arterial tree by an embolus.

Pulmonary thromboembolism—this is by far the commonest type of embolus. In most cases, the thrombotic mass originates in the deep veins of the legs above the level of the knee. After detachment, the embolic mass travels via the bloodstream to the right side of the heart and into the main pulmonary artery. Thereafter, the calibre of the blood vessels decreases progressively and the embolus eventually becomes lodged. The consequences of this depend on the volume of lung tissue subsequently deprived of blood. Emboli that occlude the main pulmonary artery or impact across the bifurcation (saddle embolus, see Fig. 3) or occlude the right or left pulmonary artery, often cause sudden death. Death is usually due to acute right heart failure. Smaller emboli can pass into and occlude smaller arteries supplying a lobe or a segment of the lung, causing severe chest pain with dyspnoea. Small emboli occluding the smaller arterioles may be clinically silent, but entrapment of multiple small emboli over the course of time eventually causes occlusion of the vascular pulmonary bed, resulting in pulmonary hypertension and cor pulmonale. Rarely, an embolus may pass through an interatrial or interventricular septal defect to gain access to the systemic circulation (paradoxical embolism).

Because of the dual blood supply to most parts of the lungs, pulmonary embolism causes infarction only when the circulation is already inadequate, e.g. patients with cardiac or respiratory disease. Infarcts are typically wedge shaped.

Most emboli eventually resolve by fibrinolysis. However, since patients who have had one pulmonary embolus are at high risk of having more, therapy with fibrinolytic agents is usually initiated. Prevention of deep-vein thrombosis is of major clinical importance.

Fat embolism—fat emboli result from fracture of bones containing fatty marrow, or by massive injury to subcutaneous fat. The globules of fat enter torn veins and become emboli.

Gas embolism—air emboli can occur after chest trauma. Undissolved nitrogen can come out of solution in divers during decompression ('decompression sickness').

Amniotic fluid embolism—this type of embolus can occur during delivery or abortion. During labour, amniotic fluid may enter torn uterine veins. Flakes of keratin and epithelial squamous cells shed from the fetal skin embolise to the lungs, where they become lodged. If the patient survives the initial crisis, thrombogenic substances contained within the amniotic fluid trigger disseminated intravascular coagulation (DIC).

Tumour embolism—clusters of tumour cells may enter the venous circulation and, if large enough, occlude the pulmonary veins.

Pulmonary hypertension

Pulmonary hypertension is defined as the point when the mean pulmonary blood pressure reaches one quarter of the systemic level. Patients present with dyspnoea and fatigue, or anginal-type chest pain. Over time, symptoms worsen and right ventricular hypertrophy develops with ensuing cor pulmonale.

Pulmonary hypertension can be primary, but it is most often secondary to other cardiopulmonary conditions such as:

- pulmonary embolism
- obstructive lung diseases
- interstitial lung diseases
- left ventricular failure
- mitral stenosis.

Pathology
Changes seen within the arteries include the deposition of atheroma, an increase in the thickness of the muscular media (medial hypertrophy) and intimal fibrosis. Changes relating to the underlying cause are also seen.

Lung tumours

Bronchogenic carcinoma

Bronchogenic carcinoma is the commonest malignancy in the UK, and has the worst prognosis. It accounts for around one-third of all cancer deaths in men, and the incidence is rising in women. Typical patients are aged between 40 and 70 years.

Aetiology
Cigarette smoking—there is overwhelming evidence implicating cigarette smoking as a major risk factor for the development of lung cancer.

Occupational hazards—there is a high correlation between asbestos exposure and the risk of lung cancer, especially adenocarcinoma. The risk is heightened dramatically if the individual also smokes. All types of radiation may be carcinogenic. There is also an increased risk of lung cancer among people who work with nickel, chromates, coal, mustard gas, arsenic, beryllium and iron.

Scarring—some lung cancers, especially adenocarcinomas, appear to arise in areas of previous scarring, e.g. old tuberculous foci. It has been proposed that scarring induces dysplasia of pneumocytes, predisposing to lung cancer in that area.

Classification
Bronchogenic carcinoma is classified according to the appearance under light microscopy:

1. Squamous cell carcinoma (25–40%)
2. Adenocarcinoma (25–40%)
3. Small cell carcinoma (20–25%)
4. Large cell carcinoma (10–15%).

Occasionally, lung carcinomas are simply classified as either small cell carcinoma or non-small cell carcinoma. The relevance of this type of classification is that small cell carcinomas are more responsive to chemotherapy than any of the other types of lung cancer.

Squamous cell carcinoma—this type of lung cancer is closely associated with smoking. The tumour commonly arises in the central bronchi and spreads locally, usually at a rapid rate. Metastases usually occur later than with the other types of lung cancer. The tumours are thought to arise from areas of squamous metaplasia through grades of dysplasia.

Adenocarcinoma—this type of cancer is usually peripheral and is sometimes associated with scarring. It is the most common type of lung cancer in women and non-smokers. Adenocarcinomas grow more slowly than the squamous cell carcinomas.

Small cell carcinoma—small cell carcinoma is a neuroendocrine tumour and is strongly related to cigarette smoking. The tumours often arise centrally in the lungs and metastasise widely but, unlike other types of lung cancer, they are sensitive to radiotherapy and chemotherapy. Small cell carcinoma is also referred to as 'oat cell' carcinoma, because the cells are thought to resemble oat grains; they are small, round to oval, and have little cytoplasm. The nuclei often appear smudged under microscopy. As these tumours originate from neuroendocrine (Kulchitsky) cells present in the bronchial epithelium, they show the following additional features:

- the cytoplasm contains neurosecretory granules similar to those seen in Kulchitsky cells
- some of these tumours secrete polypeptide hormones
- the cells stain positively for neuroendocrine markers on immunohistochemistry.

Large cell carcinoma—these are usually central, highly aggressive tumours. Histologically, the cells are highly pleomorphic with numerous bizarre mitoses. Large cell carcinoma may represent squamous cell carcinomas and adenocarcinomas that are so poorly differentiated that they can no longer be recognised.

Gross pathology

The tumour starts as an irregular thickening, which grows either exophytically (outwords into the lumen), to produce an intraluminal mass, or endophytically (into the bronchial wall), causing erosion of the bronchial wall. Spread is by local extension to neighbouring tissues, spread to lymph nodes, and distant metastases.

Clinical features

The clinical features of lung cancer are the result of local spread within the lung, direct spread to neighbouring structures, distant spread, or paraneoplastic syndromes.

Effects of local intrapulmonary spread

- cough—due to irritation of the airways
- haemoptysis—due to erosion of small blood vessels
- wheezing, stridor, atelectasis, pneumonia, brochiectasis, lung abscess—due to airway obstruction.

Effects of direct spread to neighbouring structures

- pain—with involvement of nerves, or the pleura (pleuritis)
- shortness of breath—extension to the pleura causes pleural effusions
- hoarse voice—with involvement of the recurrent laryngeal nerve
- paralysis of the diaphragm—with involvement of the phrenic nerve
- symptoms caused by a tumour in the lung apex (Pancoast's tumour)
  1. Horner's syndrome (sunken eye, small pupil, eyelid drooping and loss of sweating on the same side of the lesion) due to involvement of the sympathetic ganglia
  2. pain and weakness in the shoulder and arm due to involvement of the branchial plexus
- vena caval syndrome—characterised by facial congestion, oedema of the face, neck and upper arms, and distension of the veins in the neck and over the chest.

Effects of distant spread—depend on the sites of the secondary deposits.

Effects of the paraneoplastic syndromes—paraneoplastic syndromes are signs or symptoms in cancer patients that are not explicable in terms of local or metastatic spread of the tumour. General paraneoplastic syndromes include weight loss, fever and loss of appetite.

Paraneoplastic syndromes may be associated with the secretion of hormones (endocrinopathies). All the types of bronchogenic carcinoma can secrete hormones, including antidiuretic hormone (ADH), adrenocorticotrophic hormone (ACTH), parathormone, parathyroid hormone-related peptide, some cytokines, calcitonin, gonadotrophin and serotonin, and the syndromes associated with secretion of these hormones may become clinically apparent (e.g. development of Cushing's syndrome with the secretion of ACTH).

Other paraneoplastic syndromes that can occur include:

- Lambert–Eaton myasthenic syndrome
- peripheral neuropathy
- hypertrophic pulmonary osteoarthropathy.

Treatment and prognosis

The stage of the tumour at presentation is of prognostic significance (the tumour–node–metastasis (TNM) staging system is usually adopted), but the prognosis is generally poor. The only hope of cure is total resection of the tumour, which is only possible with peripheral tumours without metastases. Some patients with small cell carcinoma benefit from radiotherapy and chemotherapy, which can induce remission (occasionally sustained).

Neuroendocrine tumours

There are three types of malignant neuroendocrine tumours found in the lung:

- small cell carcinoma (discussed above)
- bronchial carcinoid
- large cell neuroendocrine carcinoma.

Bronchial carcinoids are considered to be tumours of low-grade malignancy and resemble carcinoid tumours found elsewhere, e.g. intestine. They are capable of producing the classic carcinoid syndrome. Growth of these tumours is slow and they may be amenable to resection. Consequently, the survival figures for bronchial carcinoids are much better than those for bronchogenic carcinoma.

Large cell neuroendocrine tumours are more aggressive than bronchial carcinoids.

Miscellaneous primary lung tumours

Included in this category of lung tumour are:

- benign and malignant tumours of salivary-gland type
- benign and malignant mesenchymal tumours
- benign and malignant lymphoreticular tumours
- lung hamartomas
- adenomas.

Metastatic lung tumours

The lung is a frequent site for metastatic neoplasms. Just about any carcinoma, sarcoma or lymphoma can spread to the lung, but those most commonly implicated are carcinomas from the breast, kidney and gastrointestinal tract. Multiple discrete tumour nodules may be scattered throughout the lungs, or if the spread is via the lymphatics, the metastatic growth may be confined to peribronchial and perivascular tissue, leading to the characteristic appearance of grey-white streaking of tumour in the lungs (lymphangitis carcinomatosis).

2.4 The pleura

Learning objectives

You should:

- Understand what is meant by the term 'pleural effusion' and know the various clinical settings in which it may arise

- Understand what is meant by the term 'pneumothorax' and know the various types

- Know about malignant mesothelioma

The structure of the pleura

The pleura are composed of two opposing layers of connective tissue lined by mesothelial cells. The visceral pleura covers the lungs and the parietal pleura lines the internal thoracic wall and covers the thoracic surface of the diaphragm, the heart and the mediastinum. The potential space between these two layers is called the pleural cavity or pleural space.

Pleural effusion

This term denotes an increased accumulation of fluid between the two layers of the pleura, causing shortness of breath. Pleural effusions can occur in the following settings:

- increased hydrostatic pressure, e.g. congestive cardiac failure
- increased capillary permeability, e.g. pneumonia, bronchogenic carcinoma, mesothelioma
- decreased intrapleural negative pressure, e.g. atelectasis
- decreased lymphatic drainage, e.g. mediastinal carcinomatosis
- decreased oncotic pressure (hypoalbuminaemia), e.g. nephrotic syndrome, liver cirrhosis.

Pleural effusions can be either inflammatory, when they are associated with a pleuritis, or non-inflammatory (see Table 5). To try to establish the cause of the effusion, a diagnostic aspiration of the pleural fluid is useful. If the fluid is a transudate (protein < 20 g L^{-1}), then heart failure or hypoalbuminaemia is the cause; if the fluid is an exudate (protein > 30 g L^{-1}), then all other causes should be considered.

Pneumothorax

Pneumothorax refers to air/gas in the pleural cavity. When severe, a pneumothorax can cause symptoms of

Table 5 Types of pleural effusion and their causes

	Type of pleural effusion	Common associations
Inflammatory	Serofibrinous effusion	Inflammation of the adjacent lung, e.g. pneumonia, lung abscess, TB, collagen vascular diseases
	Suppurative effusion (empyema, pyothorax)	Suppuration in the adjacent lung
	Haemorrhagic effusion	Neoplastic infiltration, pulmonary infarction
Non-inflammatory	Serous effusion (hydrothorax)	Cardiac failure, renal failure, liver failure
	Haemothorax	Trauma to chest wall, ruptured aortic aneurysm
	Chylothorax (lymph in the pleural space)	Obstruction of the lymphatics by tumour

respiratory distress and may be fatal. Resorption of the air in the pleural space occurs slowly, and if deemed necessary, interventional procedures may be employed to remove the air from the pleural cavity, e.g. chest drain.

Spontaneous pneumothorax

This type of pneumothorax occurs in people with pre-existing disease that causes rupture of an alveolus. It is most often seen in association with emphysema, asthma and tuberculosis.

Traumatic pneumothorax

This can occur following penetrating injuries to the chest.

Therapeutic pneumothorax

Intentional deflation of the lung was a method once used to enhance healing of tuberculous lesions.

Spontaneous idiopathic pneumothorax

This condition occurs in young healthy people, and appears to be due to rupture of small peripheral usually apical subpleural blebs. Recurrent attacks are common.

Tension pneumothorax

This term refers to when the defect responsible for the pneumothorax acts as a valve, allowing air into the pleural cavity during inspiration, but not permitting its escape during expiration. Consequently, the pressure in the pleural cavity rises swiftly and progressively. The condition is a medical emergency, and is fatal if the pressure is not relieved.

Tumours

Tumours of the pleura may be benign or malignant.

Benign

The solitary fibrous tumour of the pleura is a tumour that is often attached to the pleura by a peduncle. These benign tumours can become enormous.

Malignant

Malignant tumours of the pleura may be primary or secondary. Secondary metastatic tumours (e.g. from lung carcinomas or breast carcinomas) are much more common than primary tumours of the pleura.

Malignant mesothelioma

This term refers to a malignant tumour of mesothelial cells, and when applied to the pleura, means a primary malignant tumour of the pleura.

Aetiology—malignant mesothelioma is associated with exposure to asbestos, particularly crocidolite ('blue' asbestos) and amosite ('brown' asbestos). It should be noted, however, that for any individual asbestos worker, the risk of developing malignant mesothelioma is much lower than the risk of developing lung carcinoma.

Pathology—the tumour begins as pleural nodules that enlarge and extend over the surface of the lung, gradually encasing it. Infiltration of the chest wall and intercostal muscles by the tumour causes severe pain. Histologically, mesotheliomas may be composed of epithelial cells (epithelioid type) or spindle cells (sarcomatoid type) or a mixture of both.

Self-assessment: questions

Multiple choice questions

1. The following statements are correct:
   a. Epiglottitis is usually caused by the bacterium *Haemophilus influenzae*
   b. Squamous cell carcinoma of the larynx is strongly associated with cigarette smoking
   c. Epithelial dysplasia precedes squamous cell carcinoma of the larynx
   d. Laryngeal cancer often presents with persistent hoarseness of voice
   e. Laryngeal cancer may present with haemoptysis.

2. The following statements are correct:
   a. Smokers are at an increased risk of developing pneumonia
   b. Bronchopneumonia is characterised by consolidation of a large portion of a lobe or of an entire lobe
   c. *Pneumocystis carinii* is the organism frequently implicated in the development of bronchopneumonia
   d. Lobar pneumonia is most frequently caused by the bacterium *Streptococcus pneumoniae*
   e. Pneumonia can be treated with antibiotics and is now infrequently fatal.

3. The following statements regarding tuberculosis are correct:
   a. Since the 1980s, western countries have seen a decline in the incidence of tuberculosis
   b. Primary pulmonary tuberculosis is always symptomatic
   c. Histologically, tuberculosis is characterised by the presence of caseating granulomas
   d. Tuberculosis may affect the gastrointestinal tract
   e. Miliary tuberculosis represents lymphohaematogenous dissemination of the infection.

4. The following statements regarding obstructive airways disease are correct:
   a. In the pathogenesis of chronic bronchitis, smoking induces hypersecretion of mucus in airways
   b. In emphysema there is abnormal permanent dilation of the bronchi
   c. Emphysema may be associated with α_1-antitrypsin deficiency

   d. Asthma is characterised by irreversible bronchoconstriction
   e. Obstruction and infection are important influences in the pathogenesis of bronchiectasis.

5. Interstitial lung disease:
   a. Is associated with reduced vital capacity (VC) of the lung
   b. Is associated with reduced peak expiratory flow rate (PEFR)
   c. May be caused by inhalation of mineral dusts
   d. May lead to cardiac failure
   e. In its advanced form results in a macroscopic appearance referred to as 'honeycomb lung'.

6. The following statements are correct:
   a. The most common cause of pulmonary oedema is left ventricular failure
   b. An embolus may be a solid, liquid or gas
   c. Pulmonary thromboembolism may cause pleuritic chest pain
   d. Pulmonary thromboemboli most commonly originate from the arteries of the lower limbs
   e. Pulmonary hypertension is almost always idiopathic.

7. The following statements regarding lung cancer are correct:
   a. Smoking is associated with an increased risk of developing small cell carcinoma of the lung
   b. Non-small cell carcinomas are particularly sensitive to chemotherapy
   c. Bronchogenic carcinoma may cause development of a hoarse voice
   d. There is an association between bronchogenic carcinoma and Cushing's syndrome
   e. Lung cancer may be associated with a pleural effusion.

8. The following statements are correct:
   a. A tension pneumothorax is a medical emergency that requires immediate management
   b. Pneumonia is the likely cause of a pleural effusion that has a protein content of $< 20 \text{ g L}^{-1}$
   c. Involvement of the pleural cavity by tumour induces a haemorrhagic pleural effusion
   d. Mesothelioma is a benign tumour of the pleura
   e. Asbestos exposure is a risk factor for the development of mesothelioma.

Case histories

Case history 1

A 58-year-old man was admitted to hospital for repair of an inguinal hernia under a general anaesthetic. He smoked 10 cigarettes a day for 40 years (20 pack years). On the third postoperative day, he became pyrexial and developed a cough productive for green sputum. A blood count showed a raised white cell count with increased neutrophil polymorphs. A chest X-ray showed patchy opacities.

1. From these symptoms, signs and investigations, what is the most likely diagnosis?
2. What predisposing factors are present in this case?
3. Describe the pathological changes in the lungs.

Case history 2

A 72-year-old women presents to her GP with a persistent cough, haemoptysis, shortness of breath, weight loss and a hoarse voice. She is an ex-smoker. On clinical examination, she has finger clubbing, wasting of the small muscles of the left hand, and left-sided Horner's syndrome.

1. What is the most likely diagnosis?
2. What is the pathological basis for these signs and symptoms?
3. What further investigations should be performed?

Short note questions

Write brief notes on the following:
1. The classification and pathogenesis of emphysema.
2. Respiratory tract pathology caused by asbestos exposure.
3. The differential diagnosis of a pleural effusion.

Viva questions

1. What diseases of the respiratory tract are related to smoking?
2. What defence mechanisms are employed by the respiratory tract to reduce the risk of infection by microorganisms?

Self-assessment: answers

Multiple choice answers

1. a. **True.**
   b. **True.**
   c. **True.**
   d. **True.**
   e. **True.**

2. a. **True.** Cigarette smoke interferes with alveolar macrophage function and causes injury to the mucociliary apparatus.
   b. **False.**
   c. **False.**
   d. **True.**
   e. **False.** Despite antibiotic treatment pneumonia may still be fatal, especially in the debilitated.

3. a. **False.** Since the 1980s, western countries have seen a *rise* in the incidence of TB.
   b. **False.** Primary TB is frequently asymptomatic.
   c. **True.**
   d. **True.** Either during lymphohaematogenous dissemination or during primary infection due to ingestion of *Mycobacterium bovis*.
   e. **True.**

4. a. **True.**
   b. **False.** There is permanent dilatation of the airways distal to the terminal bronchioles.
   c. **True.**
   d. **False.** The bronchoconstriction is characteristically *reversible*.
   e. **True.**

5. a. **True.**
   b. **False.** The PEFR is usually normal.
   c. **True.**
   d. **True.** Interstitial lung disease can lead to cor pulmonale.
   e. **True.**

6. a. **True.**
   b. **True.**
   c. **True.**
   d. **False.** They most frequently originate from the *veins* of the lower limbs.
   e. **False.** Most cases of pulmonary hypertension are secondary to other pathology.

7. a. **True.**
   b. **False.** *Small cell* carcinomas are particularly sensitive to chemotherapy.

   c. **True.** If a lung tumour spreads into the mediastinum, there may be involvement of the recurrent laryngeal nerve as it passes close to the aortic arch.
   d. **True.** Some bronchogenic tumours secret hormones. Secretion of ACTH may induce Cushing's syndrome.
   e. **True.**

8. a. **True.**
   b. **False.** A protein content of $< 20 \text{ g L}^{-1}$ indicates that the effusion is a transudate. Pneumonia would cause an exudative effusion.
   c. **True.**
   d. **False.** Although the name of this tumour suggests that it is benign, mesotheliomas are in fact malignant.
   e. **True.**

Case history answers

Case history 1

1. A cough productive of green sputum associated with pyrexia is highly suspicious for pneumonia. A raised white cell count with increased neutrophil polymorphs suggests bacterial infection. Patchy opacities on the chest X-ray would support a diagnosis of bronchopneumonia in which the consolidation is patchy throughout the lung. In view of the history of recent surgery, the most likely diagnosis is postoperative pneumonia.

2. You need to know the defence mechanisms that are in operation in the respiratory tract to prevent infection, and ways in which they may be impaired predisposing individuals to pneumonia. There are several predisposing factors in this case. First, general anaesthesia would cause suppression of the cough reflex. Second, coughing increases intra-abdominal pressure and so any pain associated with the abdominal surgical wound would be increased when the patient coughs. Hence he may try to avoid coughing. Third, the patient is a smoker, and cigarette smoke interferes with alveolar macrophage function and injures the mucociliary apparatus.

3. In bronchopneumonia there is often widespread but patchy consolidation. The primary infection is centred on the bronchi, with spread to involve the adjacent bronchioles and alveolar spaces. In this case, the changes may be seen mostly in the dependent parts of the lung, where the retained secretions

would accumulate. Macroscopically, the lungs would show firm red/grey airless areas and pus may be present in the airways. Microscopically, there is acute inflammation in the airways.

Case history 2

1. This combination of symptoms in an elderly person who is an ex-smoker is highly suggestive of a malignant process. The findings on clinical examination support a diagnosis of a lung cancer. The Horner's syndrome, together with the muscle wasting seen in the hands, is particularly suggestive of an apical (Pancoast) tumour.

2. The cough may be due to distal infection, airway irritation, or airway obstruction by a tumour or lymph node mass. Haemoptysis results from ulceration of the tumour and consequent bleeding into the airway. Shortness of breath may be due to pleural effusions or obstruction of a main airway by tumour. The hoarse voice is caused by recurrent laryngeal nerve palsy secondary to mediastinal spread. Wasting of the small muscles of the hand is due to infiltration of the branchial plexus. Horner's syndrome results when there is involvement of the cervical sympathetic plexus.

3. A tissue diagnosis should be sought so that an appropriate management plan can be formulated. As stated earlier, small cell carcinomas are sensitive to chemotherapy and radiotherapy, but non-small cell carcinomas are not. Several methods may be employed. Cells in sputum, bronchoscopy-obtained bronchial brushings and washings, or pleural fluid can be examined under the microscope for any cytological features of malignancy. In the vast majority of cases small cell and non-small cell carcinomas can be distinguished. For central tumours, tissue may be obtained during bronchoscopy (yielding bronchial biopsies). Peripheral tumours may be biopsied percutaneously (yielding needle biopsies). After tissue diagnosis, further investigations are directed towards tumour staging, e.g. CT scan.

Short note answers

1. Start your answer with the definition of emphysema. Then go on to explain how emphysema is classified into four main types according to the anatomical distribution of the lesions, and the appearance of the lungs with the naked eye or hand lens. The four main types are centrilobular, panlobular, paraseptal and irregular, and you should be able to describe each of them. The pathogenesis of emphysema is not fully understood, but evidence suggests that emphysema

is due to an imbalance between protease and anti-protease activity in the lung. Hence its association with smoking (which causes increased recruitment of neutrophil polymorphs to the lung where they release elastase) and α_1-antitrypsin deficiency.

2. Exposure to asbestos is linked to the development of a number of disorders of the respiratory tract, namely pleural plaques (asymptomatic), pleural effusions, asbestosis, bronchogenic carcinoma, mesothelioma and laryngeal carcinoma. These conditions usually develop in the setting of occupational exposure to asbestos, where the fibres can be inhaled. It also seems that some extrapulmonary neoplasms may be linked to asbestos exposure, such as colon cancer. The development of colon cancer in this setting is presumably due to exposure of the bowel to asbestos (e.g. by accidental ingestion).

3. Pleural effusion denotes the presence of fluid within the pleural space. There are several causes of a pleural effusion, but they can be divided into 'inflammatory' and 'non-inflammatory', and you should know the various causes of each. Pleural effusions can be detected either during physical examination of the chest or on imaging (e.g. chest X-ray), and to determine the cause of an effusion you must extract as much information as possible from these, as well as taking a thorough history. A diagnostic tap can also be performed. The appearance of the fluid may provide clues. Note if the fluid is clear, cloudy or bloodstained, or composed entirely of blood, pus, or lymph. If the protein content is measured, you can determine whether the fluid is a transudate or an exudate—inflammatory effusions are exudates and therefore have a higher protein content. If neoplastic infiltration is suspected, the fluid can be examined under the microscope for the presence of malignant cells.

Viva answers

1. Several diseases of the repiratory tract are related to smoking. These include chronic bronchitis, emphysema, laryngeal carcinoma and bronchogenic carcinoma. Remember that smokers are also predisposed to pneumonia because cigarette smoke interferes with alveolar macrophage function and injures the mucociliary apparatus. These conditions together cause significant morbidity and mortality in the general population.

2. The respiratory tract employs several defence mechanisms to clear or destroy inhaled microorganisms. These include: nasal mucus (in

which particles are trapped); coughing and sneezing; the mucociliary apparatus (which traps particles in the lung and moves them within the mucus layer towards the nasopharynx where they are swallowed or expectorated); and alveolar clearance (particles that reach the alveoli are phagocytosed by alveolar macrophages). Pneumonia results whenever these defence mechanisms are impaired.

3 Upper gastrointestinal tract

Overview

This chapter covers the common pathology of the mouth, salivary glands, oesophagus, stomach and proximal duodenum. Inflammatory conditions of this region are frequent, and include oral ulcers, oesophagitis, gastritis and gastroduodenal (peptic) ulceration. Carcinoma of the oesophagus and stomach has a particularly poor prognosis. While the incidence of gastric cancer is decreasing in the UK, oesophageal carcinoma is rising in frequency. The role of *Helicobacter pylori* infection in gastric pathology, and the significance of lower oesophageal epithelial metaplasia (Barrett's oesophagus) will be discussed. Oral squamous cell cancer is relatively uncommon in the western world but is a major health problem in India and other parts of Asia.

PART 1: MOUTH AND SALIVARY GLANDS

3.1 Inflammation and infection

Learning objectives

You should:

- Know the common benign pathologies affecting the oral cavity
- Understand the terms leucoplakia and erythroplasia and their clinical significance

The following conditions are common in the mouth:

- non-specific ulceration ('aphthous ulcers')
- herpes simplex type 1 infection ('cold sore')
- candidiasis, especially in diabetic and immunosuppressed patients
- benign fibroepithelial polyp (reactive fibrous proliferation secondary to chronic irritation)
- cysts associated with teeth (developmental or inflammatory).

The oral mucosa can harbour several inflammatory conditions seen in the skin, such as lichen planus, bullous pemphigoid and erythema multiforme. Xerostomia (dry mouth) can be a feature of autoimmune disease in Sjögren's syndrome (see below).

Salivary gland inflammation can be due to:

- viral infection, e.g. mumps
- bacterial infection, staphylococcal and streptococcal, associated with salivary duct calculi (stones) and dehydration
- autoimmune disease.

Sjögren's syndrome results from autoimmune inflammatory damage to the salivary glands, lacrimal glands and small mucus glands of the nasal mucosa. Clinically this can present with dry mouth and dry eyes. There is a close association between Sjögren's syndrome and rheumatoid arthritis.

Leucoplakia is a clinical term describing a 'white patch' of oral mucosa. Leucoplakia does not reflect a specific pathological diagnosis and is often caused by inflammation or reactive hyperkeratosis (thickened keratin layer), but on occasion it can represent epithelial dysplasia or malignancy (Box 7). A more sinister lesion is erythroplakia, a velvety red patch of oral mucosa, which typically shows high-grade epithelial dysplasia on biopsy.

3.2 Oral and salivary gland neoplasia

Learning objectives

You should:

- Know the pathology of oral squamous cell carcinoma

- Know the common benign and malignant tumours of the salivary glands

Benign tumours of the oral cavity include squamous cell papilloma (analogous to skin lesions) and haemangiomas. Squamous cell carcinoma accounts for over 95% of oral malignancies (Table 6).

Salivary gland tumour pathology is complex, as both epithelial cells and the myoepithelial cells surrounding

---

Box 7 Causes of leucoplakia

- Candida infection
- Smoking-related keratosis
- Traumatic keratosis from rubbing denture plate
- Lichen planus
- Squamous epithelial dysplasia

---

the glands may give rise to neoplasms. Most tumours arise in the parotid gland, and over 80% of these are benign. Neoplasms arising in the submandibular, sublingual and minor salivary glands scattered throughout the oral mucosa have a much higher likelihood of being malignant (approximately 50%).

Pleomorphic adenoma

This is the commonest salivary tumour, arising most frequently in the parotid gland. The histological appearance is very variable, with epithelial glands or cell sheets, embedded in a connective tissue stroma showing myxoid changes, fibrosis, cartilaginous areas or even bone formation. Pleomorphic adenomas are benign tumours that appear well circumscribed macroscopically and do not infiltrate local structures (the facial nerve is, therefore, usually spared by pleomorphic adenomas arising in the parotid). However, there are often microscopic projections of tumour into the adjacent tissues, and attempted removal by enucleation carries a significant risk of multifocal recurrence, which can be difficult to treat. Up to 5% of pleomorphic adenomas may undergo malignant transformation to a high-grade carcinoma. The risk of malignant change is increased in long-standing adenomas.

Warthin's tumour

This tumour accounts for approximately 10% of salivary neoplasms, and arises almost exclusively in the parotid. There is a strong male preponderance. Ten per cent of tumours are bilateral, and a similar number are multifocal. The microscopic appearance is very distinctive, with a double layer of eosinophilic epithelial cells covering reactive lymphoid tissue. The eosinophilic cells (oncocytes) are the neoplastic population. Warthin's tumour is benign and malignant change does not occur.

Table 6 Cancer checklist: oral squamous cell carcinoma

Incidence	Age 50–70 years. Less than 5% of non-skin cancers in western world; up to 40% of all cancers in India
Risk factors	Smoking, alcohol, betel nut chewing (India/Asia), chronic inflammation. UV light and pipe smoking in lip carcinoma
Protective factors	Fruit and vegetable consumption
Associated lesions	Epithelial dysplasia, may be erythroplakia (over 50% progress to invasive cancer) or less frequently leucoplakia
Clinical presentation	Mass noted by patient or dentist
Location	Floor of mouth, tongue and hard palate most frequent
Macroscopic appearance	Raised firm mass ± ulceration
Histological features	Vary from well-differentiated tumours with orderly keratinisation to anaplastic (undifferentiated) tumours
Pattern of spread	Local infiltration of oral structures, regional lymph nodes, lung, liver, bone
Prognosis (per cent 5-year survival)	Dependent on site: lip 90%; anterior tongue 60%; other sites 20–30%

Salivary gland carcinoma (Table 7)

Many different histological variants are now recognised. The two commonest are:

1. **Muco-epidermoid carcinoma**—as the name implies, this carcinoma is composed of both glandular and squamous epithelium. Low-grade tumours are often partly cystic with well-differentiated glandular epithelium. High-grade carcinomas have a more solid growth pattern and are composed largely of squamous cells.
2. **Adenoid cystic carcinoma**—this malignancy appears low grade on histological grounds, but is both locally and distally invasive. Fifty per cent will metastasise, and long-term survival is poor. Adenoid cystic carcinoma is composed of regular small epithelioid cells in a cribriform ('sieve-like') architectural pattern, associated with basement-membrane-like material. Perineural invasion by the tumour is a characteristic feature.

PART 2: OESOPHAGUS, STOMACH AND PROXIMAL DUODENUM

3.3 Inflammation, infection and benign conditions

Learning objectives

You should:

- Understand gastro-oesophageal reflux disease and Barrett's oesophagus
- Know the causes and complications of acute and chronic gastritis, and of peptic ulcer disease

Oesophagitis

This disease may be due to infection, particularly by *Candida* in debilitated and immunosuppressed patients. Gastro-oesophageal reflux disease (GORD) is the commonest cause of oesophagitis in the UK, and its prevalence appears to be increasing. It is associated with sliding hiatus hernia, smoking, obesity, pregnancy and ingestion of certain foods. GORD classically presents with burning epigastric pain, which may be accentuated by bending or lying down, but is often asymptomatic. Histology shows hyperplasia of squamous oesophageal epithelium with inflammation (eosinophils, neutrophils and lymphocytes) and ulceration in more severe cases. Complications include:

- haematemesis
- anaemia
- inflammatory stricture
- Barrett's oesophagus (see below).

Other causes of oesophagitis include alcohol, corrosive chemical ingestion, chemotherapy, radiotherapy and graft-versus-host disease.

Barrett's oesophagus

This syndrome describes a metaplastic change of squamous epithelium of lower oesophagus into glandular epithelium. The metaplastic glandular epithelium may resemble gastric or small intestinal mucosa. Barrett's usually occurs in patients with more severe longstanding GORD. Endoscopically the metaplastic focus has a red, velvety appearance. Barrett's may progress to glandular dysplasia and eventually to invasive adenocarcinoma. Both Barrett's oesophagus and oesophageal adenocarcinoma have increased in incidence in recent years. For this reason, regular surveillance endoscopies are usually performed in patients with known Barrett's change, to identify high-grade

Table 7 Cancer checklist: salivary gland carcinoma

Incidence	Uncommon; adults; slight female predominance
Risk factors	Irradiation (muco-epidermoid carcinoma)
Associated lesions	Small percentage of pleomorphic adenomas undergo malignant transformation
Common clinical presentation	Mass, pain, facial nerve involvement (parotid tumours)
Location	Parotid, 15% of tumours are malignant Submandibular, 40% malignant Minor salivary glands, majority malignant
Macroscopic appearance	Variable, usually infiltrative margin
Histological features	Variable
Pattern of spread	Adenoid cystic, local perineural invasion, late dissemination to lung, liver, bone, brain (50%). Muco-epidermoid, low-grade lesions recur locally, high-grade lesions may disseminate widely
Prognosis (per cent 5-year survival)	Adenoid cystic, 60% at 5 years, but 15% at 15 years Muco-epidermoid, 50–90%, depending on grade

dysplasia and early-stage malignancy. However, the degree of increased cancer risk associated with Barrett's remains unclear, and less than half of all patients with oesophageal adenocarcinoma will describe any clinical history of reflux disease.

Achalasia

This is a motility disorder in which reduced oesophageal peristalsis and failure of relaxation of the lower oesophageal sphincter cause lower oesophagus dilatation. Resulting symptoms include dysphagia and food regurgitation. In most cases the pathogenesis is unknown. Achalasia can be secondary to Chagas' disease, caused by the protozoon *Trypanosoma cruzi* (frequent in Central America, Chagas' disease also causes acute myocarditis and chronic dilated cardiomyopathy.)

Hiatus hernia

This is a common condition in which part of the stomach herniates up through the oesophageal opening of the diaphragm and into the mediastinum (Fig. 9). The great majority are sliding, and are often associated with reflux oesophagitis. Rolling hernias are less common.

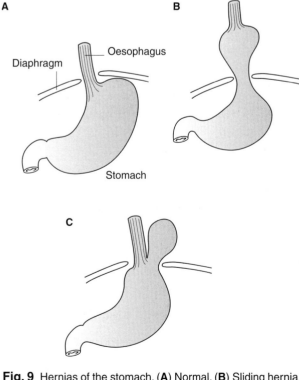

Fig. 9 Hernias of the stomach. (**A**) Normal. (**B**) Sliding hernia. (**C**) Rolling hernia.

Oesophageal varices

These are an important cause of serious haemorrhage and death in patients with portal hypertension. They are discussed further in Chapter 5.

Gastritis and benign ulcer disease

- **Gastritis**, inflammation of gastric mucosa, which may be acute or chronic
- **Gastric erosion**, superficial loss of gastric mucosal tissue, not extending beyond muscularis mucosa. Erosions are associated with acute inflammation and are transient
- **Gastric ulcer**, ulceration that extends through, and often well beyond, the mucosa, and may be acute or chronic.

Acute gastritis

Acute gastritis is most commonly due to:

- non-steroidal anti-inflammatory drugs (NSAIDs)
- excess alcohol
- heavy smoking
- 'stress' (burns, trauma, shock) causing mucosal ischaemia
- chemotherapy and radiotherapy.

Clinical consequences include haematemesis, melaena, epigastric pain, nausea and vomiting.

Acute gastric ulceration

Acute gastric ulceration can also be caused by severe stress. Sepsis, shock, trauma, burns and raised intracranial pressure are the commonest predisposing factors and up to 10% of patients admitted to intensive care units will develop acute gastric erosions or ulcers. The ulcers are small (less than 10 mm diameter), frequently multiple and occur anywhere in the stomach. The adjacent mucosa rarely shows chronic gastritis. Acute ulcers are transient lesions that heal with complete restoration of normal structure, and without scarring.

Chronic gastritis

Chronic gastritis can be classified into three major groups:

1. Autoimmune—in pernicious anaemia, with autoantibodies to gastric acid producing parietal cells in the body of the stomach.
2. Bacterial—*Helicobacter pylori* infection (most common cause of chronic gastritis, preferentially affecting the antrum).
3. Chemical—due to biliary reflux or NSAIDs.

Other causes include alcohol, smoking, Crohn's disease and graft-versus-host disease.

Chronic mucosal inflammation can lead to intestinal metaplasia and gastric atrophy, and predisposes to development of gastric carcinoma. However, chronic gastritis and *Helicobacter* infection are very common, and clearly only a small percentage of those afflicted will eventually develop malignancy. Chronic gastritis itself is often asymptomatic.

Chronic peptic ulceration

Chronic peptic ulceration occurs in the gastric antrum, but is most frequent in the proximal duodenum. Lesions are usually solitary (if multiple, think of Zollinger–Ellison syndrome, see below). Peptic ulcer disease is common in adulthood and more frequent in men than women. The pathogenesis of peptic ulceration involves breakdown of mucosal defence mechanisms and increased injurious stimuli. The majority of cases (especially duodenal ulcers) are associated with *Helicobacter pylori* chronic gastritis. Other risk factors include smoking, chronic NSAID use, liver cirrhosis, chronic lung disease, hyperparathyroidism and chronic renal failure. Significant complications of peptic ulcer include:

- haemorrhage (clinically serious in up to 33%)
- perforation with peritonitis (5%)
- gastric outlet obstruction secondary to scarring.

Malignant change does not occur in duodenal peptic ulcers and is very unusual in gastric peptic ulcers.

Recurrent peptic ulcers occur in the *Zollinger–Ellison syndrome*. Hypersecretion of gastric acid is provoked by a gastrin-secreting tumour (usually located within the pancreas). The peptic ulcers can be multiple and arise in the stomach, proximal and distal duodenum and jejunum.

3.4 Oesophageal and gastric neoplasia

Learning objectives

You should:

- Understand the pathology of gastric and oesophageal carcinoma

- Be aware of the role of *Helicobacter pylori* infection in gastric inflammation and neoplasia

Oesophagus

Benign tumours in the oesophagus are very uncommon, but can be of epithelial (squamous cell papilloma) or of connective tissue origin (lipoma, haemangioma). The

Table 8 Cancer checklist: oesophageal tumours

	Oesophageal squamous cell carcinoma	Oesophageal adenocarcinoma
Incidence	Over 50s; decreasing in incidence in western world; More common in men; high incidence in parts of China, Iran, former USSR	Increasing incidence; over 40s, more common in men
Risk factors	Smoking, alcohol (particularly spirits), ?vitamin deficiencies, ?food contamination—fungal organisms, nitrosamines	GORD, Barrett's oesophagus, smoking; obesity
Associated lesions	Chronic oesophagitis; squamous dysplasia/carcinoma-in-situ	Barrett's oesophagus
Common clinical presentation	Gradual development of dysphagia, first to solids then to liquids	As for squamous cell carcinoma
Location	Upper third 25% Middle third 50% Lower third 25%	Lower third of oesophagus
Macroscopic appearance	Polypoid usually, but can be flat or ulcerated	Variable
Histological features	Squamous differentiation, with or without keratinisation	Glandular differentiation; may be histologically indistinguishable from gastric cancer
Pattern of spread	Local submucosal spread beyond area of grossly visible tumour, can erode locally into trachea (fistula formation, aspiration pneumonia) or aorta (haemorrhage) Regional lymph nodes, liver and lung	Local invasion into stomach and through oesophageal wall into adjacent structures Regional lymph nodes, liver and lung
Prognosis (per cent 5-year survival)	5%; often advanced stage tumour at presentation	As for squamous cell carcinoma

vast majority of malignant oesophageal tumours are squamous cell carcinomas or adenocarcinomas (Table 8).

Stomach

Benign epithelial neoplastic polyps (*adenomas*) are rare in the stomach, in contrast to the colon. Over a third are associated with invasive carcinoma at the time of diagnosis, either within the polyp itself or in the adjacent mucosa. Gastric adenocarcinoma (Table 9) has classically been divided into two histological growth patterns (Fig. 10), *intestinal* type (with gland formation) and *diffuse* type (also known as 'signet-ring' carcinoma).

Lymphoma

Lymphoma can arise as a primary tumour in the stomach. There is a strong association with *Helicobacter* infection. It appears that hyperplasia of mucosal-associated lymphoid tissue (MALT) induced by chronic bacterial infection provides fertile soil for development of a monoclonal neoplastic lymphoid proliferation. In contrast to lymphomas arising in lymph nodes, MALT lymphomas tend to remain localised to their site of origin and may be amenable to surgical resection. Indeed, some apparent gastric lymphomas may regress following treatment of *Helicobacter* infection, blurring the distinction

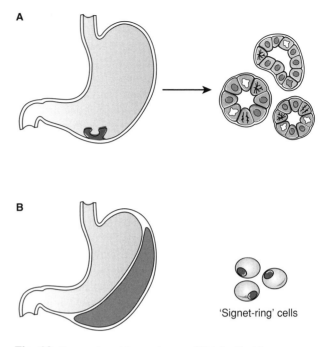

'Signet-ring' cells

Fig. 10 Types of gastric carcinoma. (**A**) Intestinal type. (**B**) Diffuse type.

between hyperplasia and neoplasia (recall that the latter is an uncontrolled proliferation, which does not regress when the precipitating stimulus is removed).

Table 9 Cancer checklist: gastric adenocarcinoma

Incidence	Geographical variation—highest in Far East, Central America, Scandinavia. Incidence of intestinal type variant has declined in UK over last 50 years
Risk factors	Chronic gastritis; dietary factors (nitrosamines, smoked/salted foods)
Protective factors	Fresh fruit and vegetable consumption
Associated lesions	*Helicobacter* gastritis, intestinal metaplasia
Common clinical presentation	Non-specific symptoms; weight loss, pain, nausea and vomiting
Location	Most frequent in antrum, but can occur anywhere
Macroscopic appearance	Polypoid, flat or ulcerated Diffuse thickening of stomach wall, 'linitis plastica', especially with signet-ring type
Histological features	Gland forming (intestinal type) or diffuse infiltration of single adenocarcinoma cells (signet-ring type)
Pattern of spread	Through serosal surface; local invasion of duodenum and pancreas Regional lymph nodes (also supraclavicular node) Peritoneal spread (especially to ovaries, resulting in Krukenberg tumour)
Prognosis (per cent 5-year survival)	Less than 5% Early gastric cancer (confined to mucosa or submucosa, with or without lymph node spread) has a better prognosis

Self-assessment: questions

Multiple choice questions

1. *Helicobacter* infection in the stomach is associated with:
   a. Gastric carcinoma
   b. Acute gastric ulceration
   c. Chronic duodenal ulceration
   d. Intestinal metaplasia
   e. Gastric lymphoma.

2. Regarding salivary gland tumours:
   a. Malignant tumours arise most commonly in the parotid gland
   b. Pleomorphic adenomas have a 20% risk of malignant transformation
   c. Facial nerve impairment is an ominous sign
   d. Adenoid cystic carcinoma has a good long-term prognosis
   e. Enucleation of pleomorphic adenoma is appropriate treatment.

3. Barrett's oesophagus:
   a. Is a dysplastic change
   b. Confers an increased risk of oesophageal squamous carcinoma
   c. Can contain small intestinal-type epithelium
   d. Can be complicated by benign oesophageal stricture
   e. Increases in frequency with increased duration of gastro-oesophageal reflux symptoms.

4. Oral leucoplakia (white mucosal patches) can be caused by:
   a. *Candida* infection
   b. Smoking
   c. Epithelial dysplasia
   d. Ill-fitting dentures
   e. Invasive carcinoma.

5. Concerning gastric cancer:
   a. It is commoner in the UK than in Japan
   b. Diffuse type (signet-ring) adenocarcinoma is decreasing in incidence
   c. Many cancers arise from pre-existing benign peptic ulcers
   d. Overall 5 year survival is 25%
   e. Histological type is the most important prognostic factor.

6. Acute gastric ulcers:
   a. Are often multiple
   b. Are common in severely ill patients
   c. Are usually > 25 mm in diameter
   d. Are confined to the antrum
   e. Usually heal without scarring.

7. Concerning chronic gastritis:
   a. Autoantibodies to gastrin-producing cells are present in autoimmune gastritis
   b. Squamous metaplasia is often seen on biopsy
   c. Chemical gastritis can be secondary to bile reflux
   d. It confers a high risk of development of gastric cancer
   e. It is frequently seen in patients taking long-term steroids.

8. Concerning squamous cell carcinoma of the mouth:
   a. The incidence is higher in the Far East than the UK
   b. Prognosis is best for anterior tumours
   c. There is an association with sun exposure
   d. The tumour rarely spreads beyond the oral cavity
   e. Erythroplakia is a high-risk factor.

Case histories

Case history 1

A 63-year-old male presents to his GP with swallowing problems. He describes gradually increasing difficulty with swallowing solid food, but no problems with liquids. He has recently lost half a stone in weight, and has a several-year history of 'heartburn'.

1. What is your differential diagnosis based on this history?
2. What changes might be present within oesophageal biopsies taken at endoscopy?

Case history 2

A 78-year-old female is admitted to hospital as an emergency with abdominal pain and haematemesis. Urgent endoscopy is performed and a 15 mm ulcer is identified in the proximal duodenum as the source of the bleeding.

1. What specific questions would you ask the patient to help establish the cause of the ulcer?
2. Why might the endoscopist take a biopsy from the stomach (rather than the duodenal lesion)?

Viva questions

1. What are the causes and complications of acute gastritis?
2. Discuss the epidemiology of upper gastrointestinal tract cancer.

Self-assessment: answers

Multiple choice answers

1. a. **True.**
   b. **False.**
   c. **True.**
   d. **True.**
   e. **True.**

2. a. **True.** Although only 10–15% of parotid tumours are malignant, neoplasms develop more frequently at this site than in the other salivary tissues, so that salivary gland cancers are still most common in the parotid.
   b. **False.** Less than 5%.
   c. **True.** As it indicates tumour infiltration of the nerve.
   d. **False.**
   e. **False.** Microscopic residual deposits cause subsequent clinical recurrence.

3. a. **False.** Barrett's is a metaplastic change; replacement of one adult differentiated epithelium by another. Although Barrett's itself is a benign process, there is a greater risk of developing glandular epithelial dysplasia and adenocarcinoma within the area of Barrett's change.
   b. **False.** It is the risk of adenocarcinoma that is increased.
   c. **True.**
   d. **True.**
   e. **True.**

4. a. **True.**
   b. **True.**
   c. **True.**
   d. **True.**
   e. **True.** Early-stage invasive carcinoma may develop within a leucoplakic patch of dysplasia or carcinoma in situ.

5. a. **False.**
   b. **False.** It is the intestinal type of adenocarcinoma that is declining in frequency.
   c. **False.**
   d. **False.** It is 5%.
   e. **False.** Surgical resectability, which is related to tumour stage, is the most important prognostic factor.

6. a. **True.**
   b. **True.**
   c. **False.**
   d. **False.**
   e. **True.** Acute gastric ulcers are usually superficial.

7. a. **False.** The antibodies present are against acid-producing parietal cells.
   b. **False.** Intestinal metaplasia may be present.
   c. **True.**
   d. **False.** Chronic gastritis is very common, and the percentage of patients developing malignancy is low.
   e. **False.** Steroids can cause acute ulceration if given in high doses. Chemical gastritis can be caused by non-steroidal anti-inflammatory drugs (NSAIDs).

8. a. **True.**
   b. **True.**
   c. **True.** For carcinoma of the lip, which shares the same risk factors as skin cancer at other sites (see Ch. 13).
   d. **False.**
   e. **True.**

Case history answers

Case history 1

1. The symptoms suggest oesophageal obstruction and are most likely to be due to a benign inflammatory stricture or a malignancy. The history of heartburn points to GORD. Another much less common possibility is achalasia. Dysphagia due to cerebrovascular accident is of sudden onset.

   Benign strictures can complicate severe oesophagitis from any cause, including physical and chemical injury (such as caustic substance ingestion, irradiation and cancer chemotherapy). Oesophageal stricture also occurs in systemic sclerosis (scleroderma).

2. In benign strictures, oesophageal mucosal biopsies may show inflammatory changes with squamous epithelial hyperplasia. Ulceration may be present. The fibrosis causing a benign stricture may not be seen histologically as the scar tissue lies deeper within the wall of the oesophagus and may not be sampled in a superficial biopsy.

   Inflammation and squamous hyperplasia would be seen in GORD. Identification of glandular epithelium within the anatomical oesophagus would signify Barrett's metaplasia.

   If a malignant tumour is present, biopsy will confirm whether this is squamous cell carcinoma, adenocarcinoma, or a more unusual tumour type (such as sarcoma or melanoma).

Even if no mass is seen, in the presence of Barrett's oesophagus there is an increased risk of malignancy and of premalignant (dysplastic) changes in the glandular epithelium. For this reason, patients known to have Barrett's change may undergo regular endoscopies, although the effectiveness of this surveillance in identifying early-stage, potentially curable, oesophageal tumours is not yet clearly established.

Case history 2

1. A careful drug history to exclude non-steroidal anti-inflammatory medication is essential. Many elderly patients may suffer with osteoarthritis and buy medications over the counter. Smoking and alcoholic liver disease are associated with peptic ulceration and the relevant history of these habits should be obtained. Other relevant medical history would include chronic lung disease, chronic renal disease and hyperparathyroidism.

2. *Helicobacter pylori* gastritis is frequently present in association with peptic duodenal ulceration. A rapid urease detection test for *Helicobacter* can be performed with the tissue sample in the endoscopy suite, or the biopsy material can be submitted for histopathological examination. Duodenal peptic ulcers do not undergo malignant transformation and can safely assumed to be benign in nature without histological confirmation.

Viva answers

1. See text, Section 3.3.

2. Important points to include would be:
   - the worldwide geographical variation in oral, gastric and oesophageal cancers
   - the changing incidence of certain cancers (increasing oesophageal adenocarcinoma, decreasing intestinal-type gastric carcinoma) and possible reasons for this (increasing incidence of GORD and Barrett's metaplasia in oesophageal adenocarcinoma; ?decreasing frequency of *Helicobacter* gastritis with improved general health and sanitation corresponding to reduced gastric cancer incidence)
   - the role of environmental factors including smoking, alcohol and dietary habits.

4 Lower gastrointestinal tract

Overview

This chapter covers pathological processes affecting the distal duodenum, jejunum, ileum, colorectum and anus. Worldwide, infective disease of the small and large intestine is one of the most important of all causes of mortality; approximately half of all deaths below the age of five are due to infectious enterocolitis. In developed countries, bowel infections are still a common cause of morbidity but are rarely fatal. Modern standards of sanitation, healthcare and nutrition have eradicated the epidemics of cholera and typhoid prevalent in the UK in previous centuries. However, civilisation comes at a price. The average diet of the developed world appears to be a contributory factor to several common large bowel diseases—in particular diverticular disease and colorectal cancer.

4.1 Inflammation and infection

Learning objectives

You should:

- Be aware of the types of pathogens that can cause enterocolitis
- Be able to describe the differences between ulcerative colitis and Crohn's disease
- Understand the pathogenesis and complications of acute appendicitis and diverticular disease

Infectious enterocolitis

Infectious diseases of the bowel most commonly present with diarrhoea, that is an increase in stool mass, stool frequency or stool fluidity. Diarrhoea can result from a number of mechanisms, shown in Table 10. The pathogen responsible—which may be bacterial, viral, parasitic, protozoal or fungal—varies with patient age, nutrition, immune status and environment, and is identifiable in only approximately half of all cases.

Viruses—Rotavirus affects primarily children aged 6 months to 2 years, and is responsible for an estimated 140 million cases of infective enterocolitis and 1 million deaths per year. Viral infection damages mature surface epithelial cells in the small intestine mucosa, which are replaced by immature secretory cells. This results in a loss of absorptive ability and increased gut secretions, producing a mixed osmotic and secretory diarrhoea (see Table 10). In older children and young adults, the majority of non-bacterial gastroenteritis is due to Norwalk-like viruses. Viral infection typically provokes cellular immunity involving cytotoxic T-lymphocytes. Biopsies of intestinal mucosa are rarely undertaken in suspected viral infection, as symptoms of vomiting and diarrhoea are often self-limiting and of short duration. However, in an immunocompetent individual, the microscopic appearance of established viral infection would characteristically include epithelial cell damage and lymphocytic infiltration of the mucosa indicative of host immune response.

Bacteria—cause disease in the gut by a number of mechanisms:

- effects of preformed bacterial toxins present in contaminated food
- toxin production by organisms within the gut
- enteroinvasive infection, in which organisms proliferate, invade and destroy the intestinal mucosal epithelium.

Enterotoxins—are polypeptides which cause diarrhoea. Some, such as cholera toxin cause massive secretion of fluid in the absence of tissue damage (secretory and osmotic diarrhoea). Cholera toxin exerts its effects by persistently activating the cytoplasmic enzyme adenylate cyclase, causing profound secretion of chloride, sodium and water.

Secretory toxins—produced by *E. coli* are the major cause of traveller's diarrhoea.

Table 10 Mechanisms and causes of diarrhoea

Type of diarrhoea	Mechanism	Major causes
Secretory diarrhoea	Stimulation of gut secretion	Viral infection Bacterial infection Neoplasms producing secretagogues
Osmotic diarrhoea	Excessive osmotic forces exerted by increased concentration of luminal solutes	Laxative therapy Malabsorbtion (many causes) Lactase deficiency
Exudative diarrhoea	Stools containing blood and inflammatory debris secondary to tissue damage	Crohn's disease Ulcerative colitis Bacterial infections Protozoal infections
Abnormal gut motility	Various causes of altered gut transit time and motility	Irritable bowel syndrome Diabetic neuropathy Post-bowel surgery

Cytotoxins, in contrast, produced for example by *Shigella* and cytotoxic strains of *E. coli*, cause tissue damage with epithelial cell necrosis and an acute inflammatory reaction. Cytotoxins usually induce 'dysentery'—low volume, painful, bloody diarrhoea.

Although bacterial infection is frequently confined to the gut, systemic disease may occasionally occur. Organisms may enter the blood stream (causing a bacteraemia), multiply within blood vessels (septicaemia) and spread to other organs (dissemination). Inflammatory mediators activated by bacterial toxins or by products of damaged host cells may result in fever, lowered blood pressure and ultimately septic shock (more fully described in *Master Medicine Pathology*, second edition), which is often fatal. Typhoid fever is the name given to the generalised illness caused by infection by *Salmonella Eyphimurium typhimurium*, which can include chronic inflammation of the biliary tree, joints, bones and meninges in addition to intestinal involvement.

Pseudomembranous colitis—is an acute infectious disease of the colorectum, which is a common cause of diarrhoea in hospitalised patients receiving broad spectrum antibiotic therapy. The organism responsible (*Clostridium difficile*) is a normal toxin-producing commensal of the gut. Antibiotic therapy appears to alter the balance of the gut flora, allowing *C. difficile* to flourish. The toxin damages the colonic mucosa, causing an acute inflammatory reaction with the formation of a typical 'pseudomembrane'. The pseudomembrane is visible endoscopically as an irregular dark yellow coating over the bowel surface; microscopically it contains mucus and acute inflammatory debris including fibrin and degenerate neutrophils. The toxin of *C. difficile* can be identified in the stool of symptomatic patients.

Acute appendicitis

Acute inflammation of the appendix is the most common acute abdominal condition requiring surgery.

It can occur at any age, although it is relatively rare in the very young and very old. Most cases are thought to arise secondary to obstruction of the appendiceal lumen by faeces. The exact sequence of events is unknown, but may involve a combination of bacterial proliferation and increased intraluminal pressure causing vascular obstruction and ischaemia. The affected appendix shows the hallmarks of acute inflammation—intense neutrophil polymorph infiltration and oedema, with tissue necrosis and peritonitis in advanced cases. The serosal surface of the organ becomes covered with an acute inflammatory exudate composed of fibrin and neutrophils. If surgery is delayed there is a risk of appendiceal rupture, with localised abscess formation or generalised peritonitis with septicaemia. Chronic inflammation is very unusual in the appendix. Small scarred appendices, presumably representing the fibrotic end stage of repeated acute inflammation, are sometimes seen in older adults.

Peritonitis

Generalised acute inflammation of the peritoneum can arise secondary to bacterial invasion or chemical irritation. Bacterial peritonitis may complicate many inflammatory processes, including acute appendicitis, cholecystitis, perforated peptic ulcer, diverticulitis, bowel ischaemia and salpingitis. Infective peritonitis may also follow abdominal trauma or medical intervention (e.g. peritoneal dialysis). Chemical inflammation of the peritoneum may occur when bile, pancreatic enzymes, foreign material or blood (endometriosis, trauma, surgery) are released into the peritoneal cavity. Healing of peritonitis can result in the formation of fibrous adhesions between bowel loops. These adhesions can subsequently cause abdominal pain and bowel obstruction.

Crohn's disease and ulcerative colitis

These two conditions are often grouped together under the term chronic idiopathic inflammatory bowel disease. As this name suggests, Crohn's disease and ulcerative colitis are of unknown aetiology, and it has been suggested that they may represent different parts of the spectrum of a single disease process. However, there are important clinical and pathological differences between these two conditions.

Crohn's disease—is a granulomatous inflammatory condition, which can affect any part of the gastrointestinal tract from mouth to anus, but most frequently involves the small intestine and colon. Annual incidence in the developed world is 1–3 per 100 000, with equal sex incidence; whites are affected more frequently than non-Caucasians. Crohn's disease often presents in the second and third decades, but can manifest at any age. In the gut, approximately 40% of cases are restricted to the small bowel, 30% involve both small and large intestines and the remaining 30% show isolated colonic disease. About one-quarter of patients have extra-intestinal involvement, which can include skin lesions, arthritis and eye disorders.

Crohn's disease is characterised by discontinuous, sharply demarcated areas ('skip lesions') of transmural chronic inflammation. Microscopically, aggregates of lymphocytes are seen in all layers of affected bowel wall. Non-necrotising granulomas, composed of epithelioid macrophages with multinucleated giant cells, are seen in approximately 60% of cases. Fissuring ulcers are another characteristic histological feature of Crohn's disease; these linear ulcers can also be seen with the naked eye, and often impart a 'cobblestone' appearance to the bowel mucosa when viewed endoscopically or in a surgical resection specimen. The intestinal wall becomes thickened by oedema in acute stages and flare-ups of Crohn's disease, and by fibrosis in chronic disease, leading to stricture formation. Extension of fissuring ulceration through to the serosal surface of the bowel can result in perforation, abscess formation, adhesions, fistulas and sinus tracts. A *fistula* is an abnormal communication between two epithelial surfaces (e.g. a colovesical fistula joins colonic mucosa to bladder mucosa). The fistulous tract itself is lined by epithelium or by granulation tissue. A *sinus* is a blind-ending tract, which connects with the skin or another epithelial surface at one end.

Crohn's disease manifests clinically with intermittent diarrhoea, fever and abdominal pain. Symptoms of the initial attack may mimic acute appendicitis. The terminal ileum is the commonest single site of disease and involvement of this region by Crohn's disease can cause symptoms relating to malabsorption. Crohn's disease typically waxes and wanes with recurrent attacks over

many years, but there are intervening symptom-free periods of remission. Later presentations include bowel obstruction secondary to fibrous stricturing and symptoms related to fistula formation. There is a slight increased risk of colorectal cancer. The features of Crohn's disease are summarised in Figure 11A.

Ulcerative colitis (UC)—is also a chronic relapsing inflammatory condition. It is slightly more common than Crohn's disease (incidence of UC is 4–6 per 100 000) but shares peak onset in early adulthood, equal frequency in males and females and predilection for whites. Unlike Crohn's disease, UC is characterised by continuous disease extending proximally from the rectum, involving a variable distance of colon up to and occasionally including the terminal ileum. Isolated small intestinal disease does not occur in UC. Inflammation is restricted to the colonic mucosa, with

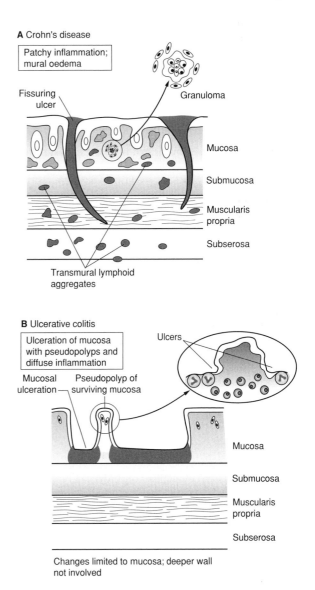

Fig. 11 (**A**) Crohn's disease and (**B**) ulcerative colitis.

occasional involvement of the submucosa. During acute attacks of colitis, there may be extensive mucosal ulceration, from which multiple islands of surviving epithelium stand proud as 'pseudopolyps'. Microscopically the lamina propria of residual mucosa shows diffuse chronic inflammation with lymphocytes and plasma cells, and acute inflammation of mucosal glandular crypts. Granulomas are characteristically absent. With progressive disease the mucosa becomes atrophic, with disruption of glandular architecture and gland loss. There is a risk of epithelial dysplasia and subsequent carcinoma developing in longstanding UC. This risk is greatest in patients having involvement of the entire large intestine (pancolitis). The features of ulcerative colitis are summarised in Figure 11B.

UC commonly manifests as recurrent attacks of bloody, mucoid diarrhoea and abdominal pain. Occasionally patients present with severe bleeding and fluid imbalance. Severe acute ulcerative colitis is one of the causes of toxic megacolon (see Box 8). As inflammation is restricted to the mucosa and submucosa, fistulae and strictures do not occur in UC.

Diverticular disease

A diverticulum is essentially a blind pouch, which is lined by epithelium and communicates with the bowel lumen. The wall of a true diverticulum contains all layers of the bowel wall (mucosa, submucosa and muscularis propria). Diverticula occur in the small intestine as the solitary Meckel's diverticulum (a remnant of the embryonic vitelline duct) or as multiple jejunal lesions. However, the distal large intestine is the most common site. Approximately half of all adults over 60 years old have developed multiple, small, flask-like or spherical outpouchings in the sigmoid colon. The diverticula extend from the luminal surface into the deep muscularis mucosa and pericolic fat, and are a frequent incidental finding on barium enema examination in elderly patients. Obstruction of a diverticulum by faeces can cause inflam-

mation (diverticulitis), pericolic abscess formation and local or generalised peritonitis. Chronic inflammation and fibrosis may complicate acute diverticulitis, leading to fistula formation and colonic stricture.

Diverticula formation occurs at points of weakness in the colonic wall where vessels and nerves penetrate the muscle coat. Low fibre diet is thought to contribute to pathogenesis; low stool bulk results in exaggerated peristalsis and increased intraluminal pressure in the affected colon. Symptomatic diverticular disease may present with cramping or continuous lower abdominal pain, constipation or alternating bowel habit, and chronic blood loss.

4.2 Ischaemia and infarction

Learning objective

You should:

- Understand the pathogenesis and clinical consequences of intestinal ischaemia

Intestinal ischaemia can be acute or chronic, and result from both arterial and venous disease. Elderly adults are most frequently affected. Atherosclerosis is often the underlying pathology. Mesenteric arteries supplying the gut may be blocked by thrombosis superimposed on atherosclerosis, or by embolisation of fragments of atheromatous plaque originating from the aorta. Non-occlusive bowel ischaemia can follow hypoperfusion due to, for example, cardiac failure, shock or dehydration. The 'watershed areas' of the colon—splenic flexure and rectum—which lie between the major arterial blood supplies are especially vulnerable. Mesenteric venous thrombosis can complicate sepsis, neoplasia, liver cirrhosis and abdominal surgery. Therapeutic radiotherapy used in the treatment of malignant disease can cause vascular damage with progressive narrowing and occlusion of arteries. Radiation enterocolitis most commonly occurs in the small intestine of patients receiving treatment for carcinoma of the cervix.

Ischaemic injury may be restricted to the mucosa and submucosa of the gut or may involve all layers of the bowel wall. In full-thickness acute bowel infarction, the serosal surface of the gut appears plum coloured due to congestion and reflow of blood into the damaged tissue. The intestinal lumen usually contains blood or blood-stained mucus. Histological changes of infarction (ischaemic necrosis) and oedema are present. Acute small bowel infarction has a high mortality, due to the short time interval between onset of symptoms and development of bowel perforation or septicaemia. The poor prognosis is partly due to coexistent cardiac and

---

Box 8 Megacolon

Definition
Marked dilatation of colon

Causes
toxic megacolon—a complication severe acute inflammation, most commonly seen in ulcerative colitis
obstruction—neoplasia, inflammatory stricture
infection—destruction of enteric nerve plexuses in Chagas' disease
congenital—Hirschsprung's disease

Clinical course
high risk of gangrene and perforation in toxic megacolon

vascular disease in the at-risk elderly population. Less severe vascular occlusion which develops gradually can present as chronic ischaemic colitis, with patchy mucosal ulceration. Chronic ischaemia involving the submucosa may heal by fibrosis, causing colonic stricture.

4.3 Immunological disorders

Learning objective

You should:

* Understand the pathology of coeliac disease and the reason for excluding gluten from the diet

Coeliac disease

Coeliac disease is a chronic inflammatory condition of the small intestinal mucosa, in which immunologically-mediated injury to the epithelium causes malabsorption. It is also known as coeliac sprue and gluten-sensitive enteropathy. The disease is relatively common in European whites (prevalence of 1 : 2000–3000). There is evidence of a genetic predisposition to coeliac disease, with family clustering and high frequency of association with certain human leucocyte antigen (HLA) alleles. Affected individuals develop an immune response to gluten, which contains the protein component gliadin in wheat and closely related grains (oat, barley and rye). Gliadin sensitive B-cells accumulate in the small intestinal mucosa on exposure to gluten, and anti-gliadin antibodies are present in the blood. Characteristically, the small bowel mucosa loses its normal villous archi-

tecture and becomes flat. Microscopically there is diffuse chronic inflammation with greatly increased numbers of lymphocytes accumulating within the surface epithelium (Fig. 12). The lamina propria contains many plasma cells. These histological abnormalities revert to normal when gluten is excluded from the diet, with subsequent improvement in clinical symptoms. There is a small long-term risk of malignancy (small intestinal lymphoma).

Graft versus host disease (GVHD)

Patients treated with donated bone marrow receive an allograft of foreign lymphocytes, which are able to mount an immune response against their new host. GVHD has acute and chronic phases. The acute phase may involve the intestinal mucosa, producing severe watery diarrhoea, intestinal haemorrhage and sepsis.

4.4 Neoplasia

Learning objectives

You should:

* Be able to define the terms polyp and adenoma

* Be able to explain the adenoma–carcinoma sequence

* Understand the risk factors for colorectal cancer, and be able to describe Dukes' staging

* Be aware of other types of tumour that occur in the colon and rectum

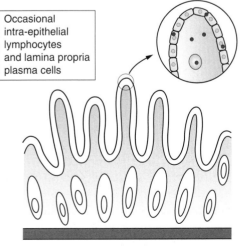

A Normal small intestine mucosa

Occasional intra-epithelial lymphocytes and lamina propria plasma cells

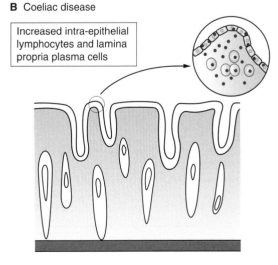

B Coeliac disease

Increased intra-epithelial lymphocytes and lamina propria plasma cells

Fig. 12 Coeliac disease.

The majority of tumours occurring in the lower gastrointestinal tract arise from the glandular epithelium of the large bowel mucosa. Colorectal adenocarcinoma is the second commonest cause of cancer mortality (after lung cancer) in the UK. The jejunum and ileum together make up 75% of the entire intestinal length but contain only 5% of intestinal tumours.

Polyps—are tissue masses, which protrude into the bowel lumen. They may be described as pedunculated (when there is a recognisable stalk) or sessile (when the polyp has a broad flat base). The word 'polyp' is not synonymous with neoplasia, as polyps may be inflammatory, hyperplastic or hamartomatous in nature, as well as neoplastic (see Box 9). Benign tumours of colonic epithelium are often polypoid in structure. Occasionally, masses arising from deeper in the bowel wall (for example, smooth muscle tumours developing in the muscularis propria) may project into the bowel lumen in a polypoid fashion.

Adenomatous polyps—benign epithelial neoplasms, very common in the colon; up to 50% of all adults over the age of 60 in the UK harbour at least one. They are classified as tubular (> 90%), tubulovillous (5–10%) or villous (1%) according to the mixture of tubular glands and villous (finger-like) projections within the polyp (Fig. 13). Adenomas are much more common in the large intestine than in the small intestine, and occur more frequently on the left side (rectum and sigmoid) than the right. Histologically, adenomas show mild, moderate or severe dysplasia. Milder degrees of cellular atypia are usual in small, pedunculated tubular adenomas, but large, sessile villous adenomas frequently show high-grade dysplasia, and up to 40% will contain invasive malignancy on microscopic examination. Most adenomas are asymptomatic and first identified on sigmoidoscopy or colonoscopic examination. Occult or overt bleeding, and rarely mucus hypersecretion per rectum can occur.

Box 9 Intestinal polyps

Metaplastic (hyperplastic) polyps
commonest polyps; arise from ? hypermaturation of glandular epithelium; very low (if any) malignant potential

Hamartomatous polyps*
Peutz–Jeghers syndrome; juvenile polyps; Cowden's syndrome

Inflammatory polyps
ulcerative colitis; Crohn's disease; diverticular disease; chronic infections

Neoplastic polyps
adenomas; adenocarcinomas

---

*Hamartoma = mass of disorganised but mature tissues, which are native to the site of origin
Peutz–Jeghers polyps arising in the jejunum and ileum consist of a branching smooth muscle core covered by small intestinal-type epithelium

The adenoma–carcinoma sequence

There is good evidence that many colorectal carcinomas evolve from pre-existing benign adenomas, which subsequently become malignant:

- populations with high prevalence of colorectal adenomas also have a high incidence of large-bowel adenocarcinoma
- the distribution of adenomas within the colon and rectum mirrors that of adenocarcinomas (left side greater than right side)
- the peak age incidence of adenomas precedes that of adenocarcinomas
- foci of invasive adenocarcinoma can be seen within some adenomatous polyps
- the risk of developing colorectal adenocarcinoma is related to the number of adenomas the patient has developed

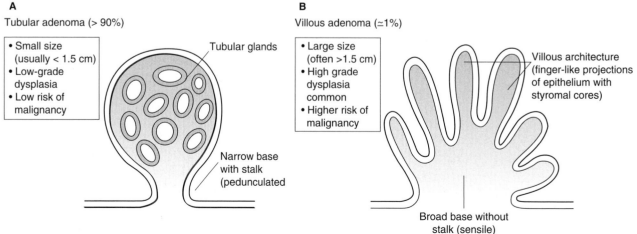

A
Tubular adenoma (> 90%)

- Small size (usually < 1.5 cm)
- Low-grade dysplasia
- Low risk of malignancy

Tubular glands

Narrow base with stalk (pedunculated

B
Villous adenoma (≈1%)

- Large size (often >1.5 cm)
- High grade dysplasia common
- Higher risk of malignancy

Villous architecture (finger-like projections of epithelium with styromal cores)

Broad base without stalk (sensile)

Fig. 13 (**A**) Tubular and (**B**) villous adenomas of the large intestine.

- removing adenomas decreases the incidence of colorectal adenocarcinoma.

Progression from the normal colonic epithelial cell to adenoma and then to carcinoma requires accumulation of DNA damage in key genes that control cellular growth, differentiation and apoptosis (Fig. 14). However, the precise sequence and nature of these multiple genetic 'hits' probably varies between individual tumours.

Colorectal cancer

Colorectal adenocarcinoma accounts for 98% of all large intestinal malignancies. Although worldwide in distribution, the incidence is much higher in North America, Australia and northern Europe than in Japan, South America and Africa. This geographical distribution suggests that differences in lifestyle have an important aetiological role. The typical western low-fibre, high-fat and high-refined-carbohydrate diet appears associated with higher risk of development of malignancy. Peak incidence of colorectal cancer is between 60 and 70 years of age. Rectal lesions are twice as common in men than women, but colonic tumours occur with equal sex incidence.

As described in the previous section, many colorectal cancers arise from adenomas. Risk of malignant transformation is greatest in large villous adenomas. Although many of these adenomas occur spontaneously, some arise in patients with inherited genetic abnormalities.

Familial adenomatous polyposis (FAP, familial polyposis coli)—is a rare autosomal dominant disorder in which patients typically develop 500–2500 adenomas within the large intestine before the age of 30. Unless prophylactic colectomy is performed at an early age, vir-

tually all patients will develop invasive malignancy in at least one of these polyps.

Another form of familial colorectal cancer accounts for around 10% of all cases, and is also associated with malignancy outside the gut (including ovarian and endometrial cancer).

Hereditary non-polyposis colorectal cancer (HNPCC)—patients have inherited mutations of DNA repair genes on chromosome 2. DNA damage can accrue unchecked throughout life and when growth-controlling genes are affected, malignancies may develop. Tumours show a preponderance for the right side of the colon, are often mucin-rich and develop 10–20 years before sporadic colorectal cancer. It is important to identify patients with suspected HNPCC so that they can be regularly examined to exclude extra-intestinal malignancies, and so that family members can be screened for the condition.

Colorectal cancer may grow into the bowel lumen as a polypoid mass, but also invades into the intestinal wall. Circumferential involvement can cause obstruction, which classically has an 'apple-core' appearance on barium enema examination. Ulceration and bleeding are common. In distal colonic and rectal lesions, fresh blood is often passed per rectum. In more proximal tumours, haemorrhage may be occult—the blood becomes altered on passage through the bowel and may not be recognised in the stool. It is not uncommon for caecal cancers to present with unexplained iron deficiency anaemia. Less specific symptoms of colorectal cancer include abdominal pain and alteration of bowel habit.

Microscopically, colorectal cancers show mucin production. They may be well, moderately or poorly differentiated (tumour grade). The stage of the tumour, that is, the extent of spread, is of great importance in prognosis. The Dukes' staging system is commonly used in the UK (Fig. 15).

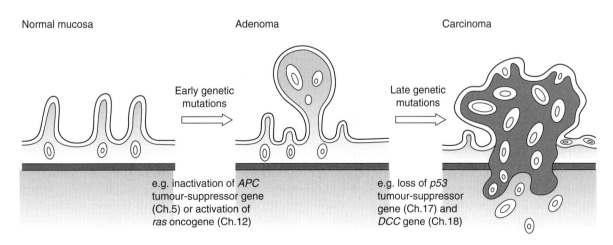

Fig. 14 The adenoma–carcinoma sequence.

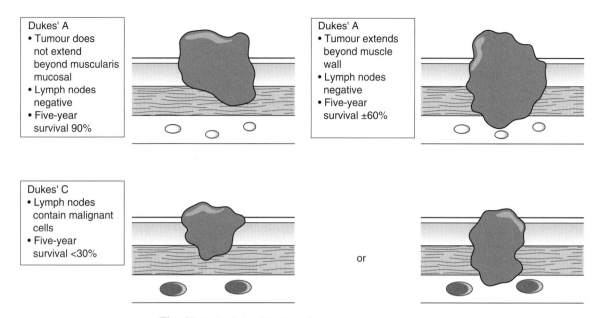

Dukes' A
• Tumour does not extend beyond muscularis mucosal
• Lymph nodes negative
• Five-year survival 90%

Dukes' A
• Tumour extends beyond muscle wall
• Lymph nodes negative
• Five-year survival ±60%

Dukes' C
• Lymph nodes contain malignant cells
• Five-year survival <30%

or

Fig. 15 Dukes' classification of colorectal adenocarcinoma.

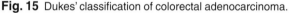

Table 11 Cancer checklist: colorectal carcinoma

Incidence	Usually over 50, unless associated with inherited genetic condition, e.g. FAP, HNPCC
Risk factors	Adenomas, FAP, HNPCC; slightly increased risk in ulcerative colitis and Crohn's disease High-fat, low-fibre diet
Protective factors	High-fibre, low-fat diet, ?aspirin
Associated lesions	Colorectal adenomas
Common clinical presentation	Change in bowel habit, rectal bleeding, iron deficiency anaemia
Location	Sigmoid, rectum, caecum (but can occur anywhere in large bowel)
Macroscopic appearance	Usually polypoid, often ulcerated
Histological features	Adenocarcinoma (gland-forming)
Pattern of spread	Lymph nodes, liver (via blood); through peritoneal surface, directly into adjacent bowel loops Lower rectal tumours can directly invade bladder and pelvic organs
Prognosis (per cent 5-year survival)	Related to stage; approximately 90% for Dukes' A, 60% Dukes' B, 30% Dukes' C

Carcinoid tumours

The normal intestinal mucosa contains a population of scattered neuroendocrine (NE) cells, which are located in the gland bases (crypts). As their name suggests, these cells show features of both neuronal and endocrine differentiation, and produce a variety of peptide hormones. Tumours arising from NE cells account for approximately 50% of all small intestinal neoplasms, and are often collectively referred to as *carcinoid* tumours. All are potentially malignant, but behaviour depends on site of origin, depth of invasion and tumour size. Gut carcinoids are most commonly seen in the appendix, and often present as an incidental finding in routine appendicectomies. Some carcinoids secrete functional hormones which produce symptoms. Examples include *gastrinomas*, which are associated with multiple gastric and duodenal ulcers (Zollinger–Ellison syndrome) and *insulinomas*, which can present with the effects of hypoglycaemia secondary to tumour production of insulin. The *carcinoid syndrome* is rare and only occurs in malignant tumours that have metastasised to the liver. Patients experience episodes of facial flushing and diarrhoea, related to hormone production by the tumour (probably excess serotonin).

Lymphoma

Intestinal involvement by malignant lymphoma may occur in widespread node-based disease or as a localised lymphoma arising within the gut itself. Primary bowel lymphomas arise from mucosal associated lymphoid tissue (MALT), and tend to remain localised to the bowel in the early stages. Primary intestinal lymphomas can be associated with immunological disorders including coeliac disease and HIV infection.

Other primary intestinal neoplasms

Mesenchymal neoplasms of the large intestine include benign tumours of fat (lipomas) and gastrointestinal stromal tumours, which may show smooth muscle or neuronal differentiation.

The lower anal canal is lined by squamous epithelium. Most malignancies of the anus resemble the squamous cell carcinomas seen elsewhere in the skin.

4.5 Miscellaneous conditions

Obstruction

Obstruction of the small and large bowel can occur in a number of pathological processes, some of which (Crohn's disease, ischaemic colitis, diverticulitis and malignant neoplasms) have already been described. The following four conditions—hernias, adhesions, intussusception and volvulus—account for around 80% of cases of bowel obstruction (Fig. 16).

Hernia—is the name given to a pouch-like peritoneal-lined sac that protrudes through a defect or weak area in the peritoneal cavity. Common sites for herniation include the inguinal and femoral canals, the umbilicus and surgical scars. The hernial sac often contains loops of small bowel, and sometimes omentum or large bowel, which can become trapped. Pressure at the neck of the hernia can impair venous return, causing stasis and oedema, and eventual infarction. Permanent trapping of bowel within the hernia is known as incarceration.

Fibrous adhesions—between intestinal loops and other peritoneal structures can follow any cause of peritoneal inflammation, and are particularly common after abdominal or pelvic surgery.

Intussusception—occurs when one segment of bowel becomes telescoped into the immediately adjacent (distal) segment. Intussusception can arise within previously normal intestine in children, sometimes in relation to hyperplastic lymphoid tissue. In adults a mass lesion (usually a neoplasm) is often found at the site of intussusception.

Volvulus—is the complete twisting of a bowel loop around its mesenteric attachment. This cause of obstruction is most frequent in the sigmoid colon of older adults.

Large intestinal haemorrhage

As mentioned earlier in this chapter, infectious colitis, diverticulitis, ulcerative colitis, Crohn's disease and colonic neoplasms may all present with rectal bleeding. Two further clinically important causes of colonic bleeding are haemorrhoids and angiodysplasia.

Haemorrhoids—are common abnormalities, consisting of dilated thick-walled veins in the anus and rectal

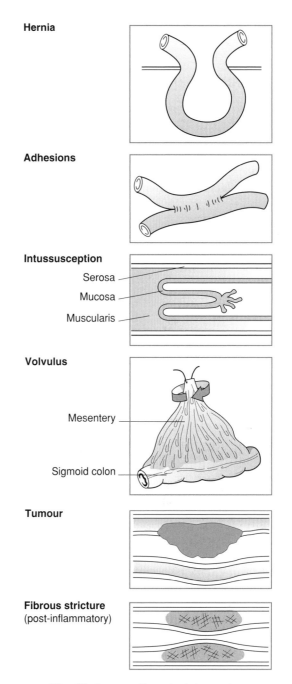

Fig. 16 Causes of intestinal obstruction.

submucosa. These abnormal vessels may protrude from the anal orifice and become traumatised, causing haemorrhage and thrombosis. Predisposing factors for developing haemorrhoids include constipation, pregnancy and portal hypertension (see Ch. 5—hepatobiliary disease).

Angiodysplasia—is a condition of unknown aetiology, characterised by the presence of dilated blood vessels in the mucosa and submucosa of the large intestine. The caecum is the most common site. Angiodysplasia accounts for up to 20% of cases of symptomatic lower intestinal haemorrhage in the elderly.

Self-assessment: questions

Multiple choice questions

1. The following are correctly paired:
   a. Ulcerative colitis—sclerosing cholangitis
   b. Diverticular disease—increased risk of malignancy
   c. Pseudomembranous colitis—*Clostridium difficile*
   d. Coeliac disease—anti-DNA antibodies
   e. Peutz–Jeghers syndrome—hamartomatous polyps.

2. Colorectal cancer:
   a. Always arises from a pre-existing benign tumour (adenoma)
   b. May present with iron deficiency anaemia
   c. Has a 5-year survival of less than 30% in the absence of lymph node involvement
   d. Occurs with increased incidence in cigarette smokers
   e. Shows squamous differentiation in 20% of cases.

3. The following statements are true:
   a. Cytotoxin-producing bacteria cause diarrhoea without tissue damage
   b. Fibrous strictures occur in ischaemic colitis
   c. Intussusception is a cause of bowel obstruction in infants
   d. Coeliac disease is characteristically associated with increased numbers of neutrophil polymorphs in the surface epithelium of the small intestine
   e. Bowel obstruction is a long-term complication of abdominal surgery.

4. Concerning small bowel infarction:
   a. It only occurs in the presence of arterial occlusion
   b. Mesenteric artery atherosclerosis is a common predisposing factor
   c. Peritonitis is a rare complication
   d. Necrosis confined to the mucosa heals by scarring
   e. The mortality rate is low.

Case histories

Case history 1

A 24-year-old female presents with several weeks' history of diarrhoea, abdominal pain and weight loss. On questioning she admits to having similar symptoms two years previously. Clinical examination reveals no abdominal abnormality, but swollen (oedematous) skin tags are noted around the anus. Stool culture is negative. Haematological investigation shows a normochromic, normocytic anaemia. Sigmoidoscopy is performed and a mucosal biopsy is taken for histology. The pathologist's report states that the appearances are consistent with Crohn's disease.

1. Which pathological features distinguish Crohn's disease from ulcerative colitis?
2. List the complications of Crohn's disease.
3. Why is the patient anaemic?

Case history 2

A 73-year-old man complains of passing blood and mucus per rectum. On sigmoidoscopy, a 4 cm polypoid lesion is seen and part of the polyp is biopsied. The pathologist reports a villous adenoma with severe dysplasia. The sigmoid colon containing the remainder of the polyp is removed. Pathological examination of the surgical resection shows invasive adenocarcinoma.

1. What is meant by dysplasia?
2. Which features of colorectal adenomas are associated with a high risk of developing invasive malignancy?
3. What pathological factors are of prognostic importance in colorectal cancer?
4. Why might postoperative measurement of blood carcinoembryonic antigen (CEA) be useful?

Short note questions

Write short notes on the following:
1. Carcinoid tumour
2. Bacterial enterocolitis
3. Colonic polyposis syndromes

Self-assessment: answers

Multiple choice answers

1. a. **True.** Extra-intestinal manifestations of ulcerative colitis include sclerosing cholangitis, an inflammatory disorder of bile ducts leading to multiple areas of fibrous stricture formation in the biliary system. Other associated conditions include arthritis and ocular inflammation.
   b. **False.** Diverticular disease and colonic cancer both occur most frequently in the distal large intestine of older adults, and may coexist in individual patients. However, there is no evidence that diverticular disease increases the risk of developing malignancy (or vice versa).
   c. **True.** Identification of *Clostridium difficile* toxin in the stool of patients with suspected antibiotic-associated diarrhoea is diagnostic of pseudomembranous colitis, even in the absence of characteristic sigmoidoscopic appearances (a reddened, ulcerated colonic mucosa with multiple yellow plaques).
   d. **False.** Coeliac disease is associated with anti-gliadin antibodies. Gliadin is a component of gluten, and treatment of coeliac disease requires removal of the offending antigen by excluding gluten from the diet. Anti-DNA antibodies are found in a number of auto-immune connective tissue diseases, particularly systemic lupus erythematosus (see Ch. 8, *Master Medicine Pathology*, second edition).
   e. **True.** Peutz–Jeghers syndrome is a rare autosomal dominant disease characterised by multiple intestinal polyps and pigmentation of mucous membranes and skin. The polyps are hamartomas (benign overgrowths of mature tissue) consisting of a smooth muscle core covered by epithelium. They arise most commonly in the small intestine but can also occur in stomach, duodenum, colon and rectum.

2. a. **False.** Many colorectal cancers can be seen to arise within a pre-existing benign tumour, usually a large villous adenoma. However, malignancies occurring in patients with hereditary non-polyposis colorectal cancer or ulcerative colitis often develop within flat mucosa that is macroscopically normal. Patients with ulcerative colitis are followed up with regular colono-scopic investigations, at which random biopsies of the intestinal mucosa can be taken for assessment of premalignant histological changes (dysplasia).
   b. **True.** Ulceration of the luminal surface of intestinal tumours can lead to chronic blood loss. This is particularly true for proximal cancers in the caecum and ascending colon, when the blood becomes altered on passage through the bowel and the patient is unaware of the haemorrhage. Tumours arising in the sigmoid colon and rectum are more likely to alert the patient to their existence by way of fresh rectal bleeding on defaecation.
   c. **False.** Tumour stage (extent of spread) is one of the most important prognostic factors for malignant disease arising at any site. Metastasis can occur via the lymphatic system, blood stream or across body cavities. For colorectal cancer, the absence of lymph-node spread in a surgical resection specimen predicts at least a 60% chance of long-term survival, providing local removal of the tumour is complete.
   d. **False.** Risk factors for large intestinal carcinoma include genetic predisposition (hereditary non-polyposis colorectal cancer and familial polyposis coli), inflammatory bowel disease (particularly ulcerative colitis) and environmental factors (high animal-fat diet).
   e. **False.** Over 98% of malignant colorectal neoplasms are adenocarcinomas. Squamous cell carcinoma occurs most frequently in the anal canal.

3. a. **False.** Cytotoxins by definition cause tissue damage. In gut infections, cytotoxins cause epithelial cell death with subsequent loss of normal intestinal absorptive function. In contrast, secretory toxins exert their effects by altering the function of viable cells (e.g. activation of adenylate cyclase by cholera toxin).
   b. **True.** Ischaemic injury to the colon may be restricted to the mucosa or extend beyond into submucosa. Chronic inflammation within the submucosa heals by fibrous scarring, which, if extensive, can lead to stricture formation.
   c. **True.** In infants and children, often no underlying cause is identified. In adults there is a much higher likelihood of a mass lesion (tumour) causing the intussusception.
   d. **False.** Coeliac disease is characterised by increased numbers of intraepithelial lymphocytes in the small intestine mucosa, along with numerous plasma cells in the lamina propria. Recall that coeliac disease is immunologically

mediated, and that plasma cells produce antibodies in immune reactions. Neutrophil polymorphs are the characteristic cell of acute inflammation.

e. **True.** Injury to the peritoneal lining of the intestine or abdominal cavity causes acute inflammation, which can undergo repair with formation of thin fibrous bands (adhesions) between bowel loops. Adhesions can follow any cause of peritonitis but are most commonly associated with previous surgery. Adhesions are a frequent cause of small intestinal obstruction.

4. a. **False.** It can follow arterial occlusion, venous thrombosis or obstruction, or generalised hypoperfusion (e.g. any cause of shock).
   b. **True.** Atherosclerosis is usually complicated by thrombosis or embolism to cause acute intestinal ischaemia.
   c. **False.** Infarction involving the full thickness of the bowel wall often results in peritonitis and perforation.
   d. **False.** If infarction is restricted to the mucosa and submucosa, it can heal by regeneration rather than repair / fibrosis (scar tissue).
   e. **False.** Small bowel infarction is a serious condition, and patients are often elderly with pre-existing cardiovascular disease.

Case history answers

Case history 1

1. Crohn's disease is characterised by chronic inflammation involving all layers of the bowel wall. Fissuring ulcers, lymphoid aggregates and non-necrotising granulomas are the classical microscopic features. The disease is segmental in distribution, with intervening areas of normal bowel in between abnormal areas ('skip lesions'). Chronic inflammation in ulcerative colitis is restricted to the mucosa. The large intestine is involved in a continuous fashion, extending proximally from the rectum.

2. Complications of Crohn's disease include abscesses, strictures and fistula formation. Perforation, toxic dilatation and carcinoma are serious but rare complications. The terminal ileum is frequently involved in Crohn's disease, causing diarrhoea, steatorrhoea (fat malabsorption) and general malabsorption. Anal disease (oedematous anal tags, fissure and perianal abscesses) is very common in colonic Crohn's disease. Ulceration is often seen in the mouth. Extragastrointestinal manifestations include arthritis, skin lesions, biliary tract inflammation and iritis.

3. Anaemia is common in Crohn's disease and is usually the normochromic normocytic anaemia of chronic disease, due to deficient erythropoiesis. Although the terminal ileum is often involved in Crohn's, megaloblastic anaemia due to vitamin B_{12} deficiency is unusual.

Case history 2

1. Dysplasia means abnormal growth. The term is usually applied to epithelium that shows many of the cytological feature of tumour cells, but without evidence of invasive malignancy. These features include hyperchromatic (darkly staining) nuclei, increased nuclear to cytoplasmic ratio, pleomorphism (variation in the size and shape of individual nuclei and cells), increased numbers of mitotic figures (often with abnormal forms), loss of polarity (orientation) of the epithelial cells and lack of maturation of the epithelium. Dysplasia in its early stages is probably reversible but many dysplastic lesions if left long enough without treatment will progress to malignancy.

2. High-risk features for development of malignancy in colorectal adenomas are large size (especially > 2 cm), severe dysplasia and villous architecture. These features often occur together.

3. The most important pathological prognostic features are the tumour grade (the degree of differentiation) and stage (the extent of spread). The depth of invasion into the bowel wall and the presence or absence of local lymph-node metastases are factors in all staging systems for colorectal cancer. Pathological assessment of the completeness of excision of a tumour in a surgical resection specimen is also a very important predictor of the likelihood of achieving cure.

4. Carcinoembryonic antigen (CEA) is a glycoprotein normally produced by gut, pancreas and liver in the embryo. It can be elevated in the serum of adults with a variety of benign and malignant diseases, including colorectal cancer. Due to the lack of specificity, measurement of blood CEA level is not a useful diagnostic test for colorectal neoplasia. However, increasing serum levels of CEA after therapy can be used as a biochemical marker of residual or recurrent disease.

Short note answers

1. Begin with a definition—carcinoid tumour is a neoplasm of neuroendocrine cells. Remember that carcinoid tumours do not just occur in the gut but can also arise in other epithelial sites, particularly lung. Many of these tumour-based questions can be approached in a similar way, by considering incidence, age, sex and geographical distribution, risk factors (including any genetic predisposition, environmental factors and occupational associations), tumour site, macroscopic and microscopic appearances, patterns and frequency of local and metastatic spread, clinical manifestations and prognosis. It is impossible (and unnecessary) to retain all this factual information for every tumour, but thinking about diseases systematically in this manner will help you to recall information and construct your answers in a logical and coherent manner.

   Carcinoids are uncommon tumours with peak incidence in the sixth decade. In the gut they arise most frequently in the small intestine. Tumours appear as small masses arising in the bowel wall, with a characteristic solid yellow cut-section appearance. Histologically they are formed of uniform epithelial-like cells arranged in a variety of architectural patterns. All carcinoids are potentially malignant but behaviour depends on site of origin, depth of local invasion and tumour size. Local lymph node spread and blood-borne liver metastasis may occur. The latter can produce the carcinoid syndrome—facial flushing, diarrhoea, bronchoconstriction, cardiac valve fibrosis—due to the systemic effects of hormones (mainly serotonin) released from tumour cells. Overall 5-year survival is greater than 50%.

2. Key points regarding bacterial enterocolitis:

   - it is common throughout the world, and an important cause of mortality in developing countries
   - pathogenesis may be due to preformed toxins in food or toxins elaborated by bacteria multiplying within the gut
   - toxins may cause symptoms by affecting gut secretion (secretory toxins) or by tissue damage (cytotoxins)
   - non-toxin producing strains of bacteria cause tissue damage by direct invasion of intestinal epithelium
   - common symptoms include fever, pain, diarrhoea and dysentery
   - a large range of organisms may cause enterocolitis; common examples include *E. coli*, *Salmonella*, *Shigella* and cholera.

3. Colonic polyposis syndromes are rare autosomally inherited diseases, characterised by multiple polyps in the large intestine, sometimes with polyps elsewhere in the gut and/or extra-intestinal manifestations. The polyps may be hamartomas (Peutz–Jeghers syndrome) or adenomas (familial polyposis coli and related conditions). It is important to identify patients with adenomatous polyposis syndromes as they are at very high risk of developing colorectal cancer, and it is necessary to screen other family members for the disease.

5

Liver, biliary system and exocrine pancreas

Overview

The liver performs many varied and vital functions. These include: the metabolism of protein, carbohydrate and fat; synthesis of proteins (including albumin, α_1-antitrypsin, transferrin and coagulation factors); detoxification of waste products and ingested chemicals; and participation in the reticuloendothelial system. Chronic liver disease, the causes and consequences of which are discussed in this chapter, most frequently results from viral or alcohol-induced injury. Genetic, autoimmune and vascular diseases also affect the liver. Primary hepatocellular carcinoma is uncommon in the UK but is very frequent in countries with high rates of hepatitis B infection. The liver is a very common site for metastatic malignancy.

The biliary system functions include digestion of dietary fat and excretion of certain metabolites via the bile. While gall-bladder stones and inflammation are very common in the western world, congenital biliary atresia and malignant disease are unusual but clinically important conditions.

The exocrine pancreas produces digestive enzymes, including lipases, amylases and trypsin. These enzymes play a role in pancreatitis, a disease that is usually precipitated by alcohol ingestion or gall stones. Pancreatic adenocarcinoma is a major cause of cancer mortality.

PART 1: LIVER

Learning objectives

You should:

- Understand the definition, causes and clinical consequences of cirrhosis

- Know the natural history of hepatitis B and C infections

- Know the pathological effects of alcohol on the liver

- Understand how therapeutic drugs can cause liver disease

- Understand the range of viral, genetic and autoimmune diseases that can cause chronic hepatitis

- Know the epidemiology and pathology of hepatocellular carcinoma

5.1 Inflammation, fibrosis, cirrhosis and liver failure

The clinical effects of cellular injury in the liver depend upon the extent of cell death and the duration of the insult. For example, infection with hepatitis A virus may cause minimal asymptomatic disease, clinically apparent acute hepatitis with jaundice or, very rarely, acute liver failure. In virtually every case, liver mass and architecture will be restored once the transient infection is cleared, and there is no residual hepatic damage. However, chronic inflammation in the liver can result in extensive fibrous tissue formation. Scarring may link portal tracts and central veins. Bands of fibrous tissue entrap regenerating nodules of hepatocytes, causing liver cirrhosis (Fig. 17). Cirrhosis is the end stage of chronic inflammatory liver disease from numerous causes, including:

- alcohol
- chronic viral hepatitis (B and C)
- biliary disease (primary and secondary biliary cirrhosis)
- haemochromatosis
- other genetic diseases (α_1-antitrypsin deficiency, Wilson's disease)
- idiopathic.

Cirrhosis—is a diffuse process and the damage is usually irreversible. The scarring disrupts and impairs blood flow through the liver, elevating the portal venous pressure (portal hypertension). As a consequence, blood flow increasingly bypasses the liver and flows through lower resistance vessels that communicate between the portal and systemic circulations. These anastomoses arise at four main sites:

1. The gastro–oesophageal junction (oesophageal varices)
2. The rectum
3. The retroperitoneum
4. The anterior abdominal wall (caput medusae).

There are two serious consequences of this vascular shunting:

1. Life-threatening haemorrhage from rupture of oesophageal varices
2. Impaired detoxification of noxious chemicals (e.g. ammonia), contributing to hepatic encephalopathy, coma and death.

Portal hypertension also causes splenomegaly and contributes to the development of ascites. Portal hypertension can be caused by other lesions that obstruct hepatic blood flow in the absence of cirrhosis, such as portal vein thrombosis and Budd–Chiari syndrome (see Section 5.3).

Cirrhosis is associated with development of hepatocellular carcinoma, although the degree of risk varies with the underlying disease.

Liver failure—can be acute or chronic, and results when hepatic functional impairment is extreme. Mortality exceeds 70%. It is often precipitated by an event such as gastrointestinal haemorrhage or infection in a patient with chronic liver disease. Acute liver failure is uncommon, but may follow viral infection, drug exposure (e.g. paracetamol overdose, halothane), toxin damage (carbon tetrachloride), acute fatty liver of pregnancy and Reye's syndrome (Section 5.3). In acute liver failure without pre-existing hepatic disease, there is extensive liver necrosis with shrinkage of the organ, and clinical features of hepatic failure—clotting deficiencies, jaundice, hepatic encephalopathy—developing over 2–3 weeks. Massive liver destruction may prove fatal without transplantation, or cause irregular scarring in survivors.

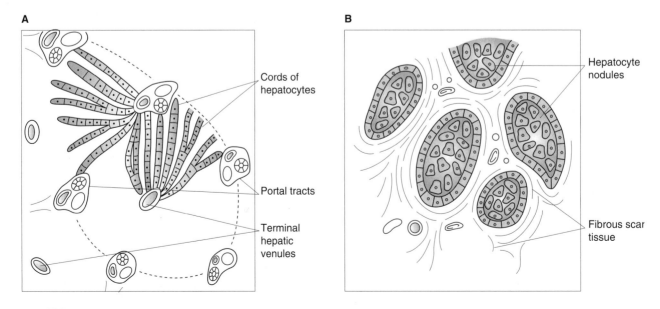

Fig. 17 Liver cirrhosis. (**A**) Normal liver—schematic acinar architecture. (**B**) Liver cirrhosis—loss of normal architecture.

Box 10 Clinical and laboratory features of liver disease

Hepatic failure
Jaundice
Encephalopathy
- drowsiness, confusion, coma
- coarse hand tremor ('liver flap')
- fetor hepaticus
Hepatorenal syndrome (renal impairment secondary to liver failure)
Ascites/oedema

Chronic liver disease
Bruising
Gynaecomastia
Testicular atrophy
Palmar erythema
Clubbing
Dupuytren's contracture (alcoholic cirrhosis)
Xanthomas (primary biliary cirrhosis)
Spider angiomas (spider naevi)
Ascites/oedema
Hypoalbuminaemia
Raised liver enzymes, coagulopathy, hyponatraemia
Raised serum ammonia in liver failure

Box 11 Acute viral hepatitis

Symptoms can include fever, fatigue, nausea, anorexia and right upper quadrant pain.
Mild hepatomegaly may be detected on examination.
Liver function tests (LFTs) are abnormal, with elevated serum liver enzymes.
If there is conjugated hyperbilirubinaemia, jaundice develops.
Increased urinary bilirubin excretion produces dark urine, while decreased biliary excretion causes pale stools.
Bile salt retention in the skin causes itching.

Infectious hepatitis

Viral infection of the liver has various clinical manifestations, according to the specific agent involved:

- asymptomatic subclinical infection with complete resolution
- acute hepatitis
- chronic hepatitis
- asymptomatic carrier state
- hepatic failure (acute or chronic)
- cirrhosis
- hepatocellular carcinoma.

Acute hepatitis

In acute viral hepatitis (Box 11) there may be isolated liver-cell necrosis or more severe bridging necrosis between portal tracts and central veins. Portal tracts are inflamed and there are increased numbers of Kupffer cells (sinusoidal macrophages). Swelling, necrosis and regeneration of hepatocytes produces architectural distortion called lobular disarray. All of these changes can revert to normal if infection is cleared.

Chronic hepatitis

Chronic hepatitis is defined as abnormal LFTs and/or clinical evidence of continuing hepatic inflammation for > 6 months. The severity of inflammation varies within and between individual cases over time. Bile-duct injury, fatty change, portal tract lymphoid aggregates and lobular inflammation are typical features of hepatitis C. Hepatitis B infected hepatocytes may show 'ground glass' pink (eosinophilic) cytoplasm. The fibrosis and hepatocyte regeneration associated with chronic inflammatory damage may develop into cirrhosis.

Chronic hepatitis is not only due to viral infection—drugs, autoimmune disease and certain genetic disorders (see later) can cause very similar histological changes. Reaching the correct diagnosis requires consideration of all the clinical, serological, biochemical and pathological findings.

Carrier state

Disease carriers harbour persistent asymptomatic infection; they may be entirely healthy or have covert subclinical chronic liver disease. A carrier can pass infective virus on to non-immune contacts. Hepatitis B, C and D infections can produce a carrier state.

Hepatic failure, *cirrhosis* and *hepatocellular carcinoma*
These are discussed elsewhere in this chapter.

Within the family of specific hepatitis viruses (Table 12), hepatitis B and C are the clinically most important causes.

Hepatitis B

Hepatitis B infection occurs worldwide, but is extremely common in southeast Asia, where the disease is frequently transmitted from mother to fetus. Exposure early in life creates a permanent carrier state in over 90% of patients. Infection in the UK is usually acquired in adult life, through sexual contact, infected needles (drug abusers and healthcare workers) or an unknown source. Needlestick injury from a hepatitis B carrier confers a 30% risk of infection. The virus is present in blood and body fluids during incubation (which can be up to six months from inoculation) and during periods of acute liver

Table 12 Hepatitis viruses

	Nature of virus	Mode of spread	Clinical disease
A	Single-stranded RNA virus	Faecal–oral spread from contaminated food and water, especially seafood	Usually self-limiting acute infection Acute liver failure occurs in <1% No chronic disease No carrier state
B	Double-stranded DNA virus	Vertical (mother to fetus), sexual contact, blood transfusion, IV drug abuse	Very high rate of carrier state if infected in early life, with frequent chronic hepatitis, cirrhosis and hepatocellular carcinoma Risk of chronic disease and malignancy is less if infection is acquired in adult life
C	Single-stranded RNA virus	Blood transfusion (haemophiliacs) and inoculation (IV drug abuse)	Up to 85% develop chronic hepatitis; up to 50% of these progress to cirrhosis +/– hepatocellular carcinoma +/– hepatic failure
D	Defective RNA virus only infective in association with HBV	Parenteral	Can co-infect with HBV (usually recover normally, but risk of severe acute hepatitis is increased) or super-infect a HBV chronic carrier, with greatly increased risk of chronic hepatitis and cirrhosis
E	Single-stranded RNA virus	Faecal–oral spread from contaminated water	Usually self-limiting but 20% mortality rate in pregnant women

inflammation. The viral antigens and host antibodies detected in the serum reflect the stage of disease and infectivity of the patient. Core antigen (HbcAg) and the related HBe antigen are infective. The presence of IgM anti-HBc indicates recent infection. As the time period from infection increases, the antibody class switches to IgG. Surface antigen (HbsAg) positivity indicates acute infection or carrier state. HbsAb appears late and indicates immunity.

Hepatitis C

Hepatitis C prevalence is uncertain, but estimated at between 0.1% and 1% of the UK population. There is an estimated 3% risk of transmission from an infected needlestick injury. Acute infection is asymptomatic in the majority. HCV antibodies are found in many patients with previously unexplained cirrhosis and hepatocellular carcinoma. Liver function tests characteristically fluctuate throughout the course of the disease, and HCV RNA is detectable despite anti-HCV antibodies (the latter do not appear to confer immunity). Liver damage in part appears immunologically mediated. Patients may benefit from immune modulation therapy with interferon. Selection for such treatment is based on histological assessment of the degree of active inflammatory damage and the extent of fibrosis in a liver biopsy specimen.

Other causes of infectious hepatitis include:

- bacterial—tuberculosis, leptospirosis
- viral—cytomegalovirus (CMV), infectious mononucleosis (EBV)
- parasitic—malaria, amoebiasis.

Hydatid disease

Hydatid disease is a systemic infection due to the canine tapeworm *Echinococcus*. While uncommon in the UK, hydatid disease occurs worldwide and incidence is increased in sheep- and cattle-farming areas. The liver is frequently involved with formation of single or multiple infected cysts, causing mass effects. There is a risk of disease dissemination or fatal anaphylactic shock if the cyst contents are liberated and care must be taken during surgical removal.

Liver abscesses

These are uncommon in the UK and are usually due to bacterial infection. Organisms reach the liver via the blood stream, biliary system or direct spread. Abscesses can be single or multiple. Surgical drainage is usually necessary. Parasitic and protozoal abscesses are more common in the developing world.

Autoimmune hepatitis

Autoimmune liver disease typically occurs in young and middle-aged adult females. Patients have a chronic hepatitis, which clinically and histologically resembles viral hepatitis, but serological tests show raised serum IgG and specific autoantibodies. The latter include antinuclear antibodies (ANA), antimitochondrial antibodies (AMA), antismooth-muscle and antimicrosomal antibodies. There is often associated extrahepatic autoimmune disease such as thyroiditis or rheumatoid arthritis.

5.2 Alcohol- and drug-related liver disease

Alcohol abuse is the major cause of chronic liver disease in the UK. Excessive alcohol intake can cause:

- fatty change (steatosis)
- alcoholic hepatitis
- cirrhosis, +/− hepatocellular carcinoma.

Fatty change—is the accumulation of fat droplets within the cytoplasm of hepatocytes, usually as a single large vacuole (macrovesicular steatosis). The change occurs throughout the liver, and may develop in chronic alcohol abuse or following 'binge' drinking in non-habituated individuals. Fatty change is reversible over several days of abstinence, but with repeated attacks, fibrosis can develop.

Alcoholic hepatitis—In alcoholic hepatitis (steato-hepatitis) fatty change is accompanied by acute inflammation, with neutrophil polymorph infiltration around degenerate and necrotic hepatocytes. Abnormal liver cells may contain condensed intracytoplasmic proteins, known as Mallory bodies. Alcoholic hepatitis is associated with developing liver fibrosis, which characteristically starts around centrilobular veins. While simple fatty change usually produces no clinical symptoms, alcoholic hepatitis presents with right upper quadrant pain and jaundice. Either condition may cause hepatomegaly.

With or without recurrent attacks of alcoholic hepatitis, individuals who maintain a high regular alcohol intake over several years are at risk of progressive fibrosis, cirrhosis and liver failure. Women appear to be at greater risk with a relatively lower alcohol intake. Coexistent liver disease, particularly haemochromatosis and hepatitis C infection can be important contributory factors in progression to cirrhosis. Current recommendations are for women to drink no more than 14–21 units of alcohol per week, and men less than 21–28 units. Moderate regular intake appears less harmful than erratic, heavy, binge drinking. Indeed, regular, low ethanol intake appears to have a protective influence in coronary heart disease!

Acute alcohol intoxication—causes injury and death through accidents, hypoglycaemia, epilepsy and direct cerebral toxicity. Chronic alcohol abuse can result in pancreatitis, cardiomyopathy, physical dependence, malnutrition and neurological disease (Wernicke–Korsakoff syndrome—confusion, ataxia and ocular disturbances due to thiamine deficiency; if untreated, severe, irreversible amnesia often results).

Hepatic fat accumulation is most frequently seen in association with ethanol but other causes include:

- non-alcoholic steatohepatitis (diabetes mellitus, obesity, drugs)
- hepatitis C infection
- drugs
- Reye's syndrome
- acute fatty liver of pregnancy.

Drugs and the liver

Drugs can cause many morphological changes in the liver; more common examples are shown in Table 13. As the histological features often mimic endogenous liver disease a thorough clinical history is essential. Mechanisms of drug damage are:

- direct toxicity
- conversion of drug to active toxin by liver
- immune-mediated (e.g. drug causes autoantibody production).

Drug damage may be *predictable*, occurring in any individual who ingests a large enough dose, or *idiosyncratic* (host dependent).

5.3 Genetic, metabolic and vascular liver disease

Haemochromatosis

Haemochromatosis is an autosomal recessive disease with excessive iron storage predominantly in the liver, pancreas, myocardium and synovial joints. The gene involved is on chromosome 6. The heterozygote rate is approximately 10% in white UK populations and the homozygote disease state is relatively common (0.5%). Gene testing can confirm suspected clinical cases of haemochromatosis and can be used to screen other family members for the disease. Men are affected more often than women, possibly due to the ameliorating effect of menstruation in reducing total body iron. Presentation is most frequent in middle-aged adults.

The typical clinical triad consists of cirrhosis, diabetes and skin pigmentation ('bronze diabetes'). Depending on the stage of disease, liver biopsy in homozygotes shows fibrosis or cirrhosis with excess iron in hepatocytes and Kupffer cells (liver macrophages). Iron is present in the form of haemosiderin pigment and appears yellow-brown on histological examination. A special stain, known as a Perl's stain, gives a bright blue colour to iron deposits and this allows the degree of iron overload to be graded microscopically. Heterozygotes for the abnormal haemochromatosis gene also show increased

Table 13 Drugs and the liver

Liver lesion	Examples of drugs responsible
Fatty change	Methotrexate, tetracycline
Hepatocyte necrosis	Paracetamol, halothane, isoniazid
Hepatitis and fibrosis	Methotrexate, amiodarone
Granulomatous inflammation	Sulphonamide antibiotics
Cholestasis	Chlorpromazine, oral contraceptive pill
Veno-occlusive disease	Cytotoxic drugs
Venous thrombosis	Cytotoxic drugs, oral contraceptive pill
Hepatocellular adenoma	Oral contraceptive pill

Box 12 Special stains

Routine histology slides are stained with haematoxylin and eosin ('H and E'). Nuclei take up the blue haematoxylin stain while cytoplasmic components show variable pink–red colouration from the eosin. When required, additional stains can be used in any tissues to demonstrate specific cell components and infectious agents. Examples include:

Periodic acid Schiff (PAS)
Stains carbohydrates magenta pink; PAS will stain glycogen in many cell types. Additional treatment with a diastase enzyme (DPAS stain) removes glycogen reactivity but allows demonstration of:

- mucin in gland-derived tumours (adenocarcinomas)
- fungi
- intracellular accumulations, such as α_1-antitrypsin.

Perl's stain
Demonstrates iron, for example in haemochromatosis. It can distinguish haemosiderin (iron-containing) pigment from melanin, both of which appear brown on H and E staining.

Congo red
Stains amyloid deposits salmon pink in normal light. When viewed with polarised light, the amyloid appears light green (see *Master Medicine Pathology*, second edition).

Ziehl–Neelsen (ZN)
Stains mycobacteria (acid fast bacilli).

Giemsa
Demonstrates *Helicobacter pylori* and *Giardia* organisms.

hepatic iron storage but not sufficient to cause significant tissue damage. The liver shows little inflammation. Cirrhosis occurring in haemochromatosis carries a very high risk of hepatocellular carcinoma, which is the leading cause of death in these patients. Complications of diabetes or of cardiac involvement (arrhythmias, cardiomyopathy) may also prove fatal. Treatment with iron chelators and regular venesection in the precirrhotic phase is successful.

Secondary causes of hepatic iron overload include severe anaemia, repeated blood transfusions and excessive dietary intake linked to use of iron cooking utensils.

α_1-Antitrypsin deficiency—is a rare autosomal recessive disease which causes emphysema (see Ch. 2) and hepatic cirrhosis. Liver biopsy shows variably sized, round intracytoplasmic globules of α_1-antitrypsin within hepatocytes, demonstrated by DPAS staining (see Box 12). Depending on the exact nature of the allele mutation, α_1-antitrypsin can present in neonates, children or adult life. In severe disease, liver transplantation is curative.

Wilson's disease—is a rare autosomal recessive disorder of copper metabolism, which affects the liver, eye and brain. The incidence is approximately 1 : 200 000. There is a decrease in the serum copper-containing protein caeruloplasmin. Histology shows increased hepatic copper, often with quite marked chronic inflammation, fibrosis and fatty change. Presentation can be at any age but is often in adolescents or young adults. Extrahepatic manifestations include a Parkinsonian movement disorder, psychiatric symptoms and iris abnormalities (Kayser–Fleischer rings; green–brown copper deposits). If diagnosed early enough, copper chelating drugs are effective. If cirrhosis intervenes, liver transplantation may be considered.

Reye's syndrome—is a rare metabolic liver disease, with fatty change and encephalopathy. Reye's syndrome usually arises in young children following a viral illness. Most patients recover but occasionally fulminant liver failure or permanent neurological deficit results. Reye's syndrome is a disease of mitochondrial metabolism and has been associated with aspirin use—because of this association, aspirin is usually contraindicated in children under 12 years of age.

Vascular disease in the liver

Venous congestion—of the liver is very common in cardiac decompensation, both right sided and congestive (biventricular). Cut section of the liver at autopsy in these patients resembles the stippled appearance of the inside of a nutmeg, hence the pathologist's descriptive phrase, 'nutmeg liver'. This appearance results from more intense congestion of blood around centrilobular veins than around portal tracts. If there has been severe hypoperfusion of the liver, centrilobular necrosis can occur—this central perivenular area is more at risk of ischaemic damage than the better oxygenated periportal zone.

Portal vein thrombosis—is uncommon. It is associated with local sepsis, liver cirrhosis, malignancy, adjacent lymphadenopathy and the postoperative state. It may present with pain, ascites, oesophageal varices or bowel infarction.

Hepatic vein thrombosis (Budd–Chiari syndrome)—occurs in thrombotic conditions (post-partum, pregnancy, polycythaemia, oral contraceptives, malignancy). It can be acute and fatal or chronic. Membranous webs, presumably representing resolved thrombus, may be seen in hepatic veins and inferior vena cava.

Veno-occlusive disease—in the UK is seen in bone-marrow transplant recipients, as a result of initial chemotherapy and radiotherapy. Intra-hepatic veins are obliterated and there is a high mortality rate, up to 50%.

5.4 Liver tumours (Table 14)

Benign liver tumours—include haemangiomas and liver-cell adenomas. The latter occur most commonly in women and are associated with oral contraceptive use. There is a risk of tumour rupture with intraperitoneal haemorrhage during pregnancy.

Hepatocellular carcinoma (HCC)—is relatively rare in the UK but represents the commonest visceral carcinoma in countries endemic for viral hepatitis. The distribution is linked to hepatitis B infection, especially if acquired by vertical transmission from mother. The incidence of HCC in the western world is likely to rise in future years due to hepatitis C infection. In UK over 85% of patients with HCC have cirrhosis (compared to 50% or less in endemic hepatitis B countries), and most patients are over 60 years of age. Aflatoxin is a chemical carcinogen associated with HCC. It is produced by *Aspergillus* fungi growing on mouldy food materials, particularly peanuts.

The majority of patients with HCC have raised serum α-fetoprotein (AFP), although this is not a specific finding. AFP can be raised in yolk-sac tumours of testis and ovary, in cirrhosis and chronic hepatitis without tumour, and in early pregnancy (fetal neural tube defects also cause elevated AFP in the mother). Patients usually die within a few months of diagnosis of hepatocellular carcinoma due to cachexia, gastrointestinal bleeding, liver failure or tumour rupture and haemorrhage.

Angiosarcoma—is a malignant vascular tumour associated with vinyl chloride and Thorotrast® (contrast agent) exposure.

Hepatoblastoma—is a malignant liver cell tumour occurring in childhood.

Metastatic malignancy—the liver is a very common site for secondary tumour spread. Breast, lung, colon and other gastrointestinal cancers metastasise most frequently, but virtually any primary site may seed to the liver. Metastases usually form multiple nodules, and may cause massive hepatomegaly.

PART 2: BILIARY DISEASE

Learning objectives

You should:

- Know the pathology and complications of gall stone disease

- Understand primary and secondary biliary cirrhosis

- Know about inflammatory and neoplastic disease of the extrahepatic bile ducts

Table 14 Cancer checklist: liver tumours

Incidence	< 2% of UK cancers; commonest visceral cancer in parts of far East with high hepatitis B prevalence
Risk factors	Cirrhosis; hepatitis B infection (especially vertical transmission); hepatitis C; aflatoxin exposure
Protective factors	Prevention of hepatitis B and C infection
Associated lesions	Chronic viral hepatitis, haemochromatosis, cirrhosis from other causes
Common clinical presentation	Abdominal pain or mass, malaise, weight loss Raised serum α-fetoprotein on monitoring of high-risk patients
Location	Single mass or multiple lesions anywhere in liver
Macroscopic appearance	Well-defined solid lesion(s) or diffusely infiltrating
Histological features	Varies from well-differentiated lesion resembling normal liver cell plates to anaplastic malignancy
Pattern of spread	Lymph nodes; vascular spread, bones, lung
Prognosis (per cent 5-year survival)	Death usual within six months of diagnosis Much better prognosis, 60%, for fibrolamellar variant (young adults, no cirrhosis and hepatitis B negative)

5.5 Inflammatory and other non-neoplastic biliary disease

Ascending cholangitis—is infection of the biliary tree, usually by gram negative gut bacteria. There is often a biliary stone or stricture causing obstruction and stasis, which predispose to infection.

Primary biliary cirrhosis (PBC)—is characterised by granulomatous inflammation and destruction of intra-hepatic bile ducts. It is an autoimmune condition with female predominance, which peaks in middle age. Symptoms include itching, jaundice and xanthomas (the latter due to cholesterol retention). Liver-function tests show a marked increase in alkaline phosphatase, and autoantibodies to mitochondria. PBC is associated with other autoimmune diseases including Sjogren's syndrome, thyroiditis and rheumatoid arthritis. Some cases will progress to cirrhosis.

Primary sclerosis cholangitis (PSC)—describes chronic inflammation with obliterative fibrosis and segmental dilatation of intra- and extrahepatic bile ducts. As with other cause of bile-duct damage, serum alkaline phosphatase is increased. Males are most frequently affected and 70% have coexistent ulcerative colitis. The aetiology of PSC is uncertain. Progressive bile-duct obstruction leads to secondary biliary cirrhosis.

Secondary biliary cirrhosis—follows prolonged extrahepatic biliary obstruction, most commonly due to gallstone impaction in the common bile duct.

Bile duct damage can also occur in viral hepatitis, drug injury and liver transplant rejection.

Gallstones—occur in 20% of the adult population, but most do not cause symptoms. Female gender, increasing age, obesity, high-fat diet, pregnancy and oral contraceptive use are risk factors for the commonest type of stone (cholesterol rich). Stone formation requires supersaturation of cholesterol in bile. Biliary stasis—due to prolonged fasting, pregnancy, rapid weight loss or parenteral nutrition—is a promoting factor. Gallstones rich in pigment material develop in patients with haemolytic anaemia. Biliary tract infection induces deconjugation of bilirubin, and the concentration of deconjugated bilirubin can exceed the low solubility. Clinical consequences of gallstones include biliary colic, obstructive jaundice and cholecystitis (Fig. 18). Gallstones are a major cause of acute pancreatitis.

Acute cholecystitis—is usually caused by impaction of a stone in the gall bladder neck or cystic duct. Bile outflow obstruction leads to chemical irritation of the

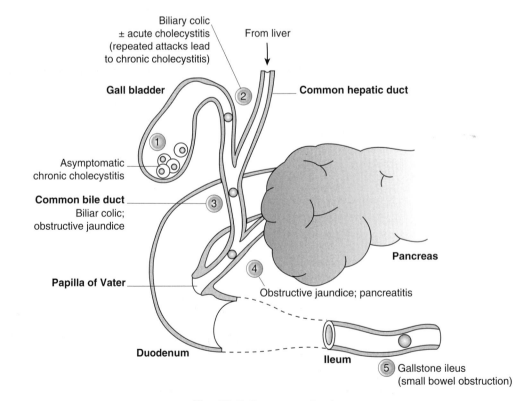

Fig. 18 Gallstone complications.

gall bladder mucosa. With increasing distension and intraluminal pressure, blood flow to the gall bladder becomes compromised and ischaemia develops. The microscopic changes are typical of acute inflammation, with oedema and neutrophil polymorph infiltration. Complications of acute cholecystitis include:

- secondary bacterial infection
- gall bladder perforation and abscess formation
- rupture with peritonitis and fistula formation between gall bladder and bowel
- gall bladder infarction.

Recurrent attacks of acute cholecystitis can progress to *chronic cholecystitis* with fibrosis and mucosal out-pouchings into the muscle layer (Rokitansky–Aschoff sinuses). Acute cholecystitis can also occur in the absence of calculi; precipitating factors include dehydration, gall bladder stasis, bile concentration ('biliary sludge') and bacterial infection. Such patients are often postoperative or have suffered severe trauma, burns, sepsis and multiple organ failure.

Extrahepatic biliary atresia—occurs 1 in 100 000 live births. Bile flow is completely obstructed due to destruction or absence of extrahepatic bile ducts in the neonatal period. The aetiology is uncertain—viral infection, genetic inheritance, and anomalous embryological development have been suggested. Untreated, cirrhosis will develop within six months. Surgical correction is not often possible as intrahepatic ducts are also involved, and transplantation may offer the only chance of survival.

5.6 Bile duct and gall bladder neoplasia

Cholangiocarcinoma—is a malignant tumour of either the intrahepatic or extrahepatic bile ducts. Associated factors include:

- Thorotrast®, a chemical formerly used in radiological imaging
- liver fluke infection (*Clonorchis sinensis*)
- gallstones, ulcerative colitis and choledochal cysts (extrahepatic cholangiocarcinoma).

Cholangiocarcinoma is usually a well-differentiated adenocarcinoma, which induces a large amount of fibrous stroma (desmoplasia), imparting a very hard consistency to the tumour. Prognosis is poor due to local invasion and irresectibility.

Carcinoma of the gall bladder—is rare; it occurs in the elderly, usually associated with gallstones. Extensive local invasion is common at presentation and these unresectable tumours have a very poor prognosis. The vast majority are adenocarcinomas.

PART 3: EXOCRINE PANCREAS

Learning objectives

You should:

- Understand the pathology and complications of pancreatitis
- Know the pathology of pancreatic carcinoma

5.7 Inflammatory disease of the pancreas

Inflammation of the pancreas can occur as a single acute attack or a chronic relapsing condition. Pancreatitis occurs most frequently in middle-aged males. Known precipitating factors of pancreatic inflammation include:

Common
- gallstones and biliary tract disease
- alcohol abuse (chronic pancreatitis, ?also acute).

Rare
- infection (mumps)
- drugs
- trauma
- shock
- localised surgical or endoscopic procedures
- congenital pancreatic abnormalities
- hypercalcaemia.

Pancreatic duct obstruction and direct injury to acinar cells appear to be involved in the initial insult. Damage to the exocrine pancreas liberates digestive enzymes—lipases, proteases and amylases—which increase the amount of tissue injury within the pancreas and adjacent organs. Raised serum amylase to greater than $5 \times$ normal is virtually diagnostic of acute pancreatitis. In severe acute haemorrhagic pancreatitis there is extensive blood vessel damage and abdominal fat necrosis. Systemic effects of enzyme release can include disseminated intravascular coagulation, adult respiratory distress syndrome (ARDS) and shock. Less serious complications are pancreatic abscess and pseudocyst formation. A pseudocyst is a collection of secretions within or outside the pancreas. The pseudocyst has a fibrous capsule but no epithelial lining. (True epithelial-lined pancreatic cysts occur in von Hippel–Lindau disease and adult polycystic kidney disease).

Repeated, often mild, acute attacks lead to chronic pancreatitis, with marked scarring of the organ and loss of exocrine and endocrine function, with development of steatorrhoea and diabetes in severe cases. Pseudo-cysts are frequent in chronic pancreatitis. There is an increased risk of pancreatic carcinoma.

5.8 Neoplastic disease of the exocrine pancreas

Benign tumours of the pancreas are often cystic, and may be composed of mucinous or serous glandular epithelium. Malignant pancreatic tumours—adenocarcinomas—almost always derive from the ductal epithelium. Most tumours arise in the proximal organ, and cause localising symptoms due to obstruction at the ampulla of Vater or distal common bile duct. The prognosis is poor, death often occurring within months of diagnosis.

Table 15 Cancer checklist: pancreatic carcinoma

Incidence	Common visceral cancer; middle-aged and older males, incidence increasing
Risk factors	Not well defined—?smoking, previous gastric surgery, chronic pancreatitis (alcohol)
Protective factors	Not known
Associated lesions	—
Common clinical presentation	Abdominal and back pain, weight loss, jaundice Migratory thrombophlebitis (10%)
Location	60% in head of pancreas, 20% diffusely involve gland
Macroscopic appearance	Hard grey/white mass
Histological features	Gland formation, with reactive, dense, fibrous tissue Perineural invasion
Pattern of spread	Extensive local spread to duodenum, bile duct, stomach, retroperitoneal organs, lymph nodes, liver
Prognosis (per cent 5-year survival)	Less than 5%

Self-assessment: questions

Multiple choice questions

1. The following diseases are associated with the development of cirrhosis:
   a. Hepatitis C
   b. Hepatitis A
   c. Haemochromatosis
   d. Haemolytic anaemia
   e. Alcoholic steatohepatitis.

2. Acute liver failure typically occurs in:
   a. Paracetamol overdose
   b. Acute viral hepatitis
   c. Primary biliary cirrhosis
   d. Reye's syndrome
   e. Budd–Chiari syndrome.

3. Regarding hepatitis B:
   a. Acute infection is usually asymptomatic
   b. Infection early in life confers a higher risk of chronic carrier state
   c. The source of infection is always identifiable
   d. HbsAg detection in the blood indicates immunity
   e. Co-infection with HDV increases the risk of severe acute hepatitis.

4. Complications of cirrhosis include:
   a. Gynaecomastia
   b. Hepatocellular carcinoma
   c. Renal failure
   d. Gastrointestinal haemorrhage
   e. Confusion.

5. The following are correctly paired:
   a. Wilson's disease—abnormal lead metabolism
   b. Haemochromatosis—hepatocellular carcinoma
   c. α_1-Antitrypsin deficiency—bronchiectasis
   d. Veno-occlusive disease—cytotoxic chemotherapy
   e. Angiosarcoma—vinyl chloride exposure.

6. Pancreatic carcinoma:
   a. Is increasing in incidence
   b. Has a 5-year survival rate of 50%
   c. Often presents with painless jaundice
   d. Is usually surgically resectable at presentation
   e. Histologically is a squamous cell carcinoma.

7. Concerning gallstones:
   a. Cholesterol is the most frequent stone component
   b. Most patients are symptomatic

   c. They are associated with gall bladder adenocarcinoma
   d. Stones can develop following prolonged fasting
   e. The incidence is increased in oral contraceptive pill users.

8. The following are causes of extrahepatic bile duct obstruction:
   a. Biliary atresia
   b. Primary biliary cirrhosis
   c. Primary sclerosing cholangitis
   d. Gallstones
   e. Pancreatic adenocarcinoma.

9. Acute cholecystitis:
   a. Can occur in the absence of gall stones
   b. Is characterised by lymphocytic infiltration of the gall bladder
   c. Can be complicated by fistula formation
   d. Frequently results in gall bladder infarction
   e. Is increased in incidence in postoperative patients.

10. The following are associated with primary biliary cirrhosis:
    a. Xanthomas
    b. Raised serum antimitochondrial antibodies
    c. Rheumatoid arthritis
    d. Granulomatous inflammation of the portal tracts
    e. Decreased serum alkaline phosphatase.

Case histories

Case history 1

A 52-year-old female presents with abdominal discomfort and increasing girth secondary to ascites. On examination there are additional signs of chronic liver disease.

1. What other physical signs of liver disease would you look for? What specific questions would you ask in the clinical history?

An ultrasound scan shows abnormal liver echogenicity suggestive of cirrhosis.

2. What further investigations would you consider?

3. What information might be provided by a liver biopsy?
4. What are the most important complications of cirrhosis?

Case history 2

> You are an occupational health physician and a venesector asks you for advice after sustaining a needlestick injury. The health care worker has been immunised against hepatitis B but is anxious about contracting hepatitis C infection.

1. What information could you give regarding the incidence, rate of transmission and rate of progression of hepatitis C infection in this situation?
2. What measures should be taken to reduce the risk of health care personnel contracting hepatitis B and C?

Case history 3

> A 44-year-old man is admitted to hospital with nausea, vomiting and abdominal pain radiating to the back. He admits to a high alcohol intake. The surgical registrar suspects acute pancreatitis and requests serum amylase, calcium, liver function tests and arterial blood gas measurement.

1. How will these investigations contribute to the patient management?

> The patient is confirmed to have acute pancreatitis. He recovers with hospital treatment and is discharged home, but returns two weeks later with further pain and vomiting. Ultrasound examination reveals a cystic mass.

2. What is the likely cause of the mass?

Viva questions

1. How would you classify tumours of the liver?
2. How does knowledge of the pathology of haemochromatosis help in the management of patients and their families?

Self-assessment: answers

Multiple choice answers

1. a. **True.**
   b. **False.** There is no chronic infective state in hepatitis A.
   c. **True.**
   d. **False.**
   e. **True.** If excess alcohol consumption continues.

2. a. **True.**
   b. **True.** Uncommon but can occur in hepatitis A (and E), very rare in B and C.
   c. **False.** Liver failure develops chronically following cirrhosis in severe cases.
   d. **True.**
   e. **True.**

3. a. **True.**
   b. **True.**
   c. **False.** Vertical transmission, sexual contact and inoculation of infected blood are the major methods of transmission but the actual source may not always be identifiable.
   d. **False.** Hepatitis B surface antigen indicates acute infection or carrier state. HbsAb indicates immunity.
   e. **True.** See Table 12.

4. a. **True.** Probably due to altered oestrogen metabolism.
   b. **True.**
   c. **True.** Decompensated cirrhosis can lead to hepatorenal syndrome, in which renal failure occurs secondary to liver failure. The mechanism is thought to involve altered renal blood flow. Kidney dysfunction is reversible if the liver failure can be successfully treated.
   d. **True.** Usually from oesophageal varices, a very important complication.
   e. **True.** If hepatic encephalopathy develops.

5. a. **False.** Copper metabolism is deranged in Wilson's disease.
   b. **True.** There is a high risk of liver cancer in patients with haemochromatosis who develop cirrhosis.
   c. **False.** The lung lesion present in α_1-antitrypsin deficiency is emphysema.
   d. **True.**
   e. **True.**

6. a. **True.**
   b. **False.** Five-year survival is less than 5%.
   c. **True.**
   d. **False.**
   e. **False.** Adenocarcinoma.

7. a. **True.**
   b. **False.** Many adults do not complain of symptoms related to their gallstones.
   c. **True.** But the risk to individual patients is very low given the high prevalence of gallstones and rarity of gall bladder cancer.
   d. **True.** Presumably due to increased bile concentration and cholesterol saturation.
   e. **True.**

8. a. **True.**
   b. **False.** This disease is confined to intrahepatic ducts.
   c. **True.**
   d. **True.**
   e. **True.** Sixty per cent of pancreatic carcinomas arise in the head of the gland and can obstruct the distal common bile duct.

9. a. **True.** But stones are present in > 90% of cases, either in the gall bladder neck or cystic duct.
   b. **False.** Neutrophil polymorphs are characteristic of acute inflammation.
   c. **True.** Between the gall bladder and intestine, usually colon.
   d. **False.** Ischaemic necrosis is a rare but serious complication leading to perforation and peritonitis.
   e. **True.**

10. a. **True.**
    b. **True.**
    c. **True.** There is an association between PBC and other autoimmune conditions.
    d. **True.**
    e. **False.** Alkaline phosphatase is raised in biliary tract damage, and may be the only abnormality in the liver function tests in PBC.

Case histories

Case history 1

1. The signs of chronic liver disease are shown in the Box 10 (page 65). Relevant information from the

clinical history would include alcohol consumption (although patients may not give an honest answer!), family history of liver disease (which may point to an inherited disease), possible exposure to hepatitis B and C and any history of autoimmune disease. As many therapeutic drugs can damage the liver in numerous ways, a careful history of recent and long-term prescribed medications is often helpful.

2. Full investigation of chronic liver disease may include:

   - liver function tests—liver enzymes released from damaged cells (γ-GT, AST and ALP), and markers of synthetic function, such as albumin
   - coagulation tests (INR)
   - viral serology—hepatitis B and C (hepatitis A does not cause chronic disease)
   - autoimmune screen—helpful for diagnosing primary biliary cirrhosis and autoimmune chronic hepatitis
   - ultrasound—to assess liver size, texture (fatty change or cirrhosis) presence of masses / cysts and examine the biliary tree for dilatation (obstruction)
   - gene analysis for haemochromatosis
   - serum protein electrophoresis for α_1-antitrypsin
   - serum caeruloplasmin measurement (Wilson's disease)
   - liver biopsy.

3. Liver biopsy is an invasive procedure which can be helpful in the investigation of:

   - unexplained hepatomegaly or abnormal LFTs
   - cirrhosis
   - tumours (primary or metastatic)
   - hepatic damage by medications—for example, methotrexate used in psoriasis
   - assessing degree of inflammation and fibrosis in hepatitis C infection, in order to select patients for interferon therapy.

   Percutaneous liver biopsy carries a very small risk of mortality but should not be undertaken in patients with abnormal clotting, obstructive jaundice or ascites. An alternative approach in high risk patients is to perform a transjugular biopsy, approaching the liver through the inferior vena cava.

4. Important complications of cirrhosis are discussed in the text (Section 5.1) but include:

   - haemorrhage from portal-systemic anastomoses, especially oesophageal varices
   - hepatic encephalopathy
   - development of hepatocellular carcinoma.

Case history 2

1. The incidence of hepatitis C in the UK is probably less than 1% of the general population but there are high-risk factors including IV drug abuse and blood transfusion prior to the introduction of hepatitis C screening of blood donations in 1991. There is an approximately 3% risk of contracting hepatitis C via a needlestick injury from an infected patient but the risk may vary according to the stage of the disease and the viral load as assessed by HCV RNA analysis using the polymerase chain reaction. The rate of progression to chronic hepatitis may be as high as 85% and up to 50% of these individuals may develop cirrhosis.

2. All heath care workers potentially exposed to blood and body fluids should be immunised against hepatitis B for their own and their patients' safety. There is no vaccination for hepatitis C, so minimising the risk of infection is vital, by wearing protective clothing including gloves and eye protection when appropriate. Open wounds must be fully covered with waterproof dressings. Any specimens of blood, body fluid or tissue sent to pathology laboratories with suspected or known infection risk must be clearly labelled as 'high risk' to protect staff—nurses, operating department assistants, porters, laboratory scientists and doctors—who may come into contact with the material. High-risk status applies to any material potentially infected by hepatitis B or C, HIV or tuberculosis. If you need advice, contact your hospital's Occupational Health Department.

Case history 3

1. The clinical history suggests an acute abdomen; the differential diagnosis would include acute pancreatitis, acute cholecystitis and a perforated peptic ulcer. Myocardial infarction must also be excluded. The investigations ordered would be appropriate to confirm a clinical diagnosis of acute pancreatitis and to assess the severity of the attack. Amylase is released from the inflamed pancreas and a serum rise to greater than five-times the normal upper limit usually indicates acute pancreatitis. However, less severe elevation of serum amylase can occur with other conditions including cholecystitis and perforated peptic ulcer. Severe attacks of acute pancreatitis may be associated with decreased serum albumin and calcium, and a lowered arterial oxygen concentration. The mortality rate in poor prognosis cases exceeds 50%.

2. The likely cause is a pancreatic pseudocyst. If large, the cyst may require drainage by aspiration or surgical excision.

Viva answers

1. Remember in viva answers to be logical, structured and emphasise the more common conditions. In the UK, liver metastases are more common than primary tumours. You could classify primary intrahepatic tumours by their cell of origin. The list below is not exhaustive but would be appropriate for this question:

Benign neoplasms
Epithelial
- hepatocellular adenoma.
Vascular (endothelium)
- haemangioma.

Primary liver malignancies
Epithelial
- hepatocellular carcinoma
- cholangiocarcinoma (arising in intrahepatic bile ducts).

Vascular (endothelium)
- angiosarcoma.

Secondary liver tumours
- from many sites, but particularly colon, upper GI tract, breast and lung.

2. The question requires you to explain the clinical implications of the pathogenesis, genetics, incidence, progression and complications of haemochromatosis. Points to include are:

- mode of inheritance (autosomal recessive)
- heterozygote carrier and homozygote population frequencies
- subclinical disease in heterozygotes
- the opportunity for familial disease screening and early diagnosis through genetic testing
- prevention of serious complications, cirrhosis and liver cancer, by early treatment aimed at reducing body iron (venesection and chelating agents)
- role of liver biopsy in assessing stage and severity of disease, and response to treatment (reduction in hepatic iron stores and cessation of disease progression).

6 Endocrine system

Overview

The endocrine system is a complex, highly integrated group of organs that have a central role in the maintenance of normal bodily functions. More specifically, the endocrine system plays a very important part in the regulation of reproduction, growth and development, maintenance of the internal environment, and energy production, utilisation, and storage. Disorders of the endocrine system are therefore important because they have far-reaching and devastating effects, which in some cases can be life-threatening (e.g. Addisonian crisis, diabetic ketoacidosis). At the heart of the endocrine system are the endocrine glands, which include the pituitary, adrenals, thyroid, parathyroids and pancreas. Endocrine glands synthesise and secrete hormones into the bloodstream, via which they are carried to distant sites to exert their effects. In this way the endocrine glands are able to influence the function of distant target organs and tissues. Disorders of the endocrine system are usually due to either overproduction or underproduction of a particular hormone, or mass lesions, and to aid understanding, the pathology will be presented in a similar scheme.

Basic principles

The ability of the various organs and tissues in the body to function in an integrated fashion is made possible by extracellular signalling. Signalling is mediated by specialised molecules, which are synthesised within the cell and secreted into the extracellular environment, where they exert their effects on other cells. There are three main signalling modalities:

1. **Paracrine**, where molecules secreted by cells exert their effects on neighbouring tissues.
2. **Autocrine**, where the secreted molecules exert their effects on the cell of origin.
3. **Endocrine**, where the secreted molecules exert their effects at distant sites that can be accessed only by the bloodstream.

Molecules that exert their effects via the endocrine modality are called hormones, and hormones are secreted and synthesised by endocrine glands. The effects of hormones are often complex. A single hormone can have different effects on several tissues, and some target tissues require the interaction of several hormones to carry out their physiological functions.

A distinguishing characteristic of the endocrine system is the feedback control of hormone production. Increased activity of a target organ downregulates the activity of the endocrine gland, a process known as negative feedback or feedback inhibition.

There are two broad categories of hormones:

1. **Peptide or amino acid derivatives**—these types of hormones bind to cell surface receptors and exert their effects by causing an increase in intracellular signalling molecules.
2. **Steroid hormones**—steroid hormones are able to diffuse across the lipid cell membrane and bind to intracellular receptors. The hormone/receptor complex then acts directly on the cell DNA.

6.1 The pituitary gland

Learning objectives

You should:

- Know the structure and function of the pituitary gland
- Know the causes of anterior pituitary hypo- and hyperfunction, and the clinical manifestations
- Know the clinical syndromes associated with disorders of ADH secretion from the posterior pituitary

Structure

The pituitary gland is located at the base of the brain within the confines of the sella turcica. It lies beneath the hypothalamus, to which it is attached by means of a stalk, and in close proximity to the optic chiasm. Despite its small size (it measures only ~ 1 cm across), the pituitary gland plays a pivotal role in the regulation of most other endocrine glands. The pituitary gland consists of two parts; the anterior pituitary (or adenohypophysis), and the posterior pituitary (or neurohypophysis) (Fig. 19).

The anterior pituitary (adenohypophysis)

The anterior pituitary constitutes 75% of the gland and is derived from an outpouching of the embryonic oral cavity known as Rathke's pouch. This part of the gland secretes six different hormones into the bloodstream. There are five different cell types in the anterior pituitary, each responsible for synthesising and secreting one or more of the six hormones. The synthesis and secretion of anterior pituitary hormones is controlled by the hypothalamus (the hypothalamic–pituitary axis). Hypothalamic neurones in the median eminence release hypothalamic releasing hormones, which are then carried to the anterior pituitary via a portal venous system in the pituitary stalk (Fig. 19). There are several types of hypothalamic releasing hormone, each acting on and controlling the functions of a specific cell type within the anterior pituitary (see Table 16). The secretion of hypothalamic releasing hormones is under neural control from other parts of the CNS, and hormonal control from the levels of anterior pituitary hormones circulating in the blood. If there are high circulating levels of a particular hormone, the secretion of the relevant hypothalamic releasing hormone is reduced (negative feedback or feedback inhibition).

Hypopituitarism

The most common causes of hypopituitarism are:

- pituitary adenoma (commonest cause)
- craniopharyngioma
- Sheehan's syndrome.

These conditions can lead to a deficiency in all of the anterior pituitary hormones (panhypopituitarism) leading to hypofunction of one or more of the target endocrine organs under pituitary control, a situation that can be life threatening.

Non-secretory pituitary adenomas—are benign tumours that may arise from any of the hormone secreting cells in the anterior pituitary.

Craniopharyngiomas—are usually benign tumours that occur most commonly in children, and are thought to arise from squamous cell rests representing the remains of Rathke's pouch.

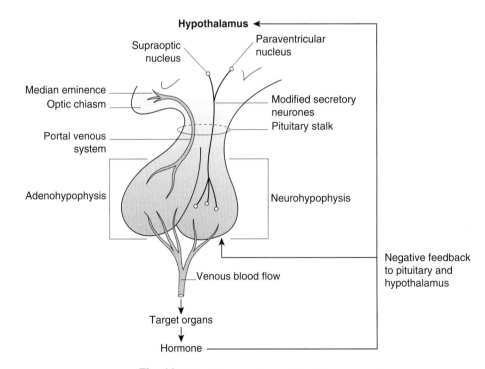

Fig. 19 The pituitary and associated tissues.

Table 16 Anterior pituitary cell types, hormone products, and controlling hypothalamic hormones

Pituitary cell type	Hormonal product	Controlling hypothalamic hormone
Somatotroph	Growth hormone (GH)	Growth hormone-releasing hormone (GHRH) Somatostatin (inhibits release of GH)
Corticotroph	Pro-opiomelanocortin (POMC) from which ACTH is a cleavage product	Corticotrophin-releasing hormone (CRH)
Gonadotroph	Follicle stimulating hormone (FSH) and luteinising hormone (LH)	Gonadotrophin-releasing hormone (GRH)
Lactotroph	Prolactin	Prolactin-inhibiting factor (PIF)
Thyrotroph	Thyroid stimulating hormone (TSH)	Thyrotrophin-releasing hormone (TRH)

Clinical presentation of these two types of tumours is related to their local effects on the surrounding tissues, which include:

- compression damage to the adjacent pituitary tissue, leading to underproduction of the adenohypophysis hormones
- compression of the optic chiasm, which leads to abnormalities in the visual fields (bitemporal hemianopia)
- symptoms of raised intracranial pressure.

Sheehan's syndrome (post-partum ischaemic necrosis)—is a condition that occurs in the post-partum period. During pregnancy, the pituitary enlarges to almost twice its normal size and becomes highly vascular. Sheehan's syndrome occurs if haemorrhage during childbirth causes a severe fall in blood pressure sufficient to cause ischaemic necrosis of the anterior pituitary, resulting in hypofunction. The posterior pituitary is usually spared. The resultant syndrome associated with anterior pituitary hypofunction is known as Simmonds' disease, the first manifestation being failure of lactation due to prolactin deficiency. The effects of the loss of TSH, LH, FSH and ACTH follow.

Clinical manifestations of hypopituitarism
Lack of growth hormone—in pre-pubertal children, lack of growth hormone causes symmetric growth retardation termed pituitary dwarfism. In this condition, sexual development may also be retarded. Lack of growth hormone in adults may cause fasting hypoglycaemia.

Lack of LH and FSH—in post-pubertal women, deficiency induces amenorrhoea, sterility, atrophy of the ovaries and external genitalia, and loss of axillary and pubic hair. In men, deficiency is manifest by decreased libido, sterility, testicular atrophy, and loss of axillary and pubic hair.

Lack of TSH—deficiency of TSH induces hypothyroidism and atrophy of the thyroid gland.

Lack of ACTH—deficiency of ACTH induces hypoadrenalism and atrophy of the adrenals.

Lack of prolactin—affected women who have just given birth find that there is failure of lactation.

Hyperpituitarism

Hyperfunction of the anterior pituitary is almost always due to a functioning adenoma. Functioning carcinomas are rare. Adenomas may produce any anterior pituitary hormone depending on their cell of origin. Clinical presentation is related to:

- overproduction of a particular hormone
- compression of the optic chiasm, causing visual abnormalities.
- raised intracranial pressure.

Somatotrophic adenomas
These adenomas lead to growth hormone overproduction. When the growth hormone excess occurs in children (before the epiphyses have closed) the result is gigantism, which is extremely rare. When the growth hormone excess occurs in adults, the resulting condition is called acromegaly. The excess growth hormone affects the viscera, bones, skin and soft tissues. The main presenting features are enlargement of the hands, feet and head with development of prominent supraorbital ridges, prominent lower jaw (prognathism) and separating of the teeth. Around a third of all acromegalic patients develop cardiac disease, which can be life-threatening.

Corticotrophic adenomas
Excess production of ACTH leads to Cushing's disease (see later).

Gonadotrophic adenomas
These rare tumours tend to secrete the hormones LH and FSH inefficiently and variably. There is often no evidence of increased gonadotroph hormone production, but there may be evidence of underproduction.

Prolactinomas

These are the most common type of pituitary tumour. Hyperprolactinaemia induces galactorrhoea in females, and hypogonadism (infertility) in males and females. Prolactinomas are an important cause of amenorrhoea in women.

Thyrotroph adenomas

These tumours cause hyperthyroidism, but they are extremely uncommon.

The posterior pituitary (neurohypophysis)

The posterior pituitary is derived from a downgrowth of the hypothalamus. Only two hormones are secreted—anti-diuretic hormone (ADH) and oxytocin. These hormones are stored within secretory granules of modified nerve fibres that originate from the supraoptic and paraventricular nuclei. These modified nerve fibres ramify in the pituitary stalk and have their terminal endings in the posterior pituitary. The stored hormones are released in response to hypothalamic stimuli.

ADH is secreted in response to raised plasma osmolarity and induces conservation of body water. It does this by causing an increase in the permeability of the renal collecting ducts, resulting in increased resorption of water and reduced urine output. The urine becomes concentrated. The secretion of oxytocin stimulates uterine smooth muscle to contract during childbirth, and causes the ejection of milk during lactation.

Disorders of the posterior pituitary are rare. The most important disorders are related to the secretion of ADH.

Decreased ADH production

Damage to the hypothalamus, for example by a tumour or trauma, causes a deficiency of ADH producing a syndrome known as diabetes insipidus, which is characterised by polyuria and hyperosmolarity of the blood leading to compensatory polydipsia (excessive drinking).

Increased or inappropriate ADH production

Inappropriate ADH production implies persistent release of ADH unrelated to the plasma osmolarity. The most common cause is ectopic production of ADH by tumours such as bronchogenic carcinoma (especially the small cell variant), and less commonly thymomas, pancreatic carcinomas and lymphomas. Other causes of inappropriate ADH production include CNS disorders (e.g. head injury, meningitis), non-neoplastic lung disorders (e.g. pneumonia, TB), and drugs.

6.2 The adrenal gland

Learning objectives

You should:

- Understand the structure and function of the adrenal glands
- Know the common disorders that can affect the adrenal medulla
- Know the disorders that can cause hypo- or hyperfunction of the adrenal cortex

Structure

The adrenal glands are located in the retroperitoneum, superomedial to the kidneys. Each is composed of two totally separate functional units; the central medulla and the peripheral cortex (Fig. 20).

The adrenal medulla

The adrenal medulla, which is derived from the embryonic neural crest, is part of the sympathetic nervous system. It consists of neuroendocrine cells (chromaffin cells) and sympathetic nerve endings. The main function of the chromaffin cells is to synthesise and secrete the catecholamines, adrenaline and noradrenaline. The adrenal medulla is the main source of endogenous adrenaline.

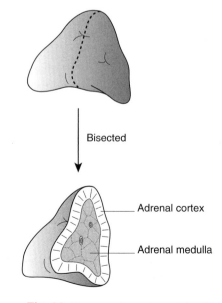

Bisected

Adrenal cortex

Adrenal medulla

Fig. 20 Diagram of an adrenal gland.

The most significant disorders arising from the adrenal medulla are neoplasms, which include phaeochromocytomas (most common), neuroblastomas, and ganglioneuromas.

Phaeochromocytoma

This is a functioning tumour derived from the chromaffin cells of the adrenal medulla, and is classified as a paraganglioma. Overproduction of catecholamines produces hypertension (which may be intermittent) associated with headaches, sweating, palpitations, pallor, anxiety and nausea. The presence of a phaeochromocytoma should be suspected in any young hypertensive patient and, although rare, is one of the curable causes of hypertension. Around 10–20% of these tumours are associated with familial syndromes such as MEN (multiple endocrine neoplasia) syndrome, von Hippel–Lindau disease, von Recklinghausen's disease, tuberous sclerosis, and Sturge–Weber syndrome. About half of these familial cases are bilateral. The diagnosis of phaeochromocytoma is based on estimating the urinary excretion of the catecholamine metabolite vanillylmandelic acid (VMA), which is at least doubled when the tumour is present.

The adrenal cortex

The adult cortex constitutes the peripheral 80% of the adrenal gland. The adrenal cortex is derived from mesoderm and synthesises and secretes the three main classes of steroid hormones: mineralocorticoids; glucocorticoids; and sex steroids. There are three functional zones of the adrenal cortex: the zona glomerulosa (10%), which lies beneath the capsule and secretes mineralocorticoids; the zona fasciculata (80%); and the zona reticularis (10%), which correspond to the middle and inner zones of the adrenal cortex and secrete glucocorticoids and sex steroids.

Glucocorticoids

These hormones have important effects on a wide range of tissues and organs. The effects include:

- increased blood sugar
- increased protein breakdown
- increased fat loss from the extremities, but fat accumulation in the trunk, neck and face.
- effects on the immune system, bone, kidneys, CNS, circulatory system, other endocrine glands and connective tissue.

The most important glucocorticoid is cortisol. The synthesis and secretion of glucocorticoids is under negative feedback control by ACTH, which is synthesised by the anterior pituitary.

Mineralocorticoids

Aldosterone is the most important mineralocorticoid. Its function is to maintain intravascular volume. When intravascular volume is decreased, aldosterone acts on renal tubules to increase the reabsorption of sodium and elimination of potassium and hydrogen ions. The retention of sodium leads to retention of water and consequent restoration of the intravascular volume. The synthesis and secretion of the mineralocorticoids is controlled by the renin–angiotensin system and *not* the pituitary (see Fig. 21).

Sex steroids

The sex steroids are involved in the development of the male and female sexual characteristics. Most of the body's sex steroids are synthesised in the gonads, but the adrenal sex steroids usually have a role in the development of some of the secondary sexual characteristics.

Adrenocortical hyperfunction (hyperadrenalism)

The clinical syndromes of cortical hyperfunction are due to excess production of one of the adrenal steroids. Cushing's syndrome is due to excess glucocorticoids, Conn's syndrome is due to excess mineralocorticoids, and adrenogenital syndromes result from excess sex steroids.

Cushing's syndrome

There are four main causes of excess circulating glucocorticoids. The commonest is administration of exogenous glucocorticoids. The three remaining causes are

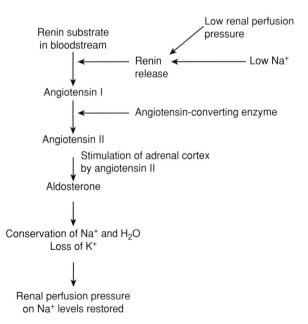

Fig. 21 The renin–angiotensin system.

related to the overproduction of endogenous glucocorticoids as follows:

- excess production of ACTH from the anterior pituitary
- over secretion of cortisol by an adrenal neoplasm
- secretion of ectopic ACTH.

Excess production of ACTH by the anterior pituitary—overproduction of ACTH by an adenoma results in bilateral adrenocortical hyperplasia and hypercortisolism. This form of Cushing's syndrome is known as Cushing's disease. Removal of the pituitary tumour is the treatment of choice. Removal of the adrenals is not advocated because this may result in the development of Nelson's syndrome, which is characterised by marked enlargement of the pituitary adenoma, high ACTH levels and skin pigmentation (due to the overproduction of melanocyte-stimulating hormone (MSH), which, as well as ACTH, is a cleavage product of POMC).

Over secretion of cortisol by an adrenal neoplasm (ACTH-independent Cushing's syndrome)—adrenal adenomas, carcinomas and cortical hyperplasia may cause autonomous production of cortisol independent of ACTH levels. If the neoplasm is unilateral, the uninvolved adrenal gland undergoes atrophy because of suppression of ACTH.

Production of ectopic ACTH—certain non-pituitary tumours, such as small cell carcinoma of the lung, may secrete ectopic ACTH, producing Cushing's syndrome.

Diagnosis of Cushing's syndrome—diagnosis depends on finding raised circulating or urinary cortisol levels. Establishing the cause of the Cushing syndrome depends on the performance of two tests (Fig. 22):

1. Levels of serum ACTH

   - low with adrenal neoplasms
   - high with pituitary adenomas and ectopic ACTH production.

2. Measurement of urinary cortisol excretion after administration of high-dose dexamethasone (a potent steroid). This is called the high-dose dexamethasone suppression test.

   - low with pituitary adenomas
   - high with ectopic ACTH production.

Primary hyperaldosteronism (Conn's syndrome)

In this condition, excess mineralocorticoid production is due to a lesion in the adrenal cortex. The commonest cause is an adenoma of the zona glomerulosa, although bilateral adrenal hyperplasia is sometimes responsible. High levels of aldosterone lead to excessive retention of sodium and water, excessive loss of potassium, and a metabolic alkalosis. The hypokalaemia may lead to muscular weakness, cardiac arrhythmias, paraesthesia and tetany. Diagnosis depends on finding raised levels of circulating aldosterone and low levels of renin (if the renin levels are raised, then the hyperaldosteronism is secondary to raised renin levels and is known as secondary hyperaldosteronism). Adrenal adenomas can be surgically excised, whereas adrenal hyperplasia can be managed medically.

Hypersecretion of the sex steroids

Disorders of sexual differentiation are known collectively as adrenogenital syndromes. There are two main causes of hypersecretion of sex steroids:

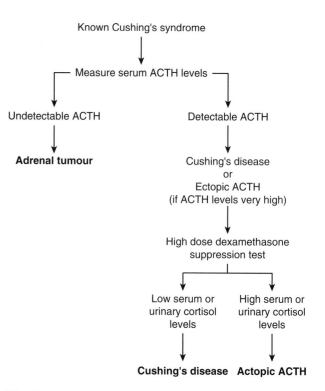

Fig. 22 Investigations to determine the cause of Cushing's syndrome.

Box 13 Clinical features of Cushing's syndrome

A wide range of clinical features, which together are termed Cushing's syndrome, result from over secretion of cortisol. These include the following:

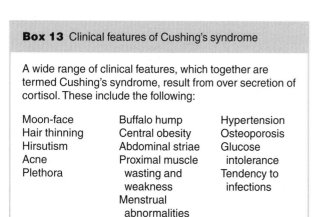

Moon-face	Buffalo hump	Hypertension
Hair thinning	Central obesity	Osteoporosis
Hirsutism	Abdominal striae	Glucose
Acne	Proximal muscle	intolerance
Plethora	wasting and	Tendency to
	weakness	infections
	Menstrual	
	abnormalities	

1. Adrenocortical neoplasms
2. A congenital enzyme deficiency in the pathways of steroid synthesis.

Adrenocortical neoplasm—adenomas or carcinomas of the adrenal cortex may secrete sex steroids (usually androgens). The effect of these androgens is to cause masculinisation in females and precocious puberty in pre-pubertal males.

Congenital enzyme defects—there is a small group of rare congenital disorders characterised by a deficiency, or total lack, of a particular enzyme involved in the synthesis of steroids. The commonest of these disorders is 21-hydroxylase deficiency. This enzyme is necessary for the synthesis of cortisol and aldosterone. Its absence leads to low levels of cortisol and consequent elevated levels of ACTH resulting in bilateral adrenocortical hyperplasia. The underproduction of mineralocorticoids is life threatening. Androgens are over secreted because they are synthesised before the metabolic block, resulting in masculinisation in females and precocious puberty in males.

Adrenocortical hypofunction (adrenocortical insufficiency)

Adrenocortical insufficiency may be due to primary adrenal disease (primary adrenocortical insufficiency) or secondary to decreased stimulation of the adrenals due to a deficiency in ACTH (secondary adrenocortical insufficiency). Insufficiency may be acute or chronic, depending on the speed of onset of the symptoms. The symptoms and signs of adrenocortical hypofunction are related to deficiencies of both mineralocorticoids and glucocorticoids.

Acute adrenocortical insufficiency

Acute primary adrenocortical insufficiency can occur in several circumstances:

- patients with chronic adrenocortical insufficiency may have an acute insufficiency crisis if an event occurs that requires an increased output of steroid hormones by the adrenals
- patients on long-term steroid treatment have suppressed adrenal glands, which are unable to respond adequately if an event occurs that requires an increased output of steroid hormones, or if the steroid treatment is withdrawn too rapidly
- destruction of the adrenal glands by haemorrhage, which can complicate bacterial (e.g. meningococcal) septicaemia (Waterhouse–Friderichsen syndrome), disseminated intravascular coagulation (DIC), and can occur in neonates following a prolonged or difficult delivery.

Affected patients develop hypovolaemic shock due to mineralocorticoid deficiency, and hypoglycaemia due to lack of glucocorticoids.

Primary chronic adrenocortical insufficiency (Addison's disease)

Addison's disease is caused by any destructive process in the adrenal cortex. Previously the commonest cause was TB of the adrenal cortex, but nowadays autoimmune destruction of the adrenal cortex is commoner. Affected patients may have autoimmune disease at other sites (e.g. diabetes, thyroiditis, pernicious anaemia). The resultant deficiency of mineralocorticoids and glucocorticoids leads to:

- weakness and fatigue
- anorexia, nausea, vomiting, and weight loss
- hypotension and dehydration
- hyperpigmentation of the skin (due to excess MSH) at pressure points and on sun exposed skin
- hyponatraemia, hyperkalaemia and hypoglycaemia.

Serum ACTH levels are high. The condition is potentially life threatening if steroids are not administered. Patients with Addison's disease may also develop an acute Addisonian crisis if exposed to any stress requiring an increased output of steroids by the adrenals (e.g. infection), with development of acute insufficiency.

To diagnose Addison's disease, ACTH stimulation tests (Synacthen tests) should be performed (Fig. 23).

- **The short Synacthen test**

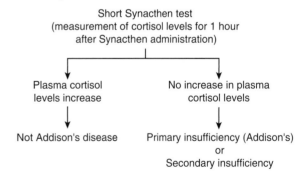

- **The long Synacthen test**

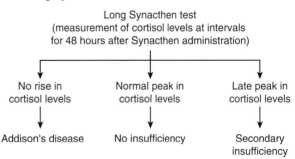

Fig. 23 Diagnosis of Addison's disease.

Synacthen is a synthetic ACTH analogue and in a normal individual, administration of Synacthen causes serum cortisol levels to rise. In the short Synacthen test, a rise in serum cortisol levels excludes Addison's disease. If there is no rise in cortisol levels, then the patient has either primary or secondary adrenocortical insufficiency, and the long Synacthen test should then be performed to establish the diagnosis.

Secondary adrenocortical insufficiency
This refers to the underproduction of adrenal steroids due to under secretion of ACTH by the pituitary. There are two main causes:

1. Primary lesions of the pituitary
2. Hypothalamic-pituitary-adrenal suppression as a result of long-term steroid therapy.

There is resultant deficiency of cortisol and sex steroids, but the aldosterone levels are normal, therefore the skin pigmentation and electrolyte disturbances typical of Addison's disease are not seen. Also, unlike the situation in Addison's disease, serum ACTH levels are low. Performance of the long Synacthen test will establish the diagnosis.

6.3 The endocrine pancreas

Learning objectives

You should:

*   Understand the structure of the pancreas and have a basic understanding of its function

*   Know the various hormones secreted by the pancreas

*   Have an understanding of the classification, pathogenesis, clinical features, and complications of diabetes mellitus, and have a basic knowledge of the theories of its pathogenesis

Structure and function

The pancreas consists of two separate functional units—the exocrine pancreas, which secretes digestive enzymes into the duodenum, and the endocrine pancreas, which secretes a number of different hormones.

The endocrine pancreas consists of ~ 1 million Islets of Langerhans, which are scattered throughout the gland. Each Islet is composed of a cluster of a number of different cell types, each cell type synthesising and secreting a different hormone (see Table 17).

Insulin and glucagon are the hormones responsible for maintaining blood sugar levels; insulin exerts a hypoglycaemic effect and glucagon exerts a hyperglycaemic effect.

The two main disorders of the Islet cells are diabetes mellitus and Islet cell tumours.

Diabetes mellitus

Diabetes mellitus is a condition characterised by an absolute or relative deficiency of insulin and/or insulin resistance, inducing hypoglycaemia.

Classification

There are two main types of diabetes mellitus:

Type I diabetes—juvenile onset diabetes; insulin-dependent diabetes (IDDM), which accounts for ~ 10% of all cases
Type II diabetes—adult onset diabetes; non-insulin-dependent diabetes (NIDDM), which accounts for 80–90% of all cases.

Gestational diabetes and maturity onset diabetes of the young (MODY) are rare causes of diabetes mellitus. MODY is due to a genetic defect in β-cell function.

Pathogenesis

Type I diabetes
Type I diabetes, which typically presents in childhood, is characterised by a complete lack of insulin. Insulin

Table 17 The cell types of the pancreas

Cell type	Hormone synthesised	Action of hormone
β (beta)	Insulin	Increases glucose entry into cells Promotes glycogen synthesis and prevents breakdown Promotes lipogenesis and prevents lipolysis
α (alpha)	Glucagon	Promotes glycogen breakdown Promotes gluconeogenesis
δ (delta)	Somatostatin	Inhibits secretion of insulin and glucagon
PP	Pancreatic polypeptide	Exerts a number of gastrointestinal effects
Enterochromaffin cells	Vasoactive intestinal polypeptide	Stimulates intestinal fluid secretion
D1	Serotonin	Potent vasodilator Increases intestinal motility

secretion is inadequate because of destruction of the β-cells in the Islets. Three separate but interrelated mechanisms appear to have a role in this destructive process:

1. Genetic susceptibility
2. Autoimmune reaction
3. Environmental event.

It has been postulated that genetic susceptibility predisposes certain individuals to the development of an autoimmune reaction against the β-cells of the Islets, and that this autoimmune reaction is triggered by an environmental event (e.g. viral infection, exposure to chemical toxins).

Type II diabetes

This type of diabetes usually presents in middle age. The precise pathogenic mechanism is unknown, but obesity and genetic factors are very important. Two mechanisms have been postulated:

1. Defective secretion of insulin by β-cells
2. Resistance of peripheral tissues to the effects of insulin.

Clinical features

Type I diabetes

The clinical features are related to increased gluconeogenesis and hyperglycaemia resulting from a lack of insulin.

Polyuria—due to glycosuria with osmotic diuresis.

Polydypsia—extracellular hyperosmolarity causes osmotic depletion of intracellular water and triggers osmoreceptors in the brain, with resultant severe thirst.

Polyphagia—breakdown of proteins and fats for gluconeogenesis causes an increased appetite.

Weight loss and weakness—despite increased dietary intake, breakdown prevails over storage.

Severe insulin deficiency may lead to diabetic ketoacidosis—lipolysis results in elevated free fatty acids, which are oxidised to produce ketone bodies in the liver. The rate of formation of ketone bodies exceeds the rate at which they are utilised, resulting in ketonuria and ketonaemia. If there is superimposed dehydration, metabolic ketoacidosis results. The condition is life threatening. Infection, which increases insulin requirements, often precedes development of diabetic ketoacidosis.

Type II diabetes

The diagnosis of Type II diabetes is usually made after routine serum or urine testing in an asymptomatic patient. The metabolic derangements are much less severe than in Type I diabetes, and metabolic ketoacidosis does not occur. Instead, patients in the decompensated state develop hyperosmolar non-ketotic coma, which results from severe dehydration due to insufficient water intake in the face of polyuria.

Other clinical features of Types I and II diabetes are related to the complications of longstanding diabetes.

Complications of diabetes mellitus

Although the two major types of diabetes have different pathogeneses and clinical presentations, the long-term systemic complications are the same and are the major causes of morbidity and mortality in these patients.

Vascular system

Atherosclerosis—patients suffer severe accelerated atherosclerosis in the aorta and large- and medium-sized arteries. Myocardial infarction, stroke, and gangrene of the lower limbs are responsible for ~ 80% of adult diabetic deaths.

Hyaline arteriolosclerosis—hyaline thickening of the wall of arterioles with narrowing of the lumen.

Diabetic microangiopathy—this is characterised by diffuse thickening of the capillary vascular basement membranes. Affected vessels are more leaky to plasma proteins. The change is most evident in the capillaries of the retina and kidney, and may account for some of the changes seen in the peripheral nerves.

Diabetic nephropathy

Glomerular changes—includes diffuse basement membrane thickening, nodular expansion of mesangial regions and exudative lesions.

Vascular changes—renal atherosclerosis and arteriolosclerosis.

Parenchymal changes—pyelonephritis with increased propensity to develop necrotising papillitis.

Diabetic retinopathy

Diabetic retinopathy can be non-proliferative (background) or proliferative. The non-proliferative changes are:

- thickening of the capillary basement membrane (microangiopathy) with development of microanurysms (dots)
- retinal haemorrhages (blots)
- retinal oedema and exudates (cotton wool spots)
- venous dilatation.

The proliferative changes are neovascularisation and fibrosis, which may lead to retinal detachment and blindness.

Diabetic neuropathy

Neuropathies seen include symmetric peripheral neuropathy, affecting both motor and sensory nerves, and autonomic neuropathy, which may cause impotence, and bladder and bowel dysfunction.

Skin complications
Include necrobiosis lipoidica diabeticorum and granuloma annulare.

Pregnancy
Pregnant diabetics are at a higher risk of developing pre-eclampsia, and tend to have large babies.

Islet tumours

These tumours are quite rare, and they can arise from any of the cell types present in the Islets. The tumours become manifest through hypersecretion of the hormone produced by the cell type from which the tumour is derived. Islet tumours may pursue a benign or malignant course. The various types are as follows:

- insulinoma (the commonest tumour; induces hypoglycaemia)
- glucagonoma (induces diabetes)
- gastrinoma (hypersecretes gastrin, which leads to hypersecretion of gastric acid. The resultant widespread peptic ulceration is known as Zollinger–Ellison syndrome)
- VIPomas (cause watery diarrhoea)
- somatostatinomas.

6.4 The thyroid gland

Learning objectives

You should:

- Know the structure and function of the thyroid gland
- Know the ways in which thyroid disorders present
- Know the major causes of hypo- and hyperthyroidism
- Know the causes of a goitre
- Know the causes of a solitary nodule in the thyroid
- Understand the classification and behaviour of thyroid carcinoma

Structure and function

The thyroid gland develops from an evagination at the root of the tongue (the foramen caecum), which grows downwards anterior to the trachea to reach its final position in front of the thyroid cartilage. During its descent, the thyroid gland is attached to the root of the tongue by means of a thyroglossal duct, which eventually undergoes atrophy. Persistence of this duct is the basis of thyroglossal cysts.

The adult thyroid gland comprises two lobes connected by an isthmus and consists of follicles lined by cuboidal epithelial cells and filled with colloid. The main function of these epithelial cells is to synthesise and secrete the two thyroid hormones—T4 (thyroxine) and T3. The secretion of T4 and T3 is under negative feedback control by TSH, which is secreted by the anterior pituitary. Scattered throughout the thyroid are C-cells, which synthesise and secrete the hormone calcitonin, which is involved in the regulation of body calcium levels.

Disorders of the thyroid manifest in four main ways:

1. Hypofunction (hypothyroidism)
2. Hyperfunction (hyperthyroidism)
3. Enlargement of the gland (goitre)
4. Solitary masses.

These groups are not mutually exclusive. For example, goitres can be associated with either hyperfunction or hypofunction of the thyroid gland, and hyperthyroidism may be associated with a goitre.

Hyperthyroidism (thyrotoxicosis)

Excess circulating T4 and T3 induces a hypermetabolic state, the resulting clinical syndrome being known as thyrotoxicosis.

Aetiology

The three commonest causes of thyrotoxicosis are as follows:

1. Graves' disease (85%)
2. Functioning adenoma
3. Toxic nodular goitre.

Graves' disease (Graves' thyroiditis)
This condition typically affects young women who present with the clinical features of thyrotoxicosis and mild goitre. If the patient develops proptosis (protrusion of the eyes) or pretibial myxoedema, the diagnosis of Graves' disease is almost certain since these changes are not seen in thyrotoxicosis due to other causes. Graves' thyroiditis is an 'organ-specific' autoimmune disease; autoantibodies bind to the TSH receptor on thyroid epithelial cells and mimic the stimulatory action of TSH. Histologically, there is an increase in the number of cells lining the follicles and a reduction in the amount of stored colloid.

Functioning adenoma
Very rarely, functioning thyroid adenomas have enough secretory activity to induce thyrotoxicosis. Such adenomas may also present as solitary thyroid masses.

Toxic nodular goitre

Rarely, one or more nodules in a multinodular goitre may develop hypersecretory activity, resulting in thyrotoxicosis.

Clinical features of thyrotoxicosis

The systemic features of thyrotoxicosis are as follows:

- eye changes (exophthalmos, lid lag, lid retraction)
- hair loss, weight loss
- anxiety, tremor, diarrhoea, warm moist hands
- cardiac manifestations (tachycardia, palpitations, atrial fibrillation)
- pretibial myxoedema (accumulation of mucopolysaccharides in the skin)
- menorrhagia, osteoporosis
- proximal myopathy.

Exophthalmos and pretibial myxoedema occur only in thyrotoxicosis due to Graves' disease.

Hypothyroidism

Insufficient circulating T4 and T3 leads to a hypometabolic state resulting in the clinical syndrome known as hypothyroidism. If hypothyroidism occurs during infancy, it results in a condition known as cretinism, in which mental and physical development is impaired. This condition is now very rare. If hypothyroidism occurs in older children or adults it results in a condition known as myxoedema, in which the skin appears oedematous and doughy due to the accumulation of mucopolysaccharides in the dermis.

Aetiology

There are many causes of hypothyroidism, but the commonest cause in adults is Hashimoto's thyroiditis. Most of the remaining cases of hypothyroidism are either radiation, surgery, or drug-induced.

Hashimoto's thyroiditis

Like Graves' disease, this condition is an 'organ-specific' autoimmune disease. Antibodies directed against thyroid tissue and thyroglobulin have been detected in patients with this condition. Hashimoto's thyroiditis may present in a number of ways:

- with **goitre**, which after time recedes due to atrophy and fibrosis of the gland as a result of autoimmune destruction
- with **hypothyroidism**
- with **thyrotoxicosis**. In the early stages of the disease, damage to the thyroid follicles may lead to a transient rise in thyroid hormone levels.

Histologically, the gland is infiltrated by lymphocytes and plasma cells. There are lymphoid aggregates, often with germinal centres. The thyroid epithelial cells become eosinophilic and granular, at which time they are termed oncocytes. In advanced cases, the gland is shrunken and fibrotic.

Clinical features of hypothyroidism

The clinical features are as follows:

- myxoedematous face
- loss of the outer third of the eyebrows
- dry hair
- hoarse voice
- slowed physical and mental activity, lethargy, weight gain
- psychosis
- cold intolerance
- constipation, muscle weakness, carpal tunnel syndrome, menstrual irregularities.

Goitre

The term goitre denotes enlargement of the thyroid gland. There are two main causes:

1. Simple and multinodular goitre
2. Inflammation of the thyroid (thyroiditis).

Simple and multinodular goitre

Simple goitres are characterised by diffuse hypertrophy and hyperplasia of the thyroid gland, without the production of nodularity. Nearly all long-standing simple goitres develop into multinodular goitres, where tracts of fibrosis separate hyperplastic areas, producing nodularity.

Simple goitres are thought to arise from over stimulation of the thyroid tissue by excess TSH. The over secretion of TSH is due to a deficiency of the thyroid hormones. The compensatory rise in TSH levels usually renders the individual euthyroid, although hypothyroidism may occur. Goitres can arise in four main settings:

1. Endemic goitres due to iodine deficiency. These are usually localised to geographic areas where the soil contains little iodine (e.g. the Derbyshire hills, some mountainous areas). Iodine is necessary for the synthesis of the thyroid hormones
2. Ingestion of certain foodstuffs. In individuals whose iodine uptake in suboptimal, ingestion of foodstuffs such as cabbage and turnips may produce a goitre
3. Rare inherited defects in thyroid hormone synthesis
4. Drug induced goitres, e.g. amiodarone, lithium.

Thyroiditis

Thyroiditis is a rare cause of goitre. There are four main forms of thyroiditis:

1. Hashimoto's thyroiditis (discussed above)
2. Subacute granulomatous (giant cell or de Quervain's) thyroiditis
3. Riedel's thyroiditis
4. Acute bacterial thyroiditis.

Subacute granulomatous thyroiditis

As its name implies, the thyroid in this condition is infiltrated by multinucleate giant cells admixed with other inflammatory cells. The cause of the condition is uncertain. Patients usually present with an abrupt onset of thyroid swelling and tenderness on palpation. There may be a fever. The condition is self-limiting.

Riedel's thyroiditis

This condition is exceptionally rare. It is characterised by replacement of the thyroid by fibrous tissue, often with involvement of adjacent tissues. The aetiology is unknown. Patients present with an enlarged thyroid, which is hard and immobile on palpation thereby mimicking carcinoma. The condition may be associated with retroperitoneal fibrosis.

Acute bacterial thyroiditis

Acute inflammation of the thyroid can result from direct bacterial spread from adjacent tissues or by blood-borne spread. Patients present with thyroid pain, tenderness and enlargement. There may be systemic features of infection. The condition usually resolves with antibiotic treatment.

Solitary masses

The differential diagnoses of solitary thyroid masses are as follows:

- one dominant nodule in a multinodular goitre
- thyroid cysts
- asymmetric enlargement due to non-neoplastic diseases (e.g. Hashimoto's thyroiditis)
- thyroid neoplasm.

Thyroid neoplasms

Thyroid neoplasms can be benign or malignant. Most thyroid tumours are non-functioning and therefore appear 'cold' on scintigraphy (i.e. they do not take up radioactive iodine). However, a minority are functioning, appearing 'warm' or 'hot' on scintigraphy and possibly causing thyrotoxicosis.

Benign

Almost all benign tumours of the thyroid gland are follicular adenomas. These tumours are well encapsulated and have an expansile growth pattern, compressing the adjacent normal thyroid tissue. These features differentiate a follicular adenoma from a dominant nodule in a multinodular goitre. Histologically, they may show a variety of appearances, the most common being a microfollicular architecture comprising multiple closely packed follicles with little colloid.

Malignant

Carcinoma of the thyroid is uncommon, and together with the fact that these tumours often have a good prognosis, they are responsible for less than 1% of all cancer deaths. Thyroid carcinoma is 2–3 times more common in females than males. The four main types of thyroid carcinoma are as follows:

- papillary carcinoma (75%)
- follicular carcinoma (10–20%)
- anaplastic carcinoma (rare)
- medullary carcinoma (5%).

Papillary carcinoma—typically occurs in women in the 3rd or 4th decade. The tumours are unencapsulated, infiltrative, and may be multifocal. Histologically, papillary carcinomas can exhibit a wide range of appearances. The diagnosis depends on the presence of certain cytological features:

- large hypochromatic nuclei termed 'Orphan Annie' nuclei
- nuclear grooves
- eosinophilic cytoplasmic inclusions
- psammoma bodies (calcified glycoprotein bodies).

Cervical lymph node metastases are present in as many as 50% of cases at presentation. However, because these tumours often pursue an indolent course, the overall prognosis is excellent.

Follicular carcinoma—occurs in older age groups. Histologically, they are solitary encapsulated tumours most commonly consisting of closely packed small follicles, and may therefore be difficult to distinguish from follicular adenomas. Invasion of the capsule or vascular invasion indicate a diagnosis of malignancy. Metastatic spread has occurred in 15% of cases at presentation, most commonly involving the lung or bones. The prognosis for these tumours is poorer than for papillary carcinomas.

Anaplastic carcinoma—tends to occur in elderly individuals. The tumours are poorly differentiated histologically, have a rapid growth rate, and metastasise widely. The prognosis is very poor.

Medullary carcinomas—are derived from the C-cells within the thyroid, and are therefore neuroendocrine tumours. Most secrete calcitonin but hyper-secretion of this hormone does not usually produce any clinical effects. Rarely, the tumour may secrete other hormones (e.g. ACTH, or 5-HT). Histologically, the tumour consists of nests or sheets of tumour cells in a characteristic amyloid stroma. These tumours may pursue an indolent or aggressive course. Most medullary carcinomas are sporadic, but around 20% are hereditary and occur as part of one of the multiple endocrine neoplasia (MEN) syndromes.

6.5 Parathyroid glands

Learning objectives

You should:

- Know the structure and function of the parathyroid glands

- Know the various subtypes of hyperparathyroidism, and their causes

- Know about hypoparathyroidism

Structure and function

Most individuals have four parathyroid glands. In the adult, the upper two glands almost always lie close to the upper posterior aspect of the thyroid gland, but the lower two may be found anywhere between the lower posterior aspect of the thyroid gland and the mediastinum. The glands are composed predominantly of chief cells, which secrete parathyroid hormone (PTH). The actions of PTH are as follows:

- mobilises calcium from bone
- increases renal tubular resorption of calcium
- promotes the production of 1,25-dihydroxyvitamin D_1 (the active form of vitamin D) in the kidney
- enhances phosphate excretion by the kidney.

Overall, serum calcium levels are controlled by the actions of three hormones—PTH, calcitonin, and vitamin D. PTH and vitamin D have a hypercalcaemic effect, and calcitonin has a hypocalcaemic effect.

The most important disorders of the parathyroids are hyperparathyroidism, hypoparathyroidism and tumours.

Hyperparathyroidism

Hyperparathyroidism can be divided into primary, secondary and tertiary types:

Primary—hypersecretion of PTH by a parathyroid lesion
Secondary—a physiological increase in PTH in response to hypocalcaemia
Tertiary—development of a hypersecretory parathyroid adenoma in an individual with longstanding secondary hyperparathyroidism.

Primary hyperparathyroidism

This condition can be caused by the following:

- an adenoma in one of the parathyroid glands (75–80%)
- hyperplasia of all of the parathyroid glands (10–15%)
- parathyroid carcinoma (< 5%).

The clinical features, with the exception of the bone changes, are due to hypercalcaemia, and are commonly summed up by the saying 'bones, stones, abdominal groans and psychic moans'.

Bone
- osteitis fibrosa cystica (Brown tumour), due to excess PTH.
Renal
- formation of calcium-containing renal stones
- nephrocalcinosis.
Gastrointestinal
- peptic ulcer
- pancreatitis
- vomiting
- abdominal pain.
Neuromuscular
- generalised weakness.
Psychiatric
- depression
- impaired memory
- emotional lability.

Secondary hyperparathyroidism (and renal osteodystrophy)

This most commonly arises in the setting of renal failure or vitamin D deficiency. In renal failure, there is loss of calcium and reduced synthesis of 1,25-dihydroxyvitamin D_1 leading to hypocalcaemia and secondary hyperparathyroidism, and there is retention of phosphate, which also induces secondary hyperparathyroidism. The result is hyperplasia of the parathyroid glands and skeletal changes comprising a mixture of osteitis fibrosa cystica (due to increased PTH-dependent osteoclastic resorption of bone) and osteomalacia (due to lack of vitamin D). The skeletal changes are referred to as renal osteodystrophy.

Hypoparathyroidism

The most common causes of hypoparathyroidism are:

- surgical removal or ablation of the parathyroid glands during thyroidectomy
- congenital absence of all of the parathyroid glands (di George syndrome)
- autoimmune destruction of the glands.

The clinical manifestations, which are due to hypocalcaemia, are:

Increased neuromuscular excitability—this is manifest by Chvostek's sign (tapping along the course of the facial nerve causes the facial muscles to twitch), Trousseau's sign (occlusion of the arteries in the forearm by inflating a blood pressure cuff induces carpal spasm), perioral paraesthesia, and, if severely hypocalcaemic, overt tetany.

Psychiatric disturbances—e.g. irritability, depression, or psychosis.

Cardiac conduction abnormalities—e.g. prolonged Q–T interval or heart block.

6.6 The multiple endocrine neoplasia (MEN) syndromes

This term refers to a group of rare inherited disorders, which are characterised by hyperplasia or tumours in several endocrine glands simultaneously. There are three MEN syndromes:

MEN I—characterised by parathyroid, pancreatic and pituitary involvement.
MEN II (or IIa)—characterised by phaeochromocytoma and medullary carcinoma, with or without parathyroid involvement.
MEN III (or IIb)—characterised by phaeochromocytoma, medullary carcinoma and mucocutaneous ganglioneuromas, with or without parathyroid hyperplasia or a marfanoid habitus.

Self-assessment: questions

Multiple choice questions

1. The following statements are correct:
   a. The anterior pituitary is derived from a downgrowth of the hypothalamus
   b. Pituitary adenomas always cause overproduction of one (or more) hormone
   c. Acromegaly is caused by overproduction of ACTH
   d. Anti-diuretic hormone is secreted from the posterior pituitary
   e. Anti-diuretic hormone may be inappropriately secreted in patients with bronchogenic carcinoma.

2. The following are associated with pituitary adenomas:
   a. Visual disturbances
   b. Headache
   c. Nausea and vomiting
   d. MEN I
   e. Sheehan's syndrome

3. The following statements are correct:
   a. Graves' disease is the most frequent cause of hyperthyroidism
   b. Graves' disease is caused by autoantibodies, which are directed against the TSH receptor
   c. Hashimoto's thyroiditis is associated with autoantibodies directed against the C-cells of the thyroid
   d. Simple and multinodular goitre are almost always associated with hyperthyroidism
   e. Ionising radiation is a major risk factor for the development of thyroid cancer.

4. The following statements are correct:
   a. Parathyroid hormone has a hypercalcaemic effect
   b. Primary hyperparathyroidism is induced by hypocalcaemia
   c. Renal failure is a common cause of secondary hyperparathyroidism
   d. Hypoparathyroidism may follow total thyroidectomy
   e. Primary hyperparathyroidism may be associated with MEN syndrome.

5. The following statements are correct:
   a. The adrenal medulla is part of the parasympathetic nervous system
   b. Phaeochromocytomas may cause secondary hypertension
   c. The most common cause of Cushing's syndrome is administration of exogenous glucocorticoids

   d. Addison's disease is associated with hyperkalaemia
   e. Secondary hyperaldosteronism may be seen in congestive cardiac failure.

6. The following statements regarding the endocrine pancreas are correct:
   a. The Islets of Langerhans are the functional unit of the endocrine pancreas
   b. Type I diabetes mellitus is more common than Type II diabetes mellitus
   c. Myocardial infarction is the most common cause of death in diabetics
   d. Diabetic microangiopathy is characterised by thickened vascular basement membranes, which renders the vessels less leaky to plasma proteins
   e. Diabetic retinopathy may cause blindness.

Case histories

Case history 1

A 40-year-old women presents to her GP with a lump in the right side of her neck. The lump has been increasing in size over the past two months. On examination, a hard nodule was felt in the right thyroid lobe and there was adjacent right-sided cervical lymphadenopathy.

1. What is the differential diagnosis of a thyroid nodule?
2. What features here are suggestive of carcinoma?
3. What investigations could be performed to help establish the diagnosis?

Case history 2

A 68-year-old diabetic, who is a frequent non-attender, attends an outpatient clinic for a routine check-up. She has been a diabetic for 16 years and requires insulin to control her diabetes. On questioning, she reveals that she is getting pain in her left calf muscles on walking. The pain comes on after a certain distance and is relieved by rest. She has also noticed some reduced visual acuity. On examination, she has an absent left dorsalis pedis pulse and the left posterior tibial and left popliteal pulses were present but weak. Routine ophthalmoscopy reveals background and proliferative retinopathy. Routine urinalysis shows moderate proteinuria.

1. What is the pathogenesis of this type of diabetes?
2. What is the cause of her leg symptoms?
3. What is proliferative retinopathy, and why is it important?
4. What are the possible causes of the proteinuria in this case?

Short note questions

Write short notes on:
1. The concept of negative feedback.
2. The major causes of Cushing's syndrome and the tests you might perform to establish the cause in any individual case.
3. Hyperparathyroidism.

Viva questions

1. What is a hormone?
2. What is Waterhouse–Friderichsen syndrome?
3. What is Graves' disease?

Self-assessment: answers

Multiple choice answers

1. a. **False.**
   b. **False.** Some adenomas are non-functioning.
   c. **False.**
   d. **True.**
   e. **True.**

2. a. **True.**
   b. **True.**
   c. **True.**
   d. **True.**
   e. **False.**

3. a. **True.**
   b. **True.**
   c. **False.**
   d. **False.**
   e. **True.**

4. a. **True.**
   b. **False.**
   c. **True.**
   d. **True.** The parathyroid glands lie close to the thyroid gland and may also be removed during surgery.
   e. **True.**

5. a. **False.** It is part of the sympathetic nervous system.
   b. **True.**
   c. **True.**
   d. **True.**
   e. **True.** In congestive cardiac failure, reduced renal perfusion causes increased renin secretion leading to secondary hyperaldosteronism.

6. a. **True.**
   b. **False.**
   c. **True.**
   d. **False.** Affected vessels are more leaky to plasma proteins.
   e. **True.**

Case history answers

Case history 1

1. The differential diagnosis of a thyroid nodule is a dominant nodule in a multinodular goitre, thyroid cyst, asymmetric enlargement due to non-neoplastic diseases and thyroid neoplasm.

2. The recent increase in the size and the presence of a hard nodule are both suggestive of carcinoma over a benign process. The presence of ipsilateral cervical lymphadenopathy suggests lymph node spread, which can be present at presentation of a thyroid carcinoma.

3. Thyroid function tests (TFTs) may be performed to establish thyroid status, which may aid diagnosis. An ultrasound scan will tell you if the mass is cystic or solid. Solid masses are more suspicious of carcinoma, but be aware that carcinoma can arise within cysts. A radioactive iodine scan will establish whether the mass is functioning ('hot' nodule) or non-functioning ('cold' nodule). Almost all thyroid carcinomas are non-functioning. Lastly, a fine-needle aspiration may be performed. This involves using a needle to aspirate the mass extracting cells, which can then be examined under the microscope for any features of malignancy.

Case history 2

1. The history indicates that this is Type II diabetes, because of the adult onset. Remember that some patients with Type II inject insulin to control their diabetes. The pathogenesis is poorly understood, but obesity and genetic factors are important.

2. Cramp-like pain in the calf muscles on walking, which comes on after a certain distance and is relieved by rest, are the classic symptoms of intermittent claudication and they indicate ischaemia of the limb. Diabetic patients are predisposed to accelerated atherosclerosis in all large- and medium-sized arteries. When the arteries supplying the limbs are affected, blood flow through them is restricted and cannot be significantly increased when demand is increased (e.g. during exercise). Hence, during exercise the limb becomes ischaemic leading to pain. The pain is then relieved by rest.

3. The proliferative changes of diabetic retinopathy are neovascularisation and fibrosis. Proliferative retinopathy is important because it can lead to retinal detachment and cause blindness.

4. The proteinuria may be due to:
   - a urinary tract infection (to which diabetic patients are predisposed)

- glomerular lesions associated with diabetic nephropathy (basement membrane thickening, expansion of mesangial regions and exudative lesions)
- glomerular damage secondary to chronic ischaemia caused by renal vascular lesions.

Short note answers

1. Negative feedback is a common means of controlling an endocrine gland's production of a hormone. As the plasma concentration of the hormone (or a substance that it regulates) rises, it increasingly inhibits its own production. An example is the hypothalamic–pituitary–thyroid axis. The initial stimulus for the production of thyroxine in the thyroid gland is secretion of thyrotrophin-releasing hormone (TRH) from the hypothalamus. The trigger for TRH secretion is a reduction in the circulating levels of thyroxine. TRH stimulates the release of thyroid-stimulating hormone (TSH) from the anterior pituitary, which in turn stimulates thyroid follicular cells to produce thyroxine. As the levels of thyroxine in the blood rise, the stimulus for TRH secretion is reduced leading to less thyroxine production by the thyroid. Another example is the β-cells of the pancreas, which secrete insulin, the actions of which remove glucose from the blood. The stimulus for insulin secretion is a rise in blood glucose levels. As the blood sugar levels drop as a consequence of the actions of insulin, the stimulus is reduced and less insulin is released.

2. Cushing's syndrome is due to excess glucocorticoids and there are a number of situations in which this can arise. The main causes are administration of exogenous glucocorticoids (e.g. people on long-term steroid treatment for chronic inflammatory conditions), overproduction of ACTH from the anterior pituitary, overproduction of cortisol by an adrenal neoplasm, and secretion of ectopic ACTH (usually by a tumour). If exogenous administration of steroids is the cause, this can usually be elicited from the drug history. To distinguish between the other three causes, a serum ACTH should be performed followed by a high-dose dexamethasone test if necessary.

3. Perhaps start by describing the function of the parathyroid glands. They are the sites of production of parathyroid hormone, which is involved in the regulation of serum calcium levels. Hyperparathyroidism denotes overproduction of parathyroid hormone, and it is divided into primary, secondary and tertiary types. Be able to describe each of these. A brief account of the consequences of hyperparathyroidism is also needed—remember 'bones, stones, abdominal groans and psychic moans'.

Viva answers

1. Hormones are substances that are synthesised and secreted by endocrine glands. Hormones exert their effects at distant sites that can be accessed only by the bloodstream.

2. This is a catastrophic condition characterised by an overwhelming bacterial infection (classically *Neisseria meningitidis* septicaemia) associated with shock, disseminated intravascular coagulation, and rapidly progressive adrenocortical deficiency with massive bilateral adrenal haemorrhages. The condition is rapidly fatal if appropriate treatment is not given immediately.

3. Graves' disease is the most common cause of hyperthyroidism. It is an 'organ specific' autoimmune disease produced by autoantibodies to the TSH receptor on thyroid follicular cells. Binding of the autoantibody stimulates the receptor and leads to increased synthesis and secretion of thyroxine. This account of the pathogenesis should be followed by a description of the clinical findings, remembering to include the presence of goitre, and that pre-tibial myxoedema and proptosis are seen only in hyperthyroidism due to Graves' disease.

7 Female breast

Overview

The female breast is a complex glandular structure, which is extremely sensitive to hormonal influences and can be affected by a number of pathological processes. Breast cancer is one of the most dreaded diseases of women and is the second most common cause of cancer death in women. Hence, malignant and premalignant breast conditions deserve considerable attention. Benign breast conditions, such as inflammatory and fibrocystic changes, are extremely common and frequently receive medical attention because they may mimic breast cancer in their clinical presentation. For these reasons, awareness of benign breast diseases is also important. The male breast is a rudimentary structure, and pathological conditions are rare.

7.1 The normal female breast

Learning objectives

You should:

- Understand the structure and function of the female breast
- Understand hormonal influences on breast tissue

Structure and function

The function of the female breast is to produce and express milk. The functional unit of the breast is called a lobule (Fig. 24), and there are numerous lobules within each breast. A lobule consists of a variable number of acini (glands) lined by secretory epithelium. The acini connect to, and drain into, a terminal duct. Each terminal duct and its acini are together referred to as the terminal duct lobular unit. The terminal ducts drain via a series of larger ducts into the lactiferous ducts and sinuses. The lactiferous ducts open onto the skin surface at the nipple. The nipple and areola are covered by stratified squamous epithelium, and the areolar skin is pigmented. Areolar glands of Montgomery produce secretions to lubricate the nipple during lactation.

The ducts and acini are lined by two cell types—an inner layer of secretory epithelium and an outer layer of myoepithelial cells. Surrounding and supporting the ducts and acini is breast stroma, which consists of loose connective tissue.

Hormonal influences on the breast

Breast tissue is sensitive to many different hormones. The breast undergoes minor changes with the menstrual cycle, more significant changes during pregnancy and lactation, and undergoes involution when hormone stimulation is withdrawn (menopausal and post-menopausal period)

Changes with the menstrual cycle

After ovulation, there is epithelial proliferation and an increase in the number of acini, and the breast stroma becomes oedematous. These changes occur under the influence of oestrogen and rising levels of progesterone. With menstruation, there is a drop in the levels of these sex steroids with consequent apoptosis of epithelial cells and disappearance of the stromal oedema. The breast becomes quiescent again until the next ovulation.

Pregnancy and lactation

A number of hormones, including oestrogen, progesterone, prolactin and growth hormone, are important in the development of the breast during pregnancy. During pregnancy, there is a marked increase in the number of acini and lobules within the breast at the expense of the stroma. The epithelial cells begin to synthesise milk, which is stored in secretory vacuoles in the cell

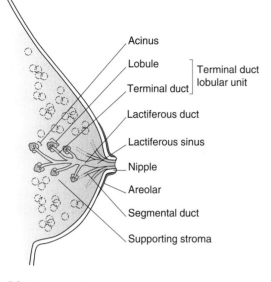

Acinus
Lobule
Terminal duct
Terminal duct lobular unit
Lactiferous duct
Lactiferous sinus
Nipple
Areolar
Segmental duct
Supporting stroma

Fig. 24 Diagrammatic representation of the structure of the adult female breast.

cytoplasm. With delivery of the baby, the levels of oestrogen and progesterone fall, and the activity of prolactin causes the secretion of milk (lactation).

When breast-feeding ceases, the breast tissue regresses back towards the prepregnancy state.

Involution

With increasing age and the reduction in the levels of circulating sex steroids, the ducts and acini begin to atrophy and the amount of breast stroma decreases. In the very elderly, the acini may be completely lost, leaving only breast ducts in a little stroma.

7.2 Benign breast conditions

Learning objectives

You should:

- Be aware of the ways that benign breast conditions can present

- Know the common inflammatory conditions of the breast

- Understand fibrocystic change

- Know the common benign breast tumours

- Know the risk of subsequent breast cancer in women with diagnosed benign breast disease

Inflammations
Acute mastitis

Acute mastitis is the most common inflammatory disorder of the breast, and is usually confined to the lactation period. During breast-feeding, the nipple can develop fissures and cracks. Via these cracks, bacteria (usually *Staphylococcus aureus*) gain access to the breast tissue. The infection is usually confined to one segment of the breast, and is manifest by oedema and erythema of the overlying skin.

If severe and untreated, the acute inflammation may progress to abscess formation.

Mammary duct ectasia

This term is used to refer to dilatation of the breast ducts. The ducts become filled with inspissated breast secretions and there is associated inflammation and fibrosis. If there is an unusually heavy infiltrate of plasma cells, the term 'plasma cell mastitis' is sometimes applied. The aetiology of mammary duct ectasia is unknown. Affected women can present with a palpable mass, skin retraction or nipple discharge, which can occasionally be blood-stained. The lesion is of clinical significance because it can be mistaken for carcinoma clinically, grossly and mammographically.

Fat necrosis

This lesion is usually related to previous trauma to the breast, although a history of trauma may not always be obtained. Histologically, there is an initial focus of necrotic fat cells and acute inflammation, which then becomes heavily infiltrated by macrophages that engulf the debris and hence develop a lipid-laden 'foamy' appearance. With healing, the focus often becomes replaced by fibrous tissue and there may be dystrophic calcification. Affected women present with a palpable breast lump or nipple retraction, raising the suspicion of carcinoma. If there is calcium deposition, lesions may also mimic carcinoma mammographically.

Granulomatous mastitis

This condition is rare. Causes include infections (e.g. TB, deep-seated fungal infections) and systemic disorders (e.g. Wegener's granulomatosis, sarcoid).

Fibrocystic changes

This term is used to refer to a wide range of morphological changes to the breast. Fibrocystic change is the commonest disorder of the breast. The exact pathogenesis remains obscure but hormonal imbalances are thought to be important. Affected women are usually aged between 30 and 55 with a marked decrease in incidence after the menopause. The clinical features vary depending on the underlying morphological changes but, in general, fibrocystic change can mimic carcinoma clinically by producing palpable lumps, nipple discharge and mammographic densities. Evidence indicates that some of these conditions are associated with an increased risk of developing carcinoma of the breast (see later).

The morphological subtypes of fibrocystic disease are listed below:

- adenosis
- cysts
- apocrine metaplasia
- fibrosis
- epithelial hyperplasia
- sclerosing adenosis
- radial scars and complex sclerosing lesions.

An individual may show one, or some, or a combination of all of these changes.

Adenosis

This term denotes an increase in the number of acini within a lobule. The gland lumina in adenosis occasionally contain calcium deposits.

Cysts

This term refers to cystic dilatation of acini or terminal ducts. Some cysts may reach a very large size (up to 2–3 cm across). The secretions within cysts may calcify.

Apocrine metaplasia

This term refers to cysts that are lined by epithelium that resembles that of apocrine sweat glands.

Fibrosis

This is probably a secondary event to rupture of cysts and it may proceed to hyalinisation.

Sclerosing adenosis

In this condition, there is an increased number of acini and increased intralobular fibrosis. The fibrosis causes marked distortion of the acini. The lesion can present as a mammographic density or a palpable mass, therefore mimicking carcinoma. Sclerosing adenosis may be mistaken for carcinoma histologically also. Radial scars and complex sclerosing lesions are morphological variants of sclerosing adenosis, and are characterised by:

- a stellate shape
- a central area of fibrosis and elastosis
- a variable degree of adenosis and distortion of acini.

Radial scar is the term reserved for lesions less than 10 mm in diameter, whereas larger lesions are called complex sclerosing lesions. They can mimic carcinoma clinically, mammographically and histologically.

Epithelial hyperplasia

Epithelial hyperplasia is defined as an increase in the number of layers of cells lining the acini or ducts, often resulting in the obliteration of their lumen. Epithelial hyperplasia is classified as being either of usual type or atypical.

Usual-type epithelial hyperplasia (mild, moderate, florid)

In this type, the proliferating epithelial cells show no atypical features. Epithelial hyperplasia is considered *mild* if the epithelium is three to four cell layers thick, *moderate* if the epithelium is more than five layers thick, and *florid* if the lumina are nearly or completely filled by epithelium.

Atypical hyperplasia

In this type, the epithelial proliferations display various degrees of cellular and architectural atypia.

There are two subtypes:

1. Atypical ductal hyperplasia
2. Atypical lobular hyperplasia.

Benign breast tumours

Fibroadenomas

Fibroadenomas are the most common benign tumour of the breast. The tumours are composed of both glandular and stromal tissue. These benign neoplasms can occur at any age, but they are most commonly seen in women under 35 years of age. Fibroadenomas are usually solitary, although in some women they may be multiple and bilateral. In younger women they present as palpable lumps (often freely mobile), and in older women they may present as mammographic densities. They can therefore mimic carcinoma clinically.

Pathology

Fibroadenomas grow within the breast as sharply circumscribed soft to firm nodules, and are usually easily enucleated at surgery. They vary in size from less than 1 cm to around 4 cm in diameter, although rarely they can reach up to 15 cm in diameter (juvenile fibroadenoma/giant fibroadenoma—see below). The cut surface is grey-white and sometimes glistening, and contains slit-like spaces. In older women, fibroadenomas can become calcified. Histologically, these tumours are well circumscribed nodules consisting of loose cellular stroma associated with breast ducts that, in longitudinal section, appear as compressed and elongated clefts.

The vast majority of fibroadenomas are benign. However, those containing cysts, sclerosing adenosis, epithelial calcification or papillary apocrine change (so-called *complex fibroadenomas*) are associated with an increased risk of developing breast cancer.

Juvenile fibroadenoma/giant fibroadenoma—These terms are interchangeable and are used to refer to a reasonably distinct type of fibroadenoma that tends to occur in adolescents (often black girls) and reaches a large size (over 10 cm in diameter). Histologically, they also tend to be rather hypercellular, but cellular atypia is not a feature.

Duct papillomas

Duct papillomas are uncommon and are usually seen in middle-aged women. They appear as outgrowths projecting into the duct lumen and consist of a fibrovascular core covered by benign breast duct epithelium. There are two types of duct papilloma:

1. **Large duct papillomas** arise within the large central breast ducts and are usually solitary. Presentation is usually with a bloodstained nipple discharge, although some present as palpable lumps or mammographic densities. They are associated with an increased risk of developing carcinoma.
2. **Small duct papillomas** arise in the smaller peripheral ducts, are often asymptomatic, and may be multiple. Multiple small duct papillomas are seen in younger patients, and are associated with an increased risk of developing breast cancer.

Adenomas

Adenomas of the breast are rare. There are three main subtypes:

1. **Tubular adenomas** are sharply circumscribed nodules composed of closely packed ductal structures with little intervening stroma.
2. **Lactating adenomas** are adenomas that arise during pregnancy and lactation.
3. **Nipple adenomas** present as nodules just under the nipple. Microscopically, they consist of

proliferating ductal structures and show a variety of growth patterns. The overlying skin may become ulcerated mimicking Paget's disease of the nipple (see below).

Benign connective tissue tumours

Any type of benign connective tissue tumour can occur in the breast, e.g. lipoma, haemangioma, leiomyoma.

The risk of invasive breast carcinoma in women with benign breast disease

Several large case-control studies have now clarified the association between benign breast abnormalities and breast cancer risk.

No increased risk:

- mastitis
- duct ectasia
- ordinary cysts
- apocrine metaplasia
- adenosis
- fibrosis
- mild usual type epithelial hyperplasia without atypia
- fibroadenoma without complex features.

Slightly increased risk (1.5–3 times):

- moderate or florid usual type epithelial hyperplasia without atypia
- radial scars/complex sclerosing lesions
- fibroadenoma with complex features
- duct papilloma.

Moderately increased risk (4–5 times):

- atypical ductal hyperplasia
- atypical lobular hyperplasia.

A family history of breast cancer increases the risk in all categories.

Some authors advocate a new classification system for benign breast disease, which reflects the above observations. Three main categories of disease are defined in this system:

1. **Non-proliferative diseases**—this category includes the entities that are associated with no increased risk of developing breast cancer
2. **Proliferative diseases without atypia**—this category includes entities that are associated with a slightly increased risk of developing breast cancer
3. **Proliferative diseases with atypia**—this category includes atypical hyperplasia.

7.3 Breast cancer

Learning objectives

You should:

- Know the risk factors for the development of breast cancer
- Know the classification of breast cancer
- Understand the behaviour and spread of breast cancer
- Know the prognostic indicators

Breast cancer is a major cause of cancer morbidity. One woman in eight will develop breast cancer in her lifetime and, of these, a third will die from the disease.

Risk factors

The cause of breast cancer is still uncertain, but a number of factors that increase the risk of developing breast cancer have been identified.

Genetic predisposition

It has long been known that there is a familial aggregation of breast cancer, and at least four genes that convey increasing susceptibility to breast cancer have been identified. These are:

- BRCA1
- BRCA2
- p53
- The ATM gene (responsible for ataxia telangiectasia).

Genetic predisposition is responsible for only 5–10% of breast cancer cases.

Age

Breast cancer is uncommon before the age of 25 years, but the incidence increases steeply with age, doubling about every 10 years until the menopause. The rise slows in the postmenopausal period.

Factors related to menses

Early age at menarche and late age at menopause are associated with an increased risk of breast cancer. These findings indicate that hormones may have an important role in the development of carcinoma of the breast.

Factors related to pregnancy

An early age at first pregnancy is associated with a decreased risk of developing breast cancer.

Demographic influences

The incidence of breast cancer in western countries is around five times higher than that in far eastern countries. Also, the rate of breast cancer is higher in women of high socioeconomic status. These differences are thought to be related to differing reproductive patterns, such as age at first birth, age at menarche and age at menopause.

Radiation

Exposure to ionising radiation increases the risk of breast cancer. The greatest risk has been found among women exposed to radiation around the menarche.

Benign breast disease

The risk of breast cancer varies according to the type of benign breast disease (see above).

Previous breast cancer

Women with breast cancer have an increased risk of developing a new primary lesion in the contralateral breast or the conserved ipsilateral breast.

Dubious risk factors

The role of oral contraceptives, hormone replacement therapy, obesity, diet and alcohol as risk factors for the development of breast cancer remains controversial and unresolved.

Distribution

Most cancers (50%) arise in the upper outer quadrant of the breast, 10% occur in each of the remaining three quadrants, and 20% occur in the central or subareolar region. Bilaterality of breast cancer occurs in 4% of cases.

Classification

Nearly all breast cancers are adenocarcinomas. Breast cancer is traditionally divided into non-invasive (in situ) carcinoma and invasive carcinoma.

Non-invasive (in situ) carcinoma

This term is used to refer to the situation where the malignant cells are confined to the ducts or acini, with no evidence of invasion by the tumour cells through the basement membrane and into the breast stroma. Women with these lesions have a markedly increased risk (8–10 times) of developing breast cancer. There are two types of non-invasive carcinoma:

1. Ductal carcinoma in situ (DCIS)
2. Lobular carcinoma in situ (LCIS).

Ductal carcinoma in situ
In this type of non-invasive carcinoma, the breast ducts contain a malignant population of cells. DCIS is usually unilateral. Bilateral disease is uncommon. Presentation can be as a nipple discharge or Paget's disease of the nipple (see later), although DCIS may present as mammographic densities because the involved ducts often contain calcifications. Around half of all mammographically detected cancers subsequently turn out to be DCIS.

Pathology—histologically, DCIS can be divided into five architectural subtypes:

1. **Comedocarcinoma**—characterised by the presence of solid sheets of high-grade malignant cells within the ducts with central necrosis. The necrosis commonly calcifies and this calcification is detected on mammography.
2. **Solid**—denotes the presence of solid sheets of malignant cells within the ducts.
3. **Cribriform**—this type is characterised by numerous gland-like structures within the sheets of malignant cells within ducts.
4. **Papillary**.
5. **Micropapillary**.

Risk of subsequent invasive cancer—evidence now indicates that many cases of low-grade DCIS and most cases of high-grade DCIS may progress to invasive carcinoma.

Lobular carcinoma in situ
In this type of non-invasive carcinoma, the malignant cells are found in the acini, although the changes seen may extend into the ducts. LCIS is often multifocal within one breast and frequently bilateral. The lesions do not present as palpable lumps and calcifications rarely occur, which means that they are rarely detected by mammography. Hence, the lesions are usually identified incidentally in biopsies taken for other breast abnormalities.

Risk of subsequent invasive cancer—around one-quarter to one-third of women with LCIS go on to develop invasive carcinoma, but unlike DCIS, both breasts are equally at risk irrespective of which side the LCIS was originally identified.

Invasive carcinoma

With invasive carcinoma, the malignant cells have breached the basement membrane of the ducts or acini, and have spread into the surrounding stromal tissue.

Classification
Invasive breast carcinoma is classified according to overall histological appearance. The various histological subtypes are listed below:

- infiltrating ductal carcinoma (85%)
- infiltrating lobular carcinoma (10%)
- mucinous carcinoma (2%)
- tubular carcinoma (2%)
- medullary carcinoma (< 1%)
- papillary carcinoma (< 1%)
- others, e.g. apocrine carcinoma, metaplastic carcinoma, neuroendocrine tumours, adenoid cystic carcinomas and squamous cell carcinoma (< 1%).

Invasive ductal carcinoma of no special type (NST)—carcinomas that cannot be classified as any other subtype are designated invasive ductal carcinoma NST. Most breast carcinomas fall into this category. Macroscopically, these tumours appear as hard grey-white nodules (scirrhous carcinoma) imparted by their densely fibrous stroma. Histologically, the stroma is infiltrated by malignant cells that can be arranged in cords, nests, tubules or irregular masses—ductal carcinomas do not display any distinctive morphological features.

Invasive lobular carcinoma—these tumours can have a scirrhous macroscopic appearance, but they are often softer and have an ill-defined infiltrating outline. Histologically, linear cords of malignant cells infiltrate a densely fibrous stroma. This linear arrangement of cells is often referred to as an 'Indian file' pattern. Carcinoma cells often form concentric rings around ducts. Signet-ring cells are common. It is important to distinguish lobular carcinoma from other types of carcinoma for the following reasons:

- invasive lobular carcinomas tend to be multicentric within the same breast
- around 20% of women with invasive lobular carcinoma in one breast are likely to have bilateral disease
- these tumours metastasise more frequently to serosal surfaces, bone marrow, CSF, and the uterus and ovaries compared to other subtypes.

Mucinous carcinoma—these tumours typically arise in older women and grow slowly over a number of years. Macroscopically, mucinous carcinomas have a soft, grey, gelatinous cut surface and are well-circumscribed. Histologically, the tumour is composed of small nests and cords of tumour cells lying in lakes of mucin. Because of the absence of densely fibrous stroma, and the fact that this type of carcinoma does not cause skin tethering or nipple retraction, mucinous carcinomas can be mistaken for benign breast lesions clinically. The prognosis for women with this type of breast cancer is better than that for invasive ductal or lobular carcinoma.

Tubular carcinoma—these tumours tend to be small (< 1 cm in diameter) and are usually detected by mammography. Affected women are younger on average. Macroscopically, tubular carcinomas are small, firm, gritty tumours with irregular outlines. Histologically, they are composed of well-formed tubules in a desmoplastic stroma. The tubules lack a myoepithelial layer, a feature that distinguishes these malignant tumours from benign breast lesions. The prognosis for patients with tubular carcinoma is excellent.

Medullary carcinoma—macroscopically, these tumours tend to have a soft, fleshy consistency and are typically well-circumscribed. Histologically, medullary carcinomas are characterised by syncytial (fused) masses of large cells with pleomorphic nuclei, numerous mitotic figures, a conspicuous lymphoplasmocytic infiltrate, and a pushing (non-infiltrating) border. Gland formation is not seen. Despite the aggressive cytological features of the tumour cells, the prognosis for patients with this type of breast cancer is significantly better than that for many of the other subtypes.

Papillary carcinoma—these tumours are rare. Microscopically, they show a papillary architecture. The prognosis is better than that of invasive ductal carcinoma.

Paget's disease of the nipple

This condition presents as roughening and reddening of the skin of the nipple and areolar, the appearances resembling eczema. Ulceration may occur. The condition is important to recognise because it is associated with underlying in-situ or invasive carcinoma of the breast. Histologically, the epidermis is infiltrated by malignant cells.

The spread of breast carcinomas

Breast carcinomas can infiltrate locally or spread via the lymphatics or bloodstream to distant sites.

Direct spread

Breast carcinomas spread locally in all directions, becoming adherent to the underlying muscle fascia of the breast or tethered to the overlying skin. The latter manifests by dimpling of the skin and nipple retraction.

Spread via lymphatics

Involvement of the breast lymphatics by carcinoma causes blockage of the lymphatic drainage with consequent lymphoedema and thickening of the overlying skin, an appearance referred to clinically as *peau d'orange*. Several groups of lymph nodes drain lymph from the breast, but the axillary lymph nodes are the commonest initial site of lymph node metastases. Around one-third of women with breast cancer will have lymph node metastases at the time of diagnosis.

Spread via the bloodstream

Once the malignant cells have developed the ability to enter the bloodstream, they can reach virtually any organ in the body, but the most frequently affected sites are the lungs, bones, liver, adrenals and brain.

Staging of breast cancer

Two main systems are used to stage breast cancer. These are the International Classification of Staging of Breast Cancer, and the TNM (tumour, node, metastasis) system. The management of the patient will depend on the stage of the disease.

Prognostic factors

A number of factors that influence the prognosis of breast cancer have been identified.

Axillary lymph node status

At present, the best prognostic indicator in patients with breast cancer is the presence or absence of metastatic tumour in the axillary lymph nodes. The prognosis is significantly worse for those who have evidence of lymph node metastases.

Tumour size

Small tumours are associated with a more favourable prognosis.

Histological grade

Many studies have shown the value of histological grade in predicting survival in breast cancer, low-grade cancers being associated with a more favourable prognosis.

Table 18 Staging of breast cancer

Stage	Extent of spread
International Classification of Staging of Breast Cancer (ICSBC):	
I	Lump with slight tethering to skin, but node negative
II	Lump with lymph node metastases or skin tethering
III	Tumour that is extensively adherent to the skin and/or underlying muscles, or ulcerating or lymph nodes are fixed
IV	Distant metastases
Tumour, Nodes, Metastases (TMN) classification:	
T1	Tumour 20 mm or less, no fixation or nipple retraction. Includes Paget's disease
T2	Tumour 20–50 mm, or less than 20 mm but with tethering
T3	Tumour greater than 50 mm but less than 100 mm; or less than 50 mm but with infiltration, ulceration or fixation
T4	Any tumour with ulceration or infiltration wide of it, or chest wall fixation, or greater than 100 mm in diameter
N0	Node-negative
N1	Axillary nodes mobile
N2	Axillary nodes fixed
N3	Supraclavicular nodes or oedema of arm
M0	No distant metastases
M1	Distant metastases

Histological subtype

Certain types of breast carcinoma have a better prognosis than others, although the significance is less important than histological grade. Tubular carcinoma (and probably mucinous, medullary and papillary carcinoma) have a more favourable prognosis than invasive ductal carcinoma of no special type.

Oestrogen receptors

Women with oestrogen receptor-positive, node-negative breast cancer have a better prognosis than those who have oestrogen receptor-negative tumours. This is probably because tumours that express oestrogen receptors are well-differentiated and low-grade and respond well to hormonal manipulation.

Other molecular markers

It has been proposed that tumour differentiation, invasion, metastasis, and growth can be inferred by measuring certain cellular markers, e.g. expression of growth factor receptors, proteinases, cell-adhesion molecules, and other products of oncogenes and tumour suppressor genes. Much of the research in this field has focused on the oncogene c-erb-B2 (also known as the *Her2/neu* gene), the protein product of which is a cell-surface growth factor receptor. Research using molecular techniques indicates that 15–20% of breast carcinomas show amplification of the c-erb-B2 gene and such cancers are referred to as 'Her2-positive'. Recent studies have shown that *Her2*-positive cancers have a poorer prognosis, shorter survival, shorter relapse time, tend to be more aggressive and respond poorly to conventional therapies. Based on this research it has now been possible to develop a treatment strategy that employs the use of a monoclonal antibody, which can block the c-erb-B2 receptor and hence reduce tumour growth. Evidence indicates that administration of this antibody to women with *Her2*-positive breast cancers may significantly improve survival.

Other malignant breast conditions

Phyllodes tumour

Like fibroadenomas, phyllodes tumours are composed of both glandular and stromal tissue, are usually solitary, and can present as palpable lumps or mammographic densities. They can occur at any age but the median age at presentation is 45 years, some 10–20 years later than that for fibroadenomas. Phyllodes tumours can only be differentiated from fibroadenomas by their microscopic appearance.

Pathology
Phyllodes tumours vary greatly in size, and they have been reported to reach up to 450 mm in diameter. They often grow as lobulated masses within the breast tissue. Microscopically, phyllodes tumours can be differentiated from fibroadenomas by the presence of stromal cellularity, mitotic figures and nuclear pleomorphism. Most are low-grade tumours, when the major problem is local recurrence. Rare high-grade tumours can behave aggressively, metastasising via the bloodstream.

Sarcomas

Sarcomas such as angiosarcoma, fibrosarcoma, liposarcoma and leiomyosarcoma are all rare.

Lymphomas

Lymphomas in the breast may be primary, but are more usually secondary to disease elsewhere in the body.

Secondary tumours

Secondary tumours to the breast are rare. Those most commonly encountered are metastases from the lung, the contralateral breast and malignant melanoma.

7.4 Diagnosis of breast lesions

When a breast lesion is suspected on clinical grounds (history and physical examination) or detected by mammography, a number of investigation methods can be employed to gain further information about the lesion and lead to a diagnosis. These are:

- ultrasonography
- fine-needle aspiration cytology
- core biopsy
- excision biopsy.

Often, a combination of modalities is employed. The value of these methods is that benign and malignant conditions may be diagnosed without the need for removal of the breast (mastectomy). In malignant cases, prognostic information may also be provided (e.g. oestrogen receptor status). Appropriate management plans can then be formulated.

7.5 The male breast

Learning objectives

You should:

- Know the two main conditions which affect the male breast
- Know the various causes of gynaecomastia

Structure

It is not necessary for the male breast to have secretory capability. Hence, it consists of ductular structures surrounded by a small amount of supporting connective tissue, but there are no acini.

Two main conditions can affect the male breast:

1. Gynaecomastia
2. Carcinoma.

Gynaecomastia

This benign condition is defined as enlargement of the male breast due to hypertrophy and hyperplasia of both ductal and stromal elements. Most cases are unilateral, but around 25% of patients show bilateral involvement.

Aetiology

Gynaecomastia is thought to occur as a result of an imbalance between oestrogens (which stimulate the breast) and androgens. The condition can occur as a normal phenomenon in adolescents and very elderly men, but it can also occur in the following situations:

Drug-induced (most common cause)
Drugs which can cause gynaecomastia include:

- oestrogens (in the treatment of prostate cancer)
- digitalis
- cimetidine
- spironolactone.

Conditions causing high oestrogen levels
- tumours of the adrenal glands
- tumours of the testis
- chronic liver disease.

Syndromes of androgen deficiency
- e.g. Klinefelter's syndrome.

Other endocrine disorders
- hyperthyroidism
- pituitary disorders.

Carcinoma

In situ and invasive carcinoma of the male breast is very rare, accounting for only 1% of all breast cancers. Risk factors (except those functionally confined to women), presentation, spread, histological subtypes and prognostic factors are similar to those seen in women. With regard to prognosis, evidence suggests that when male and female breast cancers are matched for grade and stage, the overall prognosis for men and women is the same. However, men often present at more advanced stages than women.

Self-assessment: questions

Multiple choice questions

1. The following statements are correct:
   a. Acute mastitis is most frequently seen in the early weeks of breast-feeding
   b. Mammary duct ectasia may present with a breast mass and nipple discharge
   c. Early age at first pregnancy increases the risk of developing breast cancer
   d. Breast cancer is more frequent in multiparous women than nulliparous women
   e. Men never develop breast cancer.

2. The following breast conditions are associated with an increased risk of developing breast cancer:
   a. Apocrine metaplasia
   b. Atypical hyperplasia
   c. Radial scar
   d. Duct papilloma
   e. Complex fibroadenoma.

3. The following statements are true:
   a. Most breast cancers arise in the upper outer quadrant of the breast
   b. In situ carcinoma usually presents as a breast mass
   c. Lobular carcinoma in situ is frequently multifocal and bilateral
   d. Tumour size is the most important prognostic indicator in women with breast cancer
   e. Carcinomas that are oestrogen receptor positive have a poorer prognosis than those that are oestrogen receptor negative.

4. Invasive breast cancer:
   a. Can be genetically inherited
   b. Always presents as a breast mass
   c. Most commonly metastasises to the mediastinal lymph nodes
   d. May be associated with Paget's disease of the nipple
   e. Is most frequently of ductal type histologically.

Case histories

Case history 1

A 29-year-old women presents to her GP with a lump in the right breast.

1. What is the differential diagnosis?
2. Which of these diagnoses do you think are least likely in this case, and why?
3. What further information would you seek in the history and examination in order to help determine the diagnosis?

Case history 2

A 68-year-old women presents to her GP with a lump in the right breast. She first felt the lump after she fell over a chair sustaining a blunt injury to the right breast. On examination, the right nipple is retracted and the skin of the right breast shows peau d'orange. The breast lump itself is firm and immobile. The right axillary lymph nodes are enlarged and firm.

1. What is the most likely diagnosis?
2. Describe the pathological basis of each of the examination findings?
3. What further tests might you perform?

Short note questions

Write short notes on:

1. The diagnosis of breast cancer.
2. The association between benign breast abnormalities and breast cancer risk.
3. Risk factors for the development of breast cancer.

Viva questions

1. What conditions may affect the male breast?
2. What is the rational behind mammographic breast screening?
3. What factors influence the prognosis of women with breast cancer?

Self-assessment: answers

Multiple choice answers

1. a. **True.**
    b. **True.**
    c. **False.** This is associated with a *decreased* risk.
    d. **False.** Breast cancer is more frequent in nulliparous than multiparous women.
    e. **False.**

2. a. **False.**
    b. **True.**
    c. **True.**
    d. **True.**
    e. **True.** But fibroadenomas that do not show complex features are not associated with an increased risk.

3. a. **True.**
    b. **False.**
    c. **True.**
    d. **False.** Lymph node status is the most important prognostic factor.
    e. **False.** Oestrogen receptor positive tumours have a *better* prognosis.

4. a. **True.** 5–10% of breast cancers are due to inheritance of an autosomal dominant gene. The genes *BRCA1* and *BRCA2* account for most of these cases.
    b. **False.**
    c. **False.** Breast tumours most commonly metastasise to the *axillary* lymph nodes.
    d. **True.**
    e. **True.**

Case histories

Case history 1

1. It is important to realise that the differential diagnosis for a lump in the breast includes almost the entire spectrum of breast disorders. Inflammatory lesions, fibrocystic disease, benign tumours and malignant tumours (principally invasive carcinoma) may all present as breast lumps. Remember that in-situ carcinoma does not present as a breast lump (unless it is associated with another breast lesion).

2. Taking note of the patient's age is often helpful in determining which of the differential diagnoses are more likely and which are less likely. In this case, the patient is 29 years old. Carcinoma is therefore the least likely diagnosis, although young patients may develop breast cancer, especially if there is a strong family history.

3. Acute mastitis is painful and there would usually be a history of breast-feeding. The skin of the nipple is often cracked. Mammary duct ectasia is usually seen in older women and a history of nipple discharge is common. A history of nipple discharge would also raise the possibility of a duct papilloma. Fat necrosis would follow trauma to the breast tissue. Fibrocystic disease usually causes breast 'lumpiness', and although one lump may be dominant, the lumpiness is often revealed on clinical examination. Fibroadenomas are usually solitary palpable masses, which are freely mobile. Nipple adenomas usually cause a subareolar mass. Breast cancers produce firm masses, which may be immobile due to tethering. The overlying skin may show dimpling or peau d'orange and there may be features of Paget's disease of the nipple. The axillary lymph nodes may be enlarged due to spread of the disease. A family history of breast cancer may alert you to the possibility of carcinoma in young patients presenting with breast lumps.

Case history 2

1. The fact that this lady first felt the breast lump after she sustained an injury to the breast would raise the possibility of fat necrosis. However, the clinical findings of a retracted nipple, peau d'orange, a firm immobile mass, and enlarged axillary lymph nodes are all highly suggestive of breast cancer. The preceding trauma may simply have drawn the patient's attention to her breast, and in the ensuing self-examination the lump would have been revealed.

2. Most of the features on physical examination can be explained in terms of the way that breast cancer spreads. Extension into the overlying skin causes retraction and dimpling, and tumours that have become adherent to the deep fascia of the chest wall become fixed in position (immobile).

    Involvement of the lymphatic channels around the tumour blocks drainage of the overlying skin, causing localised lymphoedema and skin thickening, referred to as peau d'orange.

    The axillary lymph nodes become enlarged and firm when there are lymph node metastases.

3. Initial further investigations are directed towards establishing a diagnosis of cancer. Several techniques may be employed, but a combination of different modalities is often necessary to make the diagnosis. These include ultrasonography, fine-needle aspiration cytology (FNA), core biopsy and, if necessary, excision biopsy. Further investigations, e.g. CT scan, are usually aimed at determining the stage of the disease.

Short note answers

1. Whenever you are asked how you might diagnose any condition, your answer must always include the three most important tools, namely: history; physical examination; and further investigations (or tests). Focus on the most important features that you would want to elicit from the history and examination, i.e. family history, the appearance of the affected breast, the nature of any breast mass and the axillary contents, and the nature of any nipple discharge. Then discuss the further tests that you might use to establish the diagnosis, i.e. ultrasonography, FNA, core biopsy, and excision biopsy. Remember that some breast cancers are detected by mammography in the National Breast Screening Programme.

2. What is wanted here is an awareness that there are certain benign breast conditions that are associated with an increased risk of developing breast cancer. Radial scars/complex sclerosing lesions, moderate to florid usual-type epithelial hyperplasia, fibroadenomas with complex features, and duct papillomas are all associated with a slightly increased risk, while atypical hyperplasia is associated with a moderately increased risk.

3. Risk factors for breast cancer include genetic predisposition, age, factors related to the menses and pregnancy, demographic influences, radiation, certain benign breast diseases, and previous breast cancer.

Viva answers

1. The two main intrinsic breast conditions that may affect the male breast are gynaecomastia and carcinoma. Try to give an account of the various causes of gynaecomastia. Carcinoma of the male breast is uncommon. However, when it occurs it usually presents at a higher stage and therefore generally has a poorer prognosis. Remember that the male breast may also be affected by pathology of the skin and soft tissue (as may the female breast).

2. Screening implies performing a test in order to detect a particular disease (most commonly cancer) in an asymptomatic but at risk population. With cancer, the idea is to detect the disease either at its pre-invasive stage, when treatment of the lesion would prevent cancer from developing, or at a stage when the cancer is small and therefore potentially curable. With breast cancer, there is a pre-invasive stage (in situ carcinoma) and small invasive tumours do have a better prognosis. Both in situ and invasive carcinoma can be detected on mammography because they induce densities, calcifications and areas of architectural distortion that can be visualised. Mammography is both sensitive and specific, but it is also acceptable, and it is, therefore, the principle investigative modality employed in the National Breast Screening Programme.

3. Several factors influence the prognosis of breast cancer. These include lymph node status, tumour size, histological grade, histological subtype, and oestrogen receptor status.

8 Female genital tract

Overview

The female genital tract comprises vulva, vagina, uterus, cervix, fallopian tubes and ovaries. Infections in this region are common. Many are relatively trivial, but pelvic inflammatory disease can cause infertility or serious intra-abdominal sepsis. Infection with certain subtypes of human papilloma virus (HPV) predisposes to dysplasia and malignancy in the cervix. Carcinoma of the ovary is the fifth most frequent cause of female cancer mortality, and often presents at an advanced state. In contrast, the cervical cytology screening programme has allowed early diagnosis of premalignant and invasive carcinomas in many cases, with a consequential fall in cervical cancer mortality of approximately 40% in the UK. Disorders relating specifically to reproductive function include endometriosis, ectopic pregnancy and hydatidiform mole.

8.1 Inflammation, infection and non-neoplastic disease

Learning objectives

You should:

- Know the common female genital tract infections
- Know about HPV-associated diseases
- Understand the pathology of endometriosis

Genital tract infection

Common causes include:

- bacteria—*Gardnerella, Gonorrhoea, Chlamydia*
- viruses—HPV, herpes simplex type 2
- fungi—*Candida albicans*
- protozoa—*Trichomonas vaginalis*.

Gardnerella—is a common cause of vaginitis.

Gonorrhoea—can infect the cervix, endometrium, fallopian tubes and ovaries.

Chlamydia trachomatis—is an intracellular pathogen that causes urethritis, cervicitis and lymphogranuloma venereum (genital ulceration with suppurative and granulomatous inflammation of pelvic, inguinal and rectal lymph nodes). Transmission to neonates during vaginal delivery can cause conjunctivitis and pneumonia.

Staphylococcus—toxic shock syndrome is a rare but serious infection caused by exotoxin producing *S. aureus*. It is associated with tampon use and presents with fever, diarrhoea and vomiting, rash and shock. Occasionally cases are fatal.

Human papilloma virus (HPV)—infects squamous epithelia at many body sites (see Box 14). Low-risk subtypes cause genital warts (condylomata acuminata); high-risk subtypes are associated with the development of cervical carcinoma. HPV changes are frequently seen in association with cervical dysplasia on tissue biopsy. HPV serotyping using the polymerase chain reaction is likely to play an important role in future cervical cancer screening programmes. Cytological features associated with HPV infection include irregular enlarged hyperchromatic nuclei surrounded by poorly staining cytoplasm (these features are known as koilocytosis), multinucleation and abnormal keratinisation.

Herpes simplex type 2—infection is relatively common in young women. Ulcerating vesicles develop on the vulva, vagina or cervix several days after sexual contact with the virus. Spontaneous healing occurs but latent infection leads to recurrent attacks. Neonatal transmission during vaginal delivery can cause severe systemic infection and neonatal death. Herpes simplex 2 is also associated with cervical carcinogenesis.

Candida—commonly causes vulvovaginitis, with intense itching and a thick white discharge. Infection is

Box 14 HPV subtype disease associations

HPV subtype	Associated lesions
1, 2, 4, 7	Benign squamous cell papillomas (viral warts)
5, 8	Cutaneous squamous cell carcinoma
6, 11	Benign anogenital warts (condylomata acuminatum)
16, 18, (31, 33, 35)	High-grade cervical epithelial dysplasia (CIN) and squamous carcinoma

associated with diabetes, oral contraceptives, immuno-suppression and pregnancy.

Trichomonas vaginalis—is a sexually transmitted infection and causes a foamy discharge, itching, dysuria and dyspareunia.

Trichomonas, *Candida* and herpes virus infections may be identified incidentally on cytological examination of routine cervical screening smears (see below).

Pelvic inflammatory disease (PID)—describes a chronic upper genital tract infection that presents as pelvic pain, fever and vaginal discharge. Causative organisms include gonococci and *Chlamydia*, although other bacteria can cause PID following termination of pregnancy or spontaneous vaginal delivery. *Actinomyces* is a common infection in users of contraceptive coils. Infection spreads from lower genital tract to the fallopian tubes and ovaries. Complications include tubo-ovarian abscess, pyosalpinx, peritonitis, intestinal obstruction and infertility.

Chronic endometritis—is identified microscopically by the presence of plasma cells in the endometrium. Chronic endometrial infection occurs:

- in association with intrauterine contraceptive devices (IUD, 'coil')
- in patients with chronic PID
- in association with retained products of pregnancy
- in tuberculosis—diagnosis can be difficult as cyclical endometrial shedding prevents the formation of typical caseating granulomas
- without other associated factors (15%).

Treatment depends on the underlying cause—antibiotics, removal or replacement of the IUD or endometrial curettage to remove retained gestational tissue.

Lichen sclerosus—is a chronic inflammatory skin condition that most commonly affects the vulva. Classically, the surface keratin is thickened, the epidermis is atrophic and the dermis is abnormally fibrotic. There is an increased risk of developing squamous cell carcinoma.

Endometriosis—is a common condition in which endometrial glands and stroma are present in organs other than the uterus (Box 15 and Fig. 25). Typical sites of endometriosis include the ovaries, fallopian tubes, uterosacral ligaments, Pouch of Douglas and cervix, but endometriosis can occur throughout the peritoneum and even within distant organs such as the lung. The process is not neoplastic but the mechanism(s) by which endometrial tissue establishes itself in these extrauterine sites remains uncertain. Theories include: endometrial metaplasia; retrograde flow through the fallopian tube at menstruation; implantation after surgery; and bloodstream spread of viable endometrial fragments. Endometriotic foci may show proliferative and secretory activity in response to oestrogen and progesterone, in the same way as normal uterine endometrium. Endometriosis in the ovary is associated with clear cell adenocarcinoma (see below). The presence of endometrial glands and stroma within the myometrium is called adenomyosis.

Polyps—are benign polypoid proliferations of glandular epithelium and stroma. They can arise in the endocervix and endometrium and may cause abnormal vaginal bleeding. Endometrial polyps occur most frequently after the menopause, and the incidence is increased in breast carcinoma patients receiving tamoxifen treatment.

Ovarian cysts—benign follicle ('follicular') and corpus luteum cysts are very common, but sometimes raise clinical suspicion of malignancy if seen on an ultrasound scan. Multiple bilateral follicular cysts, associated with ovarian enlargement, menstrual irregularities, hirsutism, obesity and infertility, are features of polycystic ovarian disease. The underlying cause appears to be abnormal release of pituitary hormones.

Box 15 Clinical notes: endometriosis

Symptoms related to cyclical bleeding and subsequent inflammation:
- Pain, often dyspareunia or dysmenorrhoea
- Ovarian cysts ('chocolate cysts' containing altered blood)
- Infertility (fallopian tube involvement)
- Haematuria (bladder endometriosis)
- Intestinal obstruction
- Endometriotic nodules in abdominal surgical scars

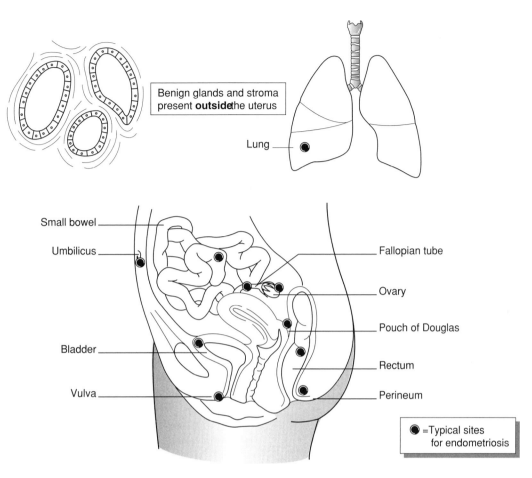

Benign glands and stroma present **outside** the uterus

Lung

Small bowel

Umbilicus

Fallopian tube

Ovary

Pouch of Douglas

Bladder

Rectum

Vulva

Perineum

= Typical sites for endometriosis

Fig. 25 Endometriosis.

8.2 Dysplasia and neoplasia

Learning objectives

You should:

- Understand the concepts of dysplasia and intraepithelial neoplasia in the female genital tract

- Understand the principles and practice of the NHS Cervical Screening Programme

- Have sufficient knowledge of neoplastic disease of the female genital tract to interpret histopathology reports of these tumours

Dysplasia means abnormal growth. Dysplastic epithelium shows morphological changes of neoplastic cells but without evidence of invasion (Fig. 26). Dysplastic changes can include:

- increased nuclear to cytoplasmic ratio
- nuclear pleomorphism (variation in size and shape)
- nuclear hyperchromatism (increased intensity of staining)
- abnormal mitoses
- abnormal cellular crowding
- failure of epithelial maturation.

Epithelial dysplasia occurs throughout the lower female genital tract:

- vulval intraepithelial neoplasia (VIN)
- vaginal intraepithelial neoplasia (VAIN)
- cervical intraepithelial neoplasia (CIN)
- cervical glandular intraepithelial neoplasia (CGIN)
- atypical endometrial hyperplasia.

The intraepithelial neoplasia of squamous epithelium in the vulva, vagina and cervix (VIN, VAIN and CIN) is numerically graded from 1 to 3, according to the severity of dysplastic changes. Thus, CIN 1 is low-grade cervical dysplasia in which the cellular abnormalities are confined to the lower third of the squamous epithelium. In CIN 3 (high-grade dysplasia, also called carcinoma-in-situ), the entire thickness of the epithelium is abnormal, showing cytological features of malignant cells. However, there is no invasion of the atypical cells

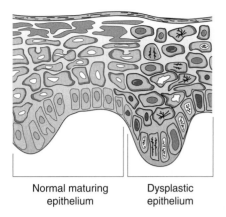

Normal maturing   Dysplastic
epithelium   epithelium

Fig. 26 Dysplastic epithelium.

beyond the epithelial basement membrane and so there is no capacity for local spread or distant metastasis. CGIN describes dysplasia of endocervical glandular epithelium, and is classified as either low or high grade.

Abnormal proliferation within the endometrium is known as hyperplasia, and occurs in response to unopposed oestrogen stimulation:

- **simple hyperplasia**—diffuse proliferation of both endometrial glands and stroma
- **complex hyperplasia**—focal glandular proliferation only, no cytological atypia
- **atypical hyperplasia**—glandular proliferation and crowding (usually focal) with atypical cytological changes.

Only atypical hyperplasia is regarded as a high-risk premalignant change. Like other adaptive tissue changes, hyperplasia remains under the control of the eliciting stimulus. If the oestrogen excess is neutralised, for example by exogenous progesterone administration, the hyperplasia will regress. Even early stage endometrial carcinoma may be effectively treated by progestogens rather than surgery.

Cervical screening

The ability to recognise the abnormal cells from dysplastic cervical epithelium forms the basis of the NHS Cervical Screening Programme. All women between the ages of 25 and 65 are invited to have a cervical smear examination every 3–5 years. A wooden spatula is used to gently scrape cells from the surface of the cervix, ensuring that the cervical os is adequately visualised and the transformation zone is sampled. The cells are smeared on to a glass slide and examined under the microscope for nuclear changes—enlargement, chromatin abnormalities and nuclear membrane irregularities—which might indicate a dysplastic or malignant lesion. The cytological changes are called dyskaryosis and graded as mild, moderate or severe. The screen-

ing programme was originally intended to identify dyskaryosis within the squamous epithelial cells, but it is also possible to detect endocervical glandular abnormalities in some cases. Smears that show changes of HPV infection in the absence of dyskaryosis are still regarded as abnormal and warrant further follow-up, in view of the association between HPV and cervical neoplasia. Cytological abnormalities that do not amount to unequivocal dyskaryosis may be described as 'borderline', and again these changes require more regular follow-up smears to exclude significant disease.

The success of the programme depends upon detecting and treating women with asymptomatic dysplastic lesions (CIN and CGIN) before they progress to invasive carcinoma. The degree of dyskaryosis in the cervical smear is an indication of the likely severity of dysplasia in the epithelium. High-grade smear abnormalities or persistent low-grade changes require colposcopic examination of the cervix by a gynaecologist, with tissue biopsy for histological confirmation of dysplasia (Fig. 27). Treatment by laser, cold coagulation or tissue resection is followed up with regular smears, until it is safe for the patient to return to routine recall.

As with all screening programmes, there are advantages and disadvantages in participation, with both false positive and false negative results possible. False positives may be caused by:

- HPV infection without dysplasia
- cervical inflammation
- degenerate cellular changes that mimic dyskaryosis.

False negatives may result from:

- failure to sample the dysplastic focus within the smear
- small numbers of dyskaryotic cells being 'missed' by the cervical screener
- dyskaryotic cells being misinterpreted by the screener or cytopathologist.

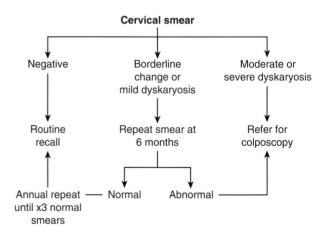

Fig. 27 Management of normal and abnormal cervical smears.

Treatment of dysplastic lesions is not without significant adverse effects, as cervical stenosis secondary to tissue resection or ablation can cause infertility. Not all patients with CIN, even of high grade, will definitely progress to invasive carcinoma if left untreated. However, the risk of a CIN lesion progressing to cancer cannot be predicted for individual patients.

Neoplasia

Vulva

Cancer is relatively uncommon; the majority are squamous cell carcinomas (>90%) and usually occur in elderly females, but the incidence is increasing in younger women. Prognosis is closely related to spread, especially to inguinal and pelvic lymph nodes. Vulval malignant melanoma is rare, but has a poor prognosis. Extramammary Paget's disease occurs in the vulva and anogenital region. This is an intraepidermal proliferation of adenocarcinoma cells, which clinically manifests as a well-demarcated, crusted, red lesion. Unlike Paget's disease of the nipple, underlying invasive malignancy is uncommon.

Vagina

Malignant neoplasms are rare. In infants the vagina is a site for embryonal rhabdomyosarcoma. There is an association between clear cell adenocarcinoma of the vagina and exposure to diethylstilboestrol during intrauterine life. Squamous cell carcinoma is the most frequent tumour in adults, but is rarely seen clinically. There is an association with both vulval and cervical carcinoma.

Cervix

Up to 90% of malignancies are squamous cell carcinomas (Table 19); the role of HPV in carcinogenesis, and the role of cervical screening in prevention of cervical cancer have already been discussed. Cervical cancers arise from the junctional region between squamous ectocervical epithelium and columnar endocervix, also known as the transformation zone. Adenocarcinoma accounts for approximately 10% of cervical malignancies, but is increasing in incidence.

Staging of cervical cancer
Stage I—confined to cervix.
Stage II—extends beyond cervix but does not involve pelvic wall or lower third of vagina.
Stage III—involvement of pelvic wall or lower third of vagina.
Stage IV—extension beyond pelvis or involvement of bladder or rectal mucosa (Table 20).

Endometrium

Endometrial adenocarcinoma is the commonest invasive tumour of the female genital tract (Table 20).

Myometrium

The commonest neoplasm arising in the female genital tract is the leiomyoma (benign smooth muscle tumour), also known as a 'fibroid'. Growth of leiomyomas is stimulated by oestrogen, hence these are tumours of reproductive life that can grow rapidly in pregnancy but may atrophy after the menopause. Leiomyomas are

Table 19 Cancer checklist: cervical squamous cell carcinoma

Incidence	age > 20, peak incidence around 40
Risk factors	HPV infection with specific subtypes—multiple sexual partners, male partner with multiple previous partners, early age of first intercourse, smoking, HIV, herpes simplex type 2
Protective factors	Celibacy, barrier contraception
Associated lesions	High grade CIN
Clinical presentation	Abnormal vaginal bleeding, pain/bleeding after sexual intercourse
Location	Initially arises in transformation zone
Macroscopic appearance	Exophytic, ulcerating or infiltrative mass
Histological features	Squamous cells +/− keratinisation
Pattern of spread	Local spread to uterine body, vagina, pelvic wall, bladder, ureters and rectum Local and distant lymph nodes Distant metastases in liver and lung
Prognosis (per cent 5-year survival)	Stage I 80–90% Stage IV 10–15% Advanced tumours often cause death through renal tract obstruction

Table 20 Cancer checklist: endometrial carcinoma

Incidence	Age > 40, usually post menopausal
Risk factors	Excessive oestrogen exposure—early menarche and late menopause, nulliparity, obesity (increased oestrogen production in peripheral fat), family history, diabetes, hypertension, oestrogen-producing tumours
Protective factors	Ovarian agenesis or removal
Associated lesions	Atypical endometrial hyperplasia
Clinical presentation	Abnormal vaginal bleeding (often post menopausal)
Location	Anywhere in endometrium
Macroscopic appearance	Polypoid or diffuse growth pattern
Histological features	Mild, moderately or poorly differentiated according to the extent of glandular and solid growth pattern
	Aggressive subtypes: clear cell carcinoma; serous papillary carcinoma
Pattern of spread	Myometrium, cervix and pelvic organs
	Lymph nodes
Prognosis (per cent 5-year survival)	Most cases are Stage I (confined to uterus) and well or moderately differentiated, with 90% survival
	Extrauterine spread, poor differentiation or aggressive histological subtypes have worse prognosis (20–50% survival)

often multiple and can reach many centimetres in diameter. They can cause pelvic pain, abnormal uterine bleeding, urinary symptoms and infertility or complications of pregnancy. Malignant smooth muscle tumours (leiomyosarcomas) are rare.

Ovary

The ovary can harbour a wide variety of benign and malignant neoplasms, the more frequent examples are listed in Table 21. Most adult tumours arise from the surface epithelium of the ovary. In children germ cell tumours predominate. Most ovarian tumours (80%) are benign. However, ovarian malignancies cause more deaths than all other female genital-tract cancers combined.

Surface epithelial tumours—are the most frequent. Histologically, they show serous, mucinous, transitional or endometrial differentiation. Benign tumours are often cystic. Malignant tumours may be partly cystic and partly solid. Tumours may affect both ovaries, especially with serous neoplasms. Prognosis of carcinomas largely depends on stage. Clinical presentation in the majority of cases is late, and many carcinomas have reached an advanced stage at diagnosis. There is also a group of 'borderline' tumours—these show cytological features of carcinoma (loss of cell polarity, hyperchromatic nuclei, abnormal mitoses) but without evidence of stromal invasion. Borderline tumours usually behave in a benign fashion or show low malignant potential.

Table 21 Ovarian tumours

Surface epithelial tumours (70%)

Benign
serous cystadenoma
mucinous cystadenoma
Brenner (transitional cell) tumour

Borderline (low malignant potential)
serous borderline tumour
mucinous borderline tumour

Malignant
serous cystadenocarcinoma
mucinous adenocarcinoma
endometrioid adenocarcinoma
clear cell carcinoma

Germ cell tumours (20%)

Benign
cystic teratoma ('dermoid cyst')

Malignant
yolk sac tumour
dysgerminoma
choriocarcinoma (non-gestational)

Stromal tumours (10%)*
fibroma, thecoma
granulosa cell tumour
Sertoli–Leydig cell tumours

*Also called sex cord–stromal tumours; most cases are benign but a small proportion of each of these lesions will show malignant behaviour.

Box 16 Clinical notes: presentation of ovarian tumours

- abdominal mass (tumour itself +/− ascitic fluid)
- pain/discomfort
- symptoms related to hormone production (abnormal vaginal bleeding in oestrogen-producing tumours; masculinisation if excess androgens are produced)
- raised serum CA125 or ovarian mass on pelvic ultrasound in patients at risk of carcinoma (e.g. families with known *BRCA1* gene)

Germ cell tumours—are a diverse group of lesions, the commonest of which is the benign dermoid cyst (mature cystic teratoma). The tumour consists of differentiated somatic tissues, and may include skin, with sebaceous glands and hair, teeth, fat, bone, cartilage, nervous tissue, respiratory epithelium and thyroid epithelium. Malignant germ cell tumours include yolk sac tumour, dysgerminoma (the female equivalent of seminoma) and choriocarcinoma (trophoblastic differentiation).

Stromal tumours—are less common. Most are benign, but they may cause symptoms due to hormone production. Granulosa cell tumours, thecomas and fibromas can secrete oestrogens, and they may be associated with endometrial hyperplasia or carcinoma. Some stromal tumours can produce androgens and clinically present with masculinisation. These include Sertoli–Leydig cell tumours and hilus cell tumours.

Metastatic tumours—form a small proportion of ovarian tumours. They may arise from primaries elsewhere in the female genital tract. The most frequent distant primary source of ovarian metastases is the breast. Bilateral ovarian enlargement due to metastatic adeno-

carcinoma from the gastrointestinal tract (particularly stomach) is known as Krukenberg's tumour.

8.3 Pathology related to pregnancy

Learning objectives

You should:

- Understand the terms pre-eclampsia, gestational trophoblastic disease and hydatidiform mole
- Know the possible causes of spontaneous abortion

Ectopic pregnancy—extrauterine implantation of the fetus occurs in approximately 1 in 150 pregnancies. The fallopian tube is by far the commonest site; predisposing factors include pelvic inflammatory disease and previous tubal surgery. Tubal pregnancy frequently ruptures within the first trimester, with serious intraperitoneal haemorrhage. Ectopic pregnancy is also associated with a greater risk of hydatidiform mole (see below).

Spontaneous abortion—early pregnancy loss (before the fetus is viable) can result from:

- chromosomal abnormalities
- congenital abnormalities
- uterine or placental malformations and abnormalities, including fibroids and cervical incompetence
- infections, including *Toxoplasma*, *Listeria*, *Mycoplasma* and viral diseases.

Table 22 Cancer checklist: ovarian malignancy

Incidence	Carcinoma > 40 years Malignant germ cell tumours < 30 years
Risk factors	Abnormal gonadal development Nulliparity Family history BRCA1 gene
Protective factors	Oral contraceptive use
Associated lesions	Breast cancer in BRCA1-related cases
Clinical presentation	Abdominal mass/pain, hormonal symptoms
Location	20–65% of carcinomas are bilateral, germ cell malignancies usually unilateral
Macroscopic appearance	Partly cystic or solid masses, papillary areas, necrosis and haemorrhage
Histological features	Very variable, according to tumour type
Pattern of spread	Into peritoneal cavity—ascites Contralateral ovary, omentum, local lymph nodes, lung, liver
Prognosis	Carcinomas dependent on stage—spread beyond ovary usually means poor outcome Some germ cell tumours—respond well to chemoradiotherapy

Pre-eclampsia—is the development of proteinuria, hypertension and oedema in late pregnancy. It is associated with young maternal age, twin pregnancy, diabetes, chronic hypertension and a history of pre-eclampsia in previous gestations. Central to the pathogenesis is defective uteroplacental blood circulation. This probably arises from failure of trophoblastic tissue to adequately invade the maternal spiral arterioles, resulting in placental ischaemia. Imbalance of arachidonic acid metabolites (prostacyclin and thromboxane) have also been identified and immune-related mechanisms may be important in some cases. Management includes monitoring, bed rest and antihypertensive medication. Delivery is curative, and may be expedited by caesarean section. Some cases may progress to eclampsia, a serious condition characterised by fits and disseminated intravascular coagulation.

Gestational trophoblastic disease—this is a group of conditions characterised by abnormal proliferation of trophoblastic tissue.

Hydatidiform mole—is composed of abnormal chorionic villi, which are enlarged and oedematous with excess cytotrophoblast and syncytiotrophoblast. There are partial and complete forms of mole. Both contain an abnormal karyotype. In complete mole, all of the genetic material is derived from paternal chromosomes (46 XX). Partial moles have triploidy with an extra set of paternal chromosomes (69 XXY). There is a marked geographical variation in incidence, with much higher rates in Asian than European or North American populations. Women over the age of 50 also have a greatly increased risk.

Molar pregnancy clinically presents in the mid-trimester of pregnancy with abnormal uterine bleeding, but earlier detection is possible with routine antenatal ultrasound. A fetus may be present in partial moles but not in complete moles. The uterus is often large for dates, and the swollen villi may be detected on scanning or on naked eye examination of aborted tissue passed vaginally. Serum levels of β-HCG are markedly elevated. Serial measurement of this hormone is used in follow-up of treated patients to detect any recurrence or malignant transformation. Occasionally the molar tissue extends deeply into the myometrium and causes uterine rupture. Although hydatidiform mole is the commonest predisposing factor to gestational choriocarcinoma, progression to this neoplasm is rare (2%).

Gestational choriocarcinoma—is a malignant tumour of trophoblast, which develops following hydatidiform mole, abortion, normal pregnancy or ectopic gestation. The malignant trophoblast does not form chorionic villus structures. Gestational choriocarcinoma metastasises widely but is very responsive to chemotherapy.

Placental site trophoblastic tumour—is a rare neoplasm derived from intermediate trophoblast. No chorionic villi structures are formed.

Self-assessment: questions

Multiple choice questions

1. The following statements are correct:
   a. Simple hyperplasia of the endometrium is usually a premalignant lesion
   b. CIN inevitably progresses to invasive carcinoma if left untreated
   c. The incidence of hydatidiform mole shows marked geographical variation
   d. Endometriosis frequently involves the ovaries
   e. Polypoid growths in the endometrium are always benign.

2. HPV infection is associated with the following diseases:
   a. Squamous cell carcinoma of the vulva
   b. Adenocarcinoma of the cervix
   c. Serous cystadenocarcinoma of the ovary
   d. Condylomata lata
   e. Endometrial hyperplasia.

3. Chronic endometritis:
   a. Is diagnosed histologically by the presence of lymphocytes in the endometrium
   b. Is associated with intrauterine contraceptive devices
   c. Can be part of pelvic inflammatory disease
   d. Can follow a normal pregnancy
   e. Is associated with endometrial carcinoma.

4. The following primary malignant tumours commonly arise in the ovary:
   a. Cystic teratoma ('dermoid cyst')
   b. Krukenberg's tumour
   c. Leiomyoma
   d. Choriocarcinoma
   e. Embryonal rhabdomyosarcoma.

5. Concerning pre-eclampsia:
   a. Symptoms begin in early pregnancy
   b. It occurs most commonly in the first pregnancy
   c. It is characterised by hypertension and haematuria
   d. The fetus may be small for dates
   e. The underlying pathology is defective uteroplacental circulation.

6. The following are correctly paired:
   a. Intrauterine contraceptive devices—*Actinomyces* infection
   b. Toxic shock syndrome—*Neisseria gonorrhoeae*
   c. Infertility—endometriosis
   d. Nulliparity—ovarian carcinoma
   e. Smoking—squamous cell carcinoma of the cervix.

Case histories

Case history 1

A 68-year-old female presents to her general practitioner with postmenopausal bleeding. She is mildly obese and diabetic. Her previous cervical smear tests have been normal. She was diagnosed with breast cancer three years ago and has been taking tamoxifen.

1. What is the likely diagnosis?
2. What diagnostic procedure should be performed?

Case history 2

A 26-year-old female attends the casualty department with acute abdominal pain. On questioning she describes her menstrual cycle as irregular. She has a previous history of pelvic inflammatory disease.

1. What differential diagnoses should you consider?
2. What immediate investigations are appropriate?

Viva questions

1. Discuss the advantages and disadvantages of a population-screening programme for cervical carcinoma.
2. How does pathological examination contribute to the management of patients with ovarian cancer?

Self-assessment: answers

Multiple choice answers

1. a. **False.** Simple hyperplasia without atypia is rarely associated with subsequent endometrial carcinoma. There is a much greater risk of atypical hyperplasia progressing to invasive malignancy.
   b. **False.** The natural history of CIN is not fully known. Some, but not all, cases of high-grade CIN will progress to invasive carcinoma over a variable period of time. Lower-grade CIN may progress, remain stable, or regress. It is not possible to predict the risk of progression for an individual patient.
   c. **True.**
   d. **True.**
   e. **False.** Most polyps in the endometrium are benign growths of endometrial glands and stroma. Submucosal leiomyomas (fibroids) can also project into the uterine cavity. However, endometrial carcinoma frequently has a partly exophytic polypoid growth pattern.

2. a. **True.** HPV is associated with squamous cell carcinoma of the vulva, vagina, cervix, anus and non-genital skin.
   b. **True.** HPV DNA can be detected with similar high frequency in both squamous and glandular carcinomas of the cervix.
   c. **False.**
   d. **False.** Condylomata lata are genital lesions seen in secondary syphilis. Condylomata acuminata are HPV-related genital warts.
   e. **False.**

3. a. **False.** Lymphocytes can be seen in normal endometrium. Plasma cells are required for the diagnosis of chronic endometritis.
   b. **True.**
   c. **True.**
   d. **True.** Retained placental material following normal vaginal delivery can become chronically inflamed.
   e. **False.**

4. a. **False.** Cystic teratomas do occur in the ovary, but these are benign germ cell neoplasms.
   b. **False.** Krukenberg's tumours are bilateral ovarian metastases, usually from gastric adenocarcinomas. The most common ovarian metastases, however, arise from primary malignancies elsewhere in the female genital tract or from the pelvic peritoneum.
   c. **False.** Leiomyomas are benign smooth muscle neoplasms, which are very common in the myometrium.
   d. **True.** Choriocarcinoma can arise as a non-gestational germ cell tumour in the ovary, or as a pregnancy-related uterine malignancy.
   e. **False.** This rare malignant skeletal muscle tumour occurs in the vagina in young children.

5. a. **False.** Symptoms begin in the third trimester.
   b. **True.**
   c. **False.** Hypertension, proteinuria and oedema are characteristic.
   d. **True.**
   e. **True.**

6. a. **True.**
   b. **False.** The causative agent is *Staphylococcus aureus*.
   c. **True.**
   d. **True.**
   e. **True.**

Case histories

Case history 1

1. Abnormal vaginal bleeding may be:
   - intermenstrual
   - post-coital
   - irregular menstrual cycles, often perimenarchal and perimenopausal
   - menorrhagia (heavy prolonged periods)
   - postmenopausal.

   There are many potential causes, including benign and malignant tumours and pregnancy-related bleeding. Abnormal bleeding during the reproductive years is most frequently related to altered oestrogen and progesterone balance (dysfunctional uterine bleeding), including anovulatory cycles and inadequate corpus luteum function. Post-coital bleeding is a classical symptom of cervical carcinoma, although benign causes are more commonly responsible. Postmenopausal bleeding—other than that related to hormone replacement therapy—suggests the presence of an endometrial polyp, endometrial hyperplasia or endometrial carcinoma.

   Relevant risk factors for carcinoma include diabetes and obesity. Tamoxifen is a drug used successfully in breast cancer; it blocks oestrogen receptors on breast tumour cells. However, tamoxifen has a stimulatory effect on the endometrium, promoting growth. An increased incidence of both endometrial hyperplasia and carcinoma has been attributed to tamoxifen use, and this may limit the length of time that the drug is given to patients who have not had a hysterectomy.

2. The nature of any endometrial pathology must be established. Ultrasound scan may demonstrate increased endometrial thickness or a mass lesion. Histological sampling is necessary for definitive diagnosis. Suction biopsy may be performed by the GP or in an out-patient clinic, but the tissue yield can be very low. More extensive material can be obtained by dilatation and curettage under general anaesthesia.

Case history 2

1. Potential serious causes of acute abdominal pain in a women of this age include appendicitis, cholecystitis and ruptured ectopic pregnancy. Other possible gynaecological causes include endometriosis, an exacerbation of pelvic inflammatory disease, ovarian torsion and 'mittelschmerz' (cramping pain experienced in the middle of the menstrual cycle, due to ovulation).

2. It is vital to ascertain whether there is any chance of pregnancy and perform a pregnancy test. Ruptured tubal ectopic pregnancy occurs in the first trimester. It is a surgical emergency, and can cause shock with life-threatening intraperitoneal haemorrhage. The patient may be unaware of their pregnancy.

Ultrasound scan helps confirm the diagnosis, as no gestational sac is identified within the uterus. The tubal abnormality might also be visualised. Often there is a little vaginal bleeding, which adds to the initial clinical suspicion of a ruptured ectopic gestation.

Viva answers

1. Be prepared to describe the pathological basis for cervical screening and to outline the management of a patient with an abnormal smear (Fig. 27). You should know potential causes for false-positive and false-negative results and ways of minimising these—such as proper training of smear takers, cytoscreeners and pathologists, and regular audit.

2. Pathological examination is necessary for accurate initial diagnosis of ovarian carcinoma, either through ovarian histology or cytology of ascitic fluid. Histological examination of cancer resection specimens provides prognostic information, particularly related to tumour stage—spread to other organs and lymph nodes—and histological tumour type. Cytological examination of peritoneal washings obtained at operation forms part of the staging investigation.

   Serum tumour markers are specific proteins elaborated by the neoplasm, which can be helpful in initial diagnosis and during follow-up of treated patients to detect recurrent disease. Markers include CA125 in surface epithelial carcinomas, α-fetoprotein in yolk sac tumour and β-HCG in choriocarcinoma.

9 Male genital tract

Overview

The male genital tract (MGT) consists principally of the penis, foreskin, testes, epididymes and prostate gland. A large range of disease processes affect the male genital tract, but inflammation and tumours are probably the most important clinically. Malignancies of the testis and prostate are particularly common tumours and it is important that you have a working knowledge of these. Sexually transmitted diseases (STDs) are also seen and may affect a variety of organs in the male genital tract. Congenital diseases are also common and vary from the relatively insignificant (overly long foreskin) to the very significant (e.g. the maldescended testis with the associated increased risk of malignancy).

9.1 The penis and scrotum

Learning objectives

You should:

* Know the basic anatomy of the penis
* Have a working understanding of the common congenital and acquired disorders, in particular inflammatory and malignant diseases

The penis is a skin-covered organ (as is the scrotum) and can therefore exhibit many of the common skin disorders (e.g. eczema / dermatitis). In addition, the penile urethra may be susceptible to tumours of the urothelium (proximally) and squamous epithelium (distally).

Congenital disorders

Abnormalities include an excessively small penis (micropenis) or a urethra that opens either on the ventral (under) surface (hypospadias) or dorsal surface (epispadias) of the penis rather than at the tip.

Acquired disorders

Inflammatory disorders

The penis, foreskin and scrotum may be subject to many inflammatory skin conditions such as eczema, psoriasis and lichen planus. In addition, more-specific inflammatory diseases may cause penile (skin) inflammation.

Granuloma annulare—is caused by the gram negative bacillus *Calymmatobacterium granulomatis*, this is a sexually transmitted disease (STD) and causes an ulcer on the glans.

Lymphogranuloma venereum—is an STD, caused by *Chlamydia trachomatis* (which also causes non-specific urethritis, NSU). Males may be asymptomatic carriers of the organism. The infection causes a spontaneously healing red papule on the penis. Enlarged lymph nodes in the groin then develop, which then become soft and attach to the overlying skin. Sinus formation occurs.

Syphilis (caused by the spirochaete, *Treponema pallidum*), herpes simplex and human papilloma virus (HPV) infection are all important causes of penile infection (see Box 17).

Peyronie's disease is a penile disease of unknown cause in which the penis becomes excessively curved or bowed due to accumulation of scar tissue (the curvature may make sexual intercourse impossible).

Tumours

The penis can be affected by both in situ and invasive (squamous) malignancies. Benign tumours of the penis are rare.

Intraepithelial neoplasia

Unfortunately, there are three very confusing historical names for intraepithelial dysplasia in the region of the penis and scrotum (see Box 18).

Box 17 Penile infections

Infection	Organism	Clinical features
SYPHILIS	*Treponema pallidum* (bacterium, spirochaete)	• Rare • Penis usually involved in *primary syphilis* ('chancre' seen—nodule on penis). Heals after about 1 month. • Penis can be involved in *secondary syphilis* (papular rash)
HERPES SIMPLEX	Herpes simplex virus (herpes virus)	• Common • Painful recurrent blisters/ulcers on penile skin • May last 2–3 weeks then resolve • Virus can remain latent in sacral sensory ganglia and reactivate/recur
HUMAN PAPILLOMA VIRUS	Human papilloma virus (HPV; papillomavirus)	• Causes condylomata acuminata ('venereal warts') • Especially type 6 + 11 • Types 16 + 18 can cause premalignant and malignant conditions
CHANCROID	*Haemophilus ducreyi*	• Rare • Penile ulceration and inguinal lymphadenopathy

Box 18 Carcinoma-in-situ of the penis

On glans	On shaft	Glans + shaft
'Erythroplasia of Queyrat'	'Bowen's disease'	Bowenoid papulosis
Red patches	Pale, thickened areas	Velvety papules (younger men) HPV-associated in most cases

Squamous cell carcinoma

This is a relatively rare tumour in western countries (and very rare in circumcised males), but may occur more frequently in parts of Asia and Africa. A poorly retracting infected foreskin and infected glans are probably risk factors. There is an association between HPV 16 and 18 infection and squamous cell carcinoma. The tumour may vary from a papillary and well-differentiated malignancy with abundant keratin formation to a solid, ulcerated, widely invasive, poorly differentiated lesion (which spreads via lymphatics to local lymph nodes).

Verrucous carcinoma—is the name given to a (very) well-differentiated, squamous cell carcinoma with surface papillae and a deep, rounded, bulbous growth pattern. It is believed to be caused by HPV.

9.2 The prostate

Learning objectives

You should:

• Understand the basic anatomical relations and zones of the prostate

• Understand benign prostatic hyperplasia and carcinoma of the prostate

The prostate is a 20 g, walnut-shaped gland located in the male perineum. The exact function of the gland is still unclear. The gland lies subjacent to the bladder and is traversed by the urethra. Any enlargement of the prostate gland, particularly that part surrounding the urethra (see Fig. 28 for zones of the prostate), can lead to reduction/obstruction in flow of urine—dribbling, hesitancy, poor stream or complete blockage (retention). The prostate is composed of glandular and fibromuscular components and it is hyperplasia/hypertrophy of both of these elements and malignancy of the glandular elements that commonly lead to urinary symptoms.

Hyperplasia of the prostate

This is such a common finding in adult males that it is often considered to be a normal part of ageing (probably about 80% of 80 year olds will have evidence of prostatic hyperplasia). The prostate has a

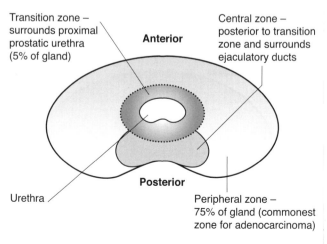

Transition zone – surrounds proximal prostatic urethra (5% of gland)

Anterior

Central zone – posterior to transition zone and surrounds ejaculatory ducts

Posterior

Urethra

Peripheral zone – 75% of gland (commonest zone for adenocarcinoma)

Fig. 28 The zones of the prostate gland.

nodular, whorled appearance to the naked eye (nodular hyperplasia). It is mainly the periurethral and transition zones that are affected. Down the microscope, the glandular and/or stromal components may be affected. The glands may become papillary in form, or cystically dilated. However, hyperplastic glands have two cell layers—an inner clear cell layer and an outer, more darkly staining, basal cell layer. Hyperplasia of the prostate is often accompanied by areas of infarction, chronic inflammation and glandular atrophy.

Acute and chronic prostatitis can also occur in the setting of UTI-type infection with organisms such as *E. coli*, *Pseudomonas* and *Klebsiella*.

Chronic granulomatous prostatitis can be due to tuberculosis but is often idiopathic and possibly due to an inflammatory response to ruptured ducts.

Carcinoma of the prostate

Carcinoma of the prostate is a very common malignancy. In the USA it is the commonest malignancy in males. The biological behaviour of this tumour is poorly understood—a significant number of latent and incidental cancers are found at autopsy or in tissue removed at operation on an apparently benign prostate (e.g. transurethral resection of the prostate, TURP). Thus, it is likely that some prostatic cancers either never progress or only do so very slowly. The disease is more common in older men (particularly those aged over 60) and is seen more often in blacks than whites or Asians. A small number of prostatic cancers appear familial. Most cases (about 70%) arise in the peripheral zone of the prostate.

Macroscopically, it is usually very difficult to see prostatic cancer (it may or may not cause gland enlargement).

Down the microscope, prostatic cancer is usually an adenocarcinoma (although leiomyosarcoma and lymphoma occur, and rhabdomyosarcoma may be seen in children). The Gleason grading system is now widely used for prostatic adenocarcinoma. This system depends on the glandular differentiation and pattern of infiltration of the tumour (see Box 19).

The higher the Gleason score (achieved by adding together the commonest two patterns or doubling a single pattern tumour) the more poorly differentiated the tumour. There is a correlation between the score of the tumour and its biological behaviour (the higher the score, the higher the cancer mortality rate). Adenocarcinoma of the prostate typically invades locally through the gland and into surrounding pelvic tissues and then by lymphatics to local/regional lymph nodes. Prostatic cancer has a propensity to metastasise via the bloodstream to bones (particularly the spine).

Box 19 Basic Gleason grading system

Gleason grade (or pattern)	Characteristics
1	UNCOMMON
	Very round, regular, monotonous, evenly spaced glands
	Well circumscribed
2	Similar to 1, BUT less circumscribed, some variation in gland size and shape
3	COMMONEST GRADE
	May be small or large glands or 'cribriform' (sieve-like) pattern
	May be marked variation in size/shape of glands
	Ragged edges and infiltrates widely
4	Glands now fused together
	Nests and streams of cells seen
5	Large sheets of malignant cells
	Necrosis may be seen
	May be very undifferentiated

Table 23 Cancer checklist: Prostatic adenocarcinoma

Incidence	age > 50 years (very common in > 80 year olds)
Risk factors	Blacks > Whites > Asians
	+family history
	?fats in diet
	?androgen-driven
Associated lesions	High grade PIN (particularly multifocal)
Clinical presentation	Incidental binding
	Urinary symptoms
Diagnosis	Per rectal examination, ultrasound scan and biopsy
	Blood levels of prostatic specific antigen (PSA)
Macroscopic	Usually invisible to the naked eye
Microscopic	Gleason scanning system (see Box 19)
Pattern of spread	Local v lymphatic v blood
Treatment	Carefully supervised 'watch and wait' (small intraprostatic lesions)
	Surgery
	Radiotherapy

9.3 The testis and epididymis

Learning objectives

You should:

- Have a working knowledge of the normal histology of the testis

- Be familiar with the basic classification of testicular tumours

The testis

Each testis is composed of densely packed, coiled, seminiferous tubules, which are lined by Sertoli cells (regulatory cells) and germ cells (which mature into spermatozoa). In the normal adult testis, luminal spermatozoa are seen. Between the tubules lies the interstitium, in which can be found Leydig cells (which secrete testosterone under the influence of luteinising hormone from the anterior pituitary gland).

Congenital abnormalities of the testis

The immature (prepubertal) testis has small seminiferous tubules, which contain mainly Sertoli cells and only a very small number of germ cells.

Cryptorchidism
In this condition, the testis (most cases are unilateral) stops somewhere along the normal pathway of descent and fails to reach the scrotum. The testis may be found in the inguinal canal or abdomen. The most serious consequence of this is the increased risk of development of testicular cancer (about 10 times that of a normal, scrotum-sited testis). Even when surgical correction occurs there is still a small increased risk of malignancy.

Torsion
Torsion of the testis, that is twisting of the spermatic cord, leading to vascular (most often venous) obstruction of the testis, is usually caused by a congenital, structural abnormality of the testis and may lead to haemorrhagic necrosis.

Inflammatory conditions

Inflammation of the epididymis is more common than the testis. There may be severe pain in the scrotal area.

Non-specific epididymitis and orchitis are usually UTI-associated. Causative bacteria include *E. coli* in older men and *Neisseria gonorrhoeae* in young adults.

Histologically, non-specific acute / acute-on-chronic inflammation may be seen, together with abscess formation and, eventually, scarring.

Granulomatous orchitis is thought to be an autoimmune reaction. The testis may be tender and granulomas are seen in and around the seminiferous tubules.

Tuberculosis (also causing a granulomatous orchitis), mumps virus and syphilis can all affect the testis.

Testicular tumours

Testicular tumours are an important cause of morbidity and mortality in young and middle-aged men. There is a wide range of tumours of the testis and the nomen-clature can be confusing and, unfortunately, different parts of the world use different systems. Most testicular tumours present as painless enlargement of the testis.

Broadly speaking, tumours of the testis can be divided into two groups:

1. Germ cell tumours (about 90%)
2. Non-germ cell tumours.

Germ cell tumours

These can be:

- seminomas
- non-seminomatous tumours
- combined seminomas and non-seminomatous tumours.

Classification of germ cell tumours of the testis
The two main classification systems are the WHO system and the British system (these are outlined in Table 24).

Both systems are based on recognition of the wide spectrum of morphological patterns seen in germ cell tumours (see Table 25). It is believed that the precursor lesion for most germ cell tumours is intratubular germ cell neoplasia. In this condition, large, pleomorphic, vacuolated, malignant cells are seen in atrophic (non-spermatozoa-producing) seminiferous tubules (often seen around invasive germ cell tumours).

Germ cell tumours tend to spread initially by lymphatics to the iliac and retroperitoneal (para-aortic) lymph nodes. Bloodstream spread occurs to the lungs, liver, bones and brain.

Clinical staging of germ cell tumour is shown in Table 26.

Other testicular tumours

These include sex cord stromal tumours, Sertoli cell tumours and lymphomas.

Table 24 Classification of germ cell tumours of the testis

British Testicular Tumour Panel	World Health Organization
Seminoma	**Seminoma**
Classical	Typical
Spermatocytic	Spermatocytic
Malignant teratoma	
Undifferentiated (MTU)	Embryonal carcinoma
Intermediate (MTI)	Embryonal carcinoma and teratoma
Differentiated (MTD)	Teratoma, mature/imature/ with malignant transformation
Trophoblastic (MTT)	Choriocarcinoma
Yolk sac tumour	**Yolk sac tumour**

Table 25 Germ cell tumours of the testis

	Seminoma	Embryonal carcinoma	Yolk sac tumour	Choriocarcinoma	Teratoma
Behaviour	Low grade malignancy	Aggressive	Variable	Very aggressive	Variable
Frequency	Commonest type of germ cell tumour		Commonest testicular tumour in infants (pure form) usually mixed with embryonal carcinoma in adults	Rare	Common. Infants to adults. Pure forms common in infants. Adults—usually mixed
Naked eye appearance	Large, white mass	Variegated appearance with haemorrhage and necrosis	Yellowish, mucinous appearance	Small haemorrhagic nodule	Large, cystic solid masses
Microscopy	Large cells with large nuclear and clear cytoplasm. Well demarcated cell membranes Fibrous septae with chronic inflammatory cells	Large, pleomorphic overlapping cells with numerous mitoses	Lacy lines of tumour cells. Pink globules (containing alpha-fetoprotein, AFP, and α_1-antitrypsin) seen in and outside cells	Cytotrophoblastic and syncytiotrophoblastic cells seen (latter contain human chorionic gonadotrophin HCG)	Haphazard arrangement of often mature tissues such as cartilage, muscle, neural tissue, fat, etc. Rarely a focus of squamous cell carcinoma or adenocarcinoma may be seen (malignant transformation)

NB. Testicular germ cell tumours secrete hormones/enzymes/proteins into the patient's blood and these can be used as a 'marker' for progression/response to treatment/relapse of the tumour. Examples include alpha-fetoprotein, human chorionic gonadotrophin and lactate dehydrogenase (LDH). Treatment/prognosis of these tumours depends on histology and extent of spread. Options include surgery alone, or with chemoradiotherapy.

Table 26 Staging of germ cell tumours

Stage	Definition
PT0	Histological scar in testis
PTis	Intratubular germ cell neoplasia
T1	Tumour confined to testis/epididymis
	No lymphatic/vascular invasion
	Tunica albuginea may be invaded
T2	As for T1, BUT lymphatic/vascular invasion seen or tumour extends through tunica albuginea and invades tunica vaginalis
T3	Tumour invades spermatic cord ± lymphatic or vascular invasion
T4	Tumour invades scrotum ± lymphatic or vascular invasion
N0	No regional lymph node metastasis
N1	Metastasis with a lymph node mass ≤ 2 cm and up to five positive nodes (≤ 2 cm)
N2	Lymph node mass > 2 cm but ≤ 5 cm, or more than five positive nodes (≤ 5 cm), or extranodal tumour spread
N3	Lymph node mass > 5 cm
M0	No distant metastases
M1	Distant metastases
M1a	Non-regional lymph nodes or lung
M1b	Other sites

NB. NX and MX not assessable.

Epididymis

The epididymis is posterolateral to the testis and functions to store, concentrate and transport spermatozoa.

The epididymis is most often affected by inflammatory conditions (epididymitis). This may then affect the testis (epididymo-orchitis). The inflammation is often bacterial in origin (*E. coli, Gonococcus* or *Chlamydia*).

Self-assessment: questions

Multiple choice questions

1. Germ cell tumours of the testis:
   a. Are most common in the over 70s
   b. May be associated with in situ malignancy
   c. Can produce HCG
   d. Are of uniformly poor prognosis
   e. Commonly spread by the lymphatics.

2. Prostatic adenocarcinoma:
   a. May be incidental
   b. Is the only cause of a raised serum PSA
   c. Is usually centrally located in the prostate gland
   d. Has a predilection for metastasising to bone
   e. Is staged using the Gleason system.

3. The following statements are correctly paired:
   a. Maldescent of the testis—increased risk of testicular lymphoma
   b. Squamous cell carcinoma of the foreskin—circumcised men
   c. Epididymitis—*E. coli* urinary tract infection
   d. Spermatocytic seminoma—widespread metastases
   e. Yolk sac tumour—α-fetoprotein production.

4. The following statements are correct:
   a. Testicular torsion is usually painless
   b. Balanitis xerotica obliterans is similar to lichen sclerosus
   c. Epispadias is a condition of the epididymis
   d. Cancer of the glans penis is usually a squamous cell carcinoma
   e. A poorly differentiated prostatic adenocarcinoma would have a Gleason score of about 8–10.

Case histories

Case history 1

A 30-year-old man noticed a steadily enlarging, painless lump in his right testis. He had no significant past medical or surgical history.

1. What are the likely differential diagnoses?
   His GP sent him for an urgent ultrasound examination and this showed a cystic and solid tumour mass. Special blood tests were performed.

2. What is the most likely diagnosis now and what 'special blood tests' would have been done?
   The following day his right testis was removed. Histology showed a malignant teratoma and areas of classical seminoma.

3. What does the term teratoma mean?

Case history 2

A 93-year-old man presented to his GP having noticed a hard, painless lump under his foreskin. He did not know how long the lump had been there. On examination, he had a craggy 15 mm mass under the foreskin.

1. What is the likely diagnosis? What are the risk factors for this?
   He was referred to a urologist who took a biopsy from the lesion. The report read:
   'This is an ulcerated, invasive, moderately differentiated squamous cell carcinoma. Tumour is seen in lymphatic channels. . . .'

2. To where is the tumour likely to spread?

Short note questions

Write short notes on:
1. Testicular swellings/tumours.
2. Prostatic adenocarcinoma.
3. Penile cancer.
4. Principles of grading and staging—use the male genital tract to illustrate your answer.

Viva questions

1. What are the risk factors for prostatic/testicular cancer?
2. What is the definition of teratoma (versus hamartoma)?
3. What are the methods of monitoring effects of treatment in prostatic and testicular cancer?

Self-assessment: answers

Multiple choice answers

1. a. **False.** Germ cell tumours of the testis are commonest in the 15–40-year-old age group. In fact, testicular tumours in men over the age of 70 are quite unusual—many turn out to be lymphomas.
   b. **True.** In many cases, In situ germ cell tumour (germ cell tumour confined inside the seminiferous tubules) will be seen around the periphery of the frankly invasive tumour. The tubules containing the tumour cells are usually atrophic (showing no spermatogenesis).
   c. **True.** Testicular seminomas may contain giant cells and syncytial-like cells (i.e. resembling normal human placental tissues) and human chorionic gonadotropin is contained in, and secreted by, these cells. This can lead to a modestly elevated level of HCG in the blood of these patients. In addition, choriocarcinoma, a highly malignant tumour made up of cytotrophoblast and syncytiotrophoblast (again tissue seen in the normal human placenta), can cause a massive outpouring of HCG into the blood stream (since urinary HCG is the basis of the pregnancy test, it is therefore possible for a man to have a positive pregnancy test). Markers like HCG can be used to monitor the success of treatment (has all the HCG-producing tumour been removed and the level therefore fallen to baseline?) and relapse (the level did fall to baseline but now it has risen again—is there a new tumour somewhere in the body?).
   d. **False.** The prognosis for many of the testicular germ cell tumours is excellent. For instance the survival for a Stage I (testis-confined) seminoma is almost 100%.
   e. **True.** Germ cell tumours spread by the lymphatics and blood stream. The common lymph node groups involved are the retroperitoneal para-aortic lymph nodes (further spread to the mediastinal and supraclavicular lymph nodes then occurs). Blood spread is to lungs, liver, central nervous system and bones.

2. a. **True.** Carcinoma of the prostate is a very common malignancy. A small, but significant, number of tumours are found incidentally (e.g. when prostatectomy tissue is examined down the microscope during life or after autopsy).
   b. **False.** An elevated PSA in the blood is not only malignancy-related. Prostatitis, and digital examination/instrumentation of the prostate are among other causes of a raised blood PSA (there is still much controversy as to whether PSA should be used as a screening test for prostatic cancer).
   c. **False.** About 70% of cases of prostatic cancer are found in the peripheral part of the gland (usually posteriorly, hence the importance of good digital rectal examination of the prostate).
   d. **True.** Prostate cancer tends to spread initially locally through the capsule into surrounding nearby structures such as the seminal vesicles and bladder. Lymphatic spread may occur to the obturator, perivesical, iliac and para-aortic lymph node groups and by the blood stream to bone (remember that cancers of the breast, kidney, thyroid, lung and prostate have a tendency to metastasise to bone). Prostatic metastases tend to induce new bone formation (i.e. they are osteoblastic).
   e. **False.** Gleason is a *grading* system NOT a *staging* system!

3. a. **False.** Abnormalities of the descent of the testis are associated with an increased risk of germ cell tumours, not lymphomas.
   b. **False.** Uncircumcised men have an increased risk of carcinoma of the foreskin/glans.
   c. **True.**
   d. **False.** Spermatocytic seminomas are a special category of seminoma. They are often found in older men and are composed of a mixed population of cells, which look like various sperm precursors. In situ germ cell tumour is not associated with these tumours, which do not metastasise.
   e. **True.** This pattern of differentiation resembles adenocarcinoma but the cells form tubules or papillae. It reflects an extraembryonic differentiation pattern. The normal human yolk sac produces α-fetoprotein (AFP) in the embryo and usually does so when malignant yolk sac tissue is produced in the testis. Again this protein will be found in the blood and can be used to monitor treatment/relapse of the tumour.

4. a. **False.** Testicular torsion is usually very painful.
   b. **True.** Balanitis xerotica obliterans (BXO) is, in fact, the male analogue of lichen sclerosus of the vulva. Neither condition is well understood. Both present as thickened, white patches and, down the microscope, show reactive/atrophic epithelial changes with a subjacent zone of hyalinised

connective tissue, below which chronic inflammation is seen. It may be a premalignant condition.

c. **False.** Epispadias and hypospadias are both conditions relating to the position of the urethral opening on the penis.

d. **True.**

e. **True.** The higher the Gleason score of a prostatic cancer, the poorer the degree of differentiation (i.e., roughly speaking, a score of 2–4 = well differentiated; 5 & 6 = moderate; and 8–10 = poorly differentiated).

Case history answers

Case history 1

1. Obviously, a full history with clinical examination is required. Often, the fact that the lump is growing and is painless is actually more worrying (and more strongly suggests cancer) than if the lump was painful (which may suggest inflammation/infection). It is probably better to assume the lump is malignant and send the patient for urgent ultrasound. This type of investigation is often conclusive as to whether the lump is benign or malignant (or inflammatory, etc.).

2. With the ultrasound results strongly suggesting this is tumour, preoperative blood tests should be done, including the 'markers' of HCG and AFP (looking for choriocarcinoma and yolk sac tumour elements in the tumour). After the operation, further imaging (of abdominal lymph node groups for instance) may be required.

3. Teratomas are tumours that show endodermal, mesodermal and ectodermal elements of differentiation. In essence, they may be *mature* (showing fully differentiated elements such as intestinal epithelium, muscle and skin), *immature* (incomplete differentiation of any of the elements of the tumour seen) or show *malignant transformation* (cancer, e.g. adenocarcinoma, seen developing in a mature teratoma). Some germ cell tumours contain both seminoma and teratoma.

Case history 2

1. This is very likely to be a squamous cell carcinoma of the glans penis. The risk factors for this tumour include:

   - uncircumcised penis
   - poor penile hygiene, with carcinogen accumulation in smegma
   - infection with HPV types 16 and 18.

2. Squamous cell carcinoma of the glans penis is usually a slow growing tumour of older men and spreads to the inguinal and iliac lymph node groups (the five-year survival rate is about 30% for tumours that have metastasised to regional lymph nodes).

Short note answers

1. With all these type of questions, it is important to set out the response in a logical fashion. Remember, common things are common. Congenital as well as acquired things should be on your list (consult surgical textbooks for comprehensive guides for examining the testis and its lumps/bumps!).

2 and 3. In these sorts of question you need to go through your 'memory jogger list' again (e.g. definition, age, sex, incidence, geography, aetiopathogenesis, macro-, micro-, spread, management) to try and shape your answer into a well-drilled, succinct response. It is worth having a set of hand-written or typed revision sheets/cards for important tumours (set out with these similar headings).

4. Applications of grading and staging is a very common question in undergraduate (and, for that matter, postgraduate) exams.

Viva answers

1. See Table 27, below.

2. A hamartoma is a mass made up of haphazardly arranged, but differentiated, tissues normally found in the area in which the mass is found. Thus, a lung hamartoma may contain a jumble of cartilage and glandular epithelium. Although it may be rapidly growing, it is not malignant.

3. Blood markers can be used (PSA in prostate cancer and AFP/HCG in testicular cancer).

Table 27 Risk factors for testicular germ cell tumours

Risk factor	Comments
Age	Peak age for germ cell tumours is 25–45 years Only yolk sac tumour is common in children
Cryptorchidism	A non-descended testis has an increased risk of developing a tumour
Genetics	Some testicular tumours are familial
Abnormally formed gonad	Testicular dysgenesis predisposes to malignancy

10 Urinary tract

Overview

The urinary tract comprises the kidneys, ureters, bladder and urethra. In males, the prostate gland surrounds a small proportion of the mid-to-lower urethra. This chapter will discuss the pathology of the kidney, ureter, bladder and urethra. Chapter 9 deals with the pathology of the prostate, testis, penis, foreskin and scrotum (i.e. the male genital tract). Some of the pathological processes of the urinary tract are very common (e.g. urinary tract infection), but some are rare (e.g. glomerulonephritis). Urine, the modified ultrafiltrate of blood produced by the kidneys, is often used to assess the general health of a person. There are many simple, colour-based 'stick tests' that enable patients and doctors to monitor substances that may leak into the urine (e.g. glucose, blood, protein).

10.1 The kidneys

Learning objectives

You should:

- Understand that many of the broader subsets of kidney disease do not fit conveniently into simple classification systems (e.g. 'inflammatory disease'). This is because diseases like glomerulonephritis and tubulointerstitial disease often have a complex aetiopathogenesis and histological appearance, which may involve two or more pathological processes, e.g. local inflammation and immunological reactions

- Know that renal diseases can be simply classified as medical, e.g. glomerulonephritis, where therapy usually relies on pharmacological treatments, or surgical, e.g. tumours or large urinary-tract stones, where an operation is often involved in the management of the patient

- Be aware that medical diseases of the kidney (and particularly the glomerulus) are often complex with a confusing nomenclature. It is much more important that you have a working understanding of the underlying basic pathological processes, rather than that you try to memorise the classification systems involved.

Structure and function

Each kidney lies in the upper retroperitoneum and has a large number of complex functions including salt and water balance and pH homeostasis. The kidneys receive about 25% of the cardiac output. With the naked eye, the kidney is seen to have a tough external capsule covering an outer 'rind' of cortex, which itself covers the inner medulla (see Fig. 29). Histologically, the kidney is made up of four discrete, but interdependent, compartments:

- glomeruli
- tubules
- interstitium
- vessels.

It is probably easiest to tackle each compartment in turn.

Glomeruli

Despite the confusing nomenclature surrounding the pathologies that affect it, the glomerulus is a relatively simple structure. The glomerulus is essentially a highly specialised, incredibly leaky, sieve under very high hydrostatic pressure. It is composed of tiny, anastomosing capillaries held together by a specialised matrix and covered by two layers of epithelium (see Fig. 30). The glomerular capillary wall is the main filtration barrier of the glomerulus and has a unique structure, directly related to its function.

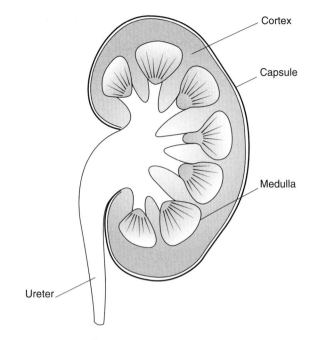

Fig. 29 Structure of the kidney.

reversible (clinically and histologically). However, chronic glomerular diseases can lead to scarring of the glomeruli, death of nephrons and eventually renal failure.

Tubules

The kidney is made up of about one million nephrons, each of which is composed, simplistically, of a glomerulus and its attached tubule (into which the filtrate from the glomerular sieve percolates). This tubule is hollow and is lined, along its complex, writhing course, by epithelial cells. Essentially, the structure of the tubular epithelial cell varies with its function (usually related to its position along the course of the tubule). The proximal tubular cells reabsorb much of the sodium, water, glucose and protein that filters through the glomerulus. It is not surprising, therefore, that their structure (microvilli projecting into the tubular lumen to increase surface area and plentiful mitochondria providing energy for absorption pumps) is much more complex than many distal tubular cells (flat, nondescript cells that may function only to 'line' the tubule and make it watertight). The specialised function and microanatomy of the proximal tubular cells can make them more susceptible to certain cellular insults such as ischaemia/poisons.

Interstitium

Previously thought to be an inert, fibrous compartment of the kidney that binds the glomeruli, tubules and vessels together, we now realise that the interstitium is very important in renal function. Indeed, scarring of the interstitium is important in the degree of impairment of

There are some general 'rules' that apply to many of the diseases that affect the glomerulus:

1. Most primary glomerular diseases are mediated by the immune system (and involve the deposition of immunoglobulins and/or complement in some part of the glomerular structure).
2. Often, glomerular diseases will present with proteinuria (if heavy, the nephrotic syndrome) or haematuria.
3. Some diseases that affect the glomerulus are relatively acute/sudden in onset and are entirely

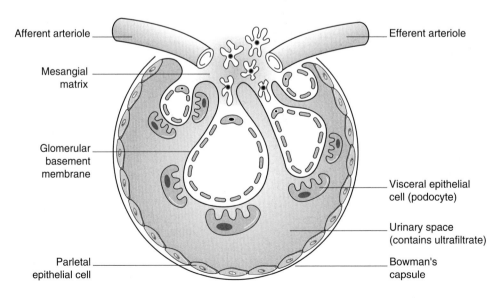

Fig. 30 Ultrastructure of the glomerulus.

renal function and progression of renal disease (see below). The cortical interstitium is very inconspicuous in the normal kidney (the tubules are virtually back-to-back), but contains peritubular capillaries and fibroblast-like cells (these latter cells communicate with each other and with their neighbouring tubular epithelial cells by means of growth factors and other molecules). In the medulla, however, the amount of interstitium increases and the tubules are more separated from each other (Fig. 31).

There are some general 'rules' that apply to many of the diseases affecting the tubules and interstitium:

1. Most diseases that affect the tubules and/or interstitium are mediated by ischaemia, toxins or infection.
2. Many diseases of the tubules and/or interstitium present as acute renal failure or abnormalities of urine volume/concentration/electrolytic composition.
3. Diseases of the tubules are potentially entirely reversible. The tubular epithelial cells are stable cells and surviving cells can, therefore, mitose and regenerate and replenish their numbers/make up new tubules. However, diseases targeting the interstitium may lead to scarring and loss of renal function.

Vessels

Combined, the kidneys weigh only a fraction of the total body weight, yet they receive 25% of the cardiac output (the cortex is much more vascular than the medulla). The kidney receives its blood supply from the main renal artery, which subdivides into anterior and posterior branches at the hilum of the kidney. There is then progressive subdivision of the arterial supply until small afferent arterioles enter the glomerulus. Efferent arterioles are formed by merging of the glomerular capillaries. These efferent arterioles form tiny calibre

plexuses of vessels, which surround cortical tubules (peritubular capillaries) and are found in the medulla (these arterial 'vasa recta' ultimately become the venous vasa recta and drain into the systemic venous system via the intrarenal veins/main renal vein).

It is important to remember that the glomerulus is a leash of capillary-sized vessels, therefore diseases that affect capillaries (e.g. vasculitis) are likely to affect the glomerulus.

The compartments of the kidney, although structurally separate, are intimately interrelated and interdependent. This means that pathology in one compartment (particularly chronic, scarring disease) will almost inevitably lead to scarring/loss of function in the other compartments. For example, chronic glomerular disease, which leads to scarring of the glomerulus, will cause atrophy of the attached tubule, scarring in the interstitium (mediated by the fibroblast-like cells) and loss of the specialised capillary plexuses. This is one of the reasons that nephrologists try to biopsy patients early in the course of their renal disease. If the disease is a chronic (potentially scarring-type) process, eventually, as nephrons are lost and the interstitium fibroses, the kidney will become a shrivelled, scarred structure and the compartment of origin of the disease will not be evident (and the initial compartment target of the disease process may be very important in the treatment/prognosis of the disease).

10.2 Congenital renal disease

Learning objectives

You should:

- Have a working knowledge of the embryology of the kidney and urinary tract

- Be able to apply this to the more common abnormalities

There are numerous possible congenital abnormalities of the kidneys from non-formation of one kidney (unilateral agenesis), which is compatible with a normal life (and may only be discovered incidentally at autopsy) to congenital absence of both kidneys, which usually leads to death in utero. Sometimes the upper or lower poles of the kidneys are fused (forming a so-called 'horseshoe kidney'). This type of kidney malformation may be found in fetuses/children who have chromosomal abnormalities such as Turner's syndrome (45 X). Congenital cystic disease of the kidney is clinically very important (see Fig. 32).

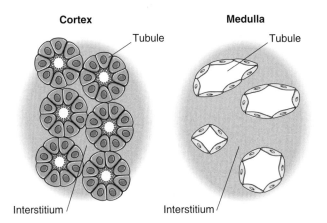

Fig. 31 The relationship between the tubules and interstitium.

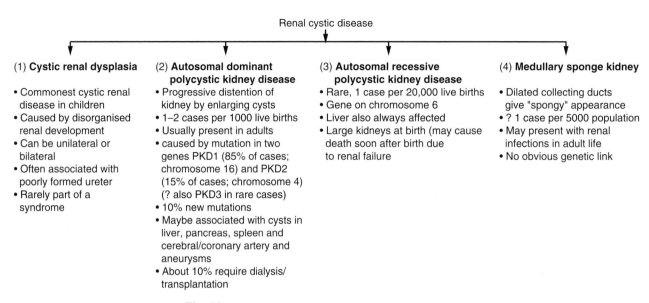

Renal cystic disease

(1) Cystic renal dysplasia

- Commonest cystic renal disease in children
- Caused by disorganised renal development
- Can be unilateral or bilateral
- Often associated with poorly formed ureter
- Rarely part of a syndrome

(2) Autosomal dominant polycystic kidney disease

- Progressive distention of kidney by enlarging cysts
- 1–2 cases per 1000 live births
- Usually present in adults
- caused by mutation in two genes PKD1 (85% of cases; chromosome 16) and PKD2 (15% of cases; chromosome 4) (? also PKD3 in rare cases)
- 10% new mutations
- Maybe associated with cysts in liver, pancreas, spleen and cerebral/coronary artery and aneurysms
- About 10% require dialysis/ transplantation

(3) Autosomal recessive polycystic kidney disease

- Rare, 1 case per 20,000 live births
- Gene on chromosome 6
- Liver also always affected
- Large kidneys at birth (may cause death soon after birth due to renal failure

(4) Medullary sponge kidney

- Dilated collecting ducts give "spongy" appearance
- ? 1 case per 5000 population
- May present with renal infections in adult life
- No obvious genetic link

Fig. 32 Common congenital cystic diseases of the kidney.

10.3 Acquired renal disease

Learning objectives

You should:

- Understand the four compartments of the kidney
- Realise their interdependence and understand the basic principles of the diseases targeting each of them

Glomerular disease

Glomerular diseases (glomerulonephritis / glomerulo-nephritides; glomerulopathy / glomerulopathies) are often caused by the immune system. Chronic glomerular disease is an important cause of chronic renal failure (CRF) worldwide. Severe chronic renal failure has a high morbidity and mortality and renal function often needs to be maintained by artificial means, either haemodialysis or peritoneal dialysis, or by kidney transplantation from a living or dead person (living-related or cadaveric transplantation). There are numerous glomerulonephritides and their nomenclature is confusing (Fig. 33).

Primary glomerulonephritis—is essentially a disease process in which the glomerulus is mainly or exclusively affected (i.e. no non-renal organs are involved), e.g. membranous glomerulonephritis.

Secondary glomerulonephritis—by contract, involves the glomerulus being affected as part of a widespread, multisystem disease, e.g. diabetes mellitus, amyloidosis and systemic lupus erythematosus (SLE), all of which can affect many organs including the lung, liver, kidney, etc.).

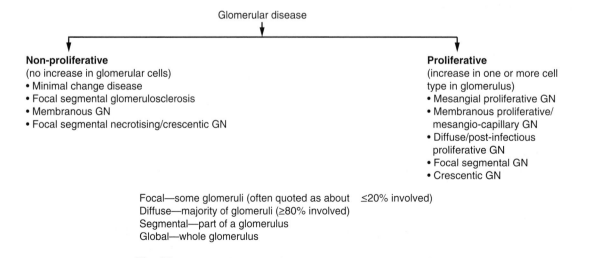

Glomerular disease

Non-proliferative
(no increase in glomerular cells)
- Minimal change disease
- Focal segmental glomerulosclerosis
- Membranous GN
- Focal segmental necrotising/crescentic GN

Proliferative
(increase in one or more cell type in glomerulus)
- Mesangial proliferative GN
- Membranous proliferative/ mesangio-capillary GN
- Diffuse/post-infectious proliferative GN
- Focal segmental GN
- Crescentic GN

Focal—some glomeruli (often quoted as about ≤20% involved)
Diffuse—majority of glomeruli (≥80% involved)
Segmental—part of a glomerulus
Global—whole glomerulus

Fig. 33 Example of the classification of glomerulonephritis (GN).

Aetiopathogenesis of primary glomerulonephritis

Most forms of primary glomerular disease appear to be mediated, in some way, by the immune system. Unfortunately, in most cases, we do not know what causes the immune 'attack'. However, a number of 'tests' are performed on renal biopsies and this has helped in our understanding of glomerular disease. The biopsy is stained with a number of 'routine' stains (e.g. haematoxylin and eosin) and 'special stains', e.g. Congo red for amyloid and Martius yellow–scarlet–blue (MSB) for fibrin, which allow recognition of the nucleus and cytoplasm of cells, as well as the deposition of matrix and the presence of necrosis when looking at the biopsy down the light microscope. In addition, and importantly in defining the aetiopathogenesis of glomerular disease, highly specialised immunohistological techniques (e.g. immunoperoxidase or immunofluorescence) are used, which allow human immunoglobulin and complement components to be visualised in the biopsy. Electron microscopy (EM) is also performed, and gives very high magnification of the renal structures (and particularly the glomerulus) allowing extremely accurate assessment of the pathological processes, including the site of deposition of the immune complexes.

Using these immunological and ultrastructural techniques (and a wealth of information from experimental models of glomerular disease), it is apparent that there are several possible mechanisms by which immune-mediated glomerular disease occurs:

Pre-formed circulating immune complexes—(made up of antibody and antigen) may lodge in any part of the glomerulus and set up a chain of reactions leading to a change in the fine structure/charge of the glomerulus, with altered function. This type of scenario probably occurs in SLE (where the antigen that sets up this reaction is likely to be normal nuclear-associated protein) and some glomerular diseases associated with infections (e.g. hepatitis B; here the foreign antigen is part of the virus).

Immune complexes may be formed in the glomerulus —(i.e. in-situ immune complex formation rather than circulating immune complexes). In this case, antibodies against certain components of the glomerulus are found in the circulation and these attack normal constituents of the glomerulus (e.g. antiglomerular basement membrane disease; in this disease, antibodies attack part of the Type IV collagen molecule in the glomerular basement membrane). Alternatively, the antibodies may 'home in' on proteins that have become stuck in the glomerulus because of their physicochemical properties (e.g. certain parts of bacterial cell walls may have a positive charge, bind to negative charges in the glomerulus and then be attacked by antibodies).

No immune complexes—it is now well established that certain glomerular diseases (e.g. minimal change disease) show no evidence of immune complex deposition (using the immunohistological/ultrastructural techniques described above). It is postulated that these diseases may be mediated by T-cells or macrophages (or, more specifically, signalling molecules produced by these cells).

Types of glomerulonephritis

As can be seen from Figure 33, there are numerous forms of glomerular disease and it is beyond the scope of this book to detail them all. However, four types of glomerulonephritis will be discussed in an attempt to illustrate important aspects of glomerular pathology:

1. Post-infectious glomerulonephritis
2. Minimal change disease
3. Membranous glomerulonephritis
4. IgA disease.

Post-infectious glomerulonephritis (PIG)

Often considered to be the prototypic glomerular disease, PIG can occur after a very large number of infections (mainly bacterial). Classically, the disease occurs in children/young adults and follows a sore throat caused by a Group A β-haemolytic *Streptococcus*. There is a time lag of about 1–2 weeks between the sore throat (often a very bad one) and a feeling of being unwell with the appearance of red- or cola-coloured urine (macroscopic haematuria), poor urine output (oliguria) and a mild-to-moderate elevation of protein excretion (proteinuria). Some patients have high blood pressure (the combination of haematuria, oliguria and hypertension is known as the nephritic syndrome).

Renal biopsy will usually show enlarged, hypercellular glomeruli, which contain numerous neutrophils and increased numbers of swollen endothelial cells with proliferating mesangial cells. Immunohistological stains reveal IgG, IgM and C3 in glomerular capillary walls and mesangial regions and electron microscopy (EM) will show these immune deposits as electron dense (black) humps on the epithelial side of the glomerular basement membrane (GBM) as well as deposits in the subendothelial and mesangial regions.

Interestingly, the vast majority of patients will get entirely better—the hypercellular glomeruli will return to normal (cell death by apoptosis) and the deposits will be cleared by phagocytosis (mesangial cells are phagocytic). A very small number of (often older) patients may develop very profound renal failure and go on to have chronic renal failure with the need for dialysis/transplantation.

Minimal change disease (MCD)

This is the commonest cause of the nephrotic syndrome in children (especially in 2–5 year olds). Nephrotic syndrome is defined as heavy protein loss in the urine with low levels of albumin in the blood and peripheral oedema as a consequence of the reduced colloid osmotic pressure. Down the microscope, this disease is characterised by normal-looking glomeruli (the tubules, interstitium and vessels are also usually normal). Classically, immunohistological stains are negative (i.e. there are no immune complexes in the glomeruli). The only significant finding is foot process fusion (spreading of the pedicels, leading to apparent loss of the 'feet' on which the podocyte stands on the GBM), seen on EM (this is actually a non-specific finding as foot process fusion is seen in most glomerular diseases where there is heavy proteinuria). In the majority of patients, there is a very good response to oral corticosteroid administration (although the disease may recur when the steroids are reduced/withdrawn).

Membranous glomerulonephritis (MGN)

MGN is the commonest cause of the nephrotic syndrome in adults. In established MGN, light microscopy classically shows glomeruli with thick capillary walls. The glomerulus is otherwise normal. A special silver deposition stain will show epithelial-directed 'spikes' poking out from the glomerular basement membrane. Immunohistologically, there is immunoglobulin (often IgG) and complement (C3) deposition along/in the capillary walls. EM reveals variably-sized subepithelial or intramembranous electron-dense deposits (see Fig. 34). The 'spikes' seen on light microscopy represent 'fingers' and 'tongues' of glomerular basement membrane insinuating up between the deposits. The disease is idiopathic in about 85% of patients, but can be associated with drugs (e.g. penicillamine), tumours (e.g. lung cancer), infections (e.g. HIV and hepatitis B), and SLE. Prognosis depends, at least in part, on the underlying disease, but at least one-third of idiopathic patients will eventually require dialysis or transplantation.

IgA disease (IgAD)

A relatively recently described glomerulonephritis (by Berger in 1967), IgAD is thought to be the most common glomerulonephritis in the world. It tends to affect young men and may present as macroscopic haematuria, which comes on at almost the same time as an upper respiratory tract infection (compare PIG). By light microscopy, the glomeruli show a variable increase in mesangial cells (this may affect only part of some glomeruli, i.e. be a focal and segmental process). By immunohistological techniques the expanded, hypercellular mesangial regions are seen to be full of granules of IgA (often accompanied by C3) and EM confirms mesangial electron-dense deposits. The cause of the IgA deposition is still uncertain (but it is likely to be related to increased mucosal IgA production/decreased hepatic metabolism). Initially, it was thought that IgAD was a recurrent, but benign, process. However, it is now known that a significant number of patients will ultimately require long-term dialysis or transplantation.

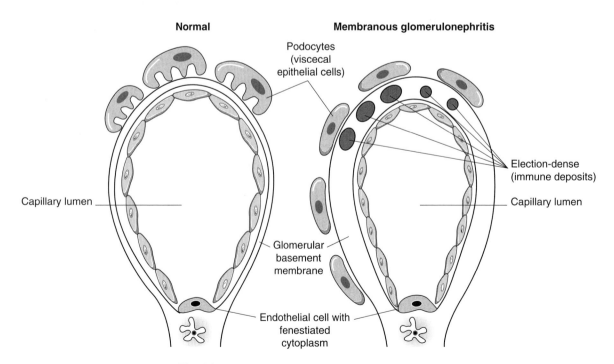

Fig. 34 Deposits in membranous glomerulonephritis.

Tubular disease

Probably the most important tubular disease in clinical practice is acute tubular necrosis (ATN). ATN is the commonest cause of acute renal failure (ARF). As the name suggests, there is death of tubular epithelial cells. However, tubular epithelial cells are stable cells. These cells are normally in the G0 phase of the cell cycle and will only become actively mitotic if stimulated to do so. ATN is such a stimulus, causing preserved epithelial cells to mitose. There are two main categories of ATN:

1. Nephrotoxic
2. Ischaemic.

Nephrotoxic ATN—can be caused by a very wide range of drugs, chemicals and poisons. Examples include: gentamicin, an antibiotic used widely in hospitals; contrast media used for radiological investigations, such as an intravenous pyelogram (IVP) used for examining renal and urinary tract structures; toxins such as ethylene glycol, used in antifreeze solutions; and substances found in some types of mushroom.

Ischaemic ATN—is most often associated with 'shock' (particularly related to burns, sepsis or haemorrhage).

The actual pathogenesis of the ARF in ATN is still uncertain; theories range from physical obstruction of tubular lumina (by shedding of dead cells/debris) to alterations in intrarenal vascular tone and glomerular ultrafiltration (see physiology textbooks for details).

Interstitial disease

It is important to realise the very close relationship between the interstitium and the tubules. The intimacy of the relationship is shown by the fact that even in ATN, a tubule-centred disease process, there is often (reactive) oedema and mild inflammation in the interstitium. It is no surprise, therefore, that in disease processes which target the interstitium, some form of tubular damage can often be seen. Interstitial diseases (interstitial nephritis or tubulointerstitial disease) are usually subdivided into acute and chronic processes.

Acute interstitial nephritis (AIN)

The patient may present with ARF. There is expansion of the interstitium by oedema and inflammatory cells. Often neutrophils (acute inflammatory cells) are quite sparse and the dominant cells are actually lymphocytes, plasma cells and eosinophils. There is acute damage to tubules. The causes of AIN include:

- drugs, e.g. non-steroidal anti-inflammatory drugs (NSAIDs) and antibiotics, especially penicillins (in drug-induced AIN eosinophils are often very conspicuous)
- infections (acute pyelonephritis should be excluded, see below), e.g. leptospirosis.

A significant number of cases will be idiopathic.

Chronic interstitial nephritis (CIN)

The patient is likely to suffer from chronic renal failure (CRF). Rather non-specific features are seen histologically with small, shrunken (atrophic) tubules, interstitial chronic inflammation and scarring. Causes include:

- progression of AIN
- toxic damage, e.g. by mercury, lead or lithium
- chronic pyelonephritis (see below)
- tuberculosis.

Vascular disease

The kidney is not protected from systemic vascular diseases (it is important to remember that the kidney contains a wide range of vessels from large renal arteries to the tiny glomerular and peritubular capillaries). Hypertension, vasculitis, emboli and diabetes mellitus will all affect the kidney (see Chapters 1 and 6 for further details).

Thrombotic microangiopathies (e.g. haemolytic uraemic syndrome and thrombotic thrombocytopenic purpura) are so-called because these diseases affect small vessels and lead to thrombus formation. The 'trigger factor' may be an infection or an inborn abnormality in the clotting/anti-clotting cascades, which leads to endothelial cell injury with subsequent platelet aggregation.

Pyelonephritis

Pyelonephritis literally means inflammation of the renal pelvis and kidney and is best considered as a separate entity (rather than being classified as a specific tubular, interstitial or tubulointerstitial disease). Classically, it is subdivided into acute and chronic forms:

Acute pyelonephritis (APN)—acute pus-forming inflammation of the renal pelvis and kidney. This occurs in the context of urinary tract infection (UTI), see Box 20. The diagnosis of APN is made by clinico-pathological-radiological methods (the renal pelvis may appear thickened and distorted).

Most commonly, bacterial colonisation of the distal urinary tract (urethra and bladder in women, bladder in men) can lead to ascending infection with infected urine refluxing up the ureters into the kidney itself (particularly to the poles of the kidney). The common organisms include *E. coli*, *Proteus* species and *Enterobacter*. Patients often present with loin pain, fevers, rigors and pain on micturition (dysuria).

Rarely, haematogenous spread of organisms can lead to them settling in the renal pelvis/kidney and setting up an inflammatory response. This most often occurs in septicaemia or infective endocarditis, when infected emboli from the heart valves may lodge in small-calibre renal vessels.

Down the microscope, pus may be seen in the renal tubules with oedema and (acute) inflammation of the interstitium. Tubular necrosis may be seen, but the glomeruli are usually normal. Severe, untreated disease may lead to abscess formation in the renal pelvis/kidney (pyonephrosis), death of the renal papillae (papillary necrosis) and even perinephric abscess formation. The inflammation in APN usually responds to the appropriate antibiotic, but repeated (untreated) attacks can lead to renal scarring and chronic pyelonephritis (see below).

Chronic pyelonephritis (CPN)—this diagnosis is made by patho-radiological means. Classically, the radiological appearances are of deformed, scarred kidneys/kidneys with blunted calyces and histologically there is tubular atrophy or dilatation (with large hyaline casts) and chronic interstitial inflammation/scarring. CPN is an important cause of CRF. Some authorities subdivide CPN into obstructive- and reflux-associated (see Fig. 35 and section on the bladder below).

Renal stones

Stones (calculi) are a relatively common problem in the urinary tract and occur most commonly in the kidneys, ureters or bladder. They can cause problems such as pain, bleeding and obstruction. Most stones (75%) are calcium-containing, and associated with hypercalcaemia/hypercalciuria. A minority (about 15%) are composed of magnesium ammonium phosphate, urate or cystine.

Tumours of the kidney

Benign tumours

See Table 28.

Malignant tumours

The two most important malignant tumours of the kidney are renal cell carcinoma and transitional cell carcinoma.

Renal cell carcinoma
This is the commonest renal malignancy (85% of all renal cancers) and may occur in young patients in the setting of genetic syndromes such as von Hippel–Lindau syndrome (when the tumour may be multiple and bilateral and the patients are usually carefully screened for the tumour). In sporadic (i.e. non-familial) cases, the tumour may be picked up during investigation for other diseases (e.g. abdominal ultrasound scan done for abdominal pain). The tumour may cause haematuria or paraneoplastic symptoms such as fever and polycythaemia or hypercalcaemia. The tumour is more common in males and has a peak incidence in the fifth and sixth decades. Macroscopically, the tumour is most often well circumscribed, yellow, with areas of haemorrhage, necrosis and cyst formation. Histologically, there are several subtypes, but the commonest is the clear cell (conventional) renal cell carcinoma. Renal cell carcinomas tend to spread by the blood stream and may spread up the inferior vena cava as far as the right atrium.

The prognosis depends on factors such as the size, nuclear grade and local/distant spread of the tumour.

Transitional cell carcinoma
This tumour arises in the renal pelvis from the urothelium, and makes up about 10% of all renal cancers. The tumour may present with haematuria or obstruction of the kidney. The tumour is mainly found in older

---

Box 20 Urinary tract infections (UTIs)

Definition	Infection of any part of the urinary tract; commonly bladder (cystitis) and kidney (pyelonephritis)
Types	UTIs may be asymptomatic or, more usually, symptomatic (pain, frequency of micturition, fevers)
Sex predilection	Females (rarely male infants/older males)
Organisms	Most often bacteria, commonly gut/perineal organisms (*E. coli*, *Proteus*, *Klebsiella*)
Predisposing factors	Urological procedures/operations (e.g. catheterisation of bladder) Obstruction to outflow Pregnancy Congenital abnormalities of the genital tract (posterior urethral valves in young boys) Vesicoureteric reflux (pyelonephritis) Diabetes mellitus Immunosuppression
Pathology	Congestion/granularity of bladder/kidney Pus formation Neutrophils in urine/tissues
Sequelae	May lead to chronic cystitis or pyelonephritis

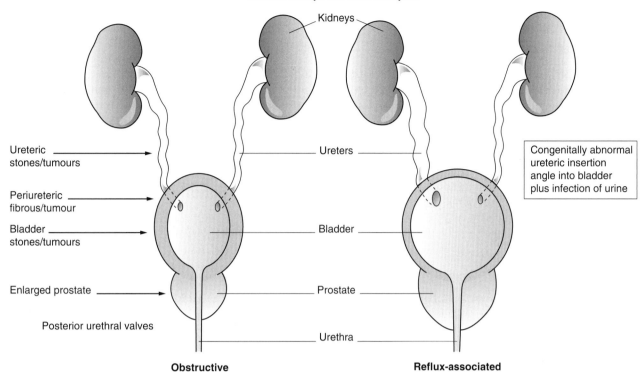

Scarred kidneys with blunted calyces

Kidneys

Ureteric stones/tumours

Periureteric fibrous/tumour

Bladder stones/tumours

Enlarged prostate

Posterior urethral valves

Ureters

Congenitally abnormal ureteric insertion angle into bladder plus infection of urine

Bladder

Prostate

Urethra

Obstructive

Reflux-associated

Fig. 35 Chronic pyelonephritis (CPN).

patients. Histologically, tumours may vary from well differentiated, non-invasive, papillary tumours to poorly differentiated, solid lesions, which widely invade the wall of the renal pelvis and/or the kidney.

The prognosis will depend particularly on the stage of the tumour (see also bladder tumours).

Wilms' tumour (nephroblastoma)
In children this is the commonest malignant tumour of the kidney. The tumour is derived from the embryonic components of the kidney and occurs mainly in young children (less than 5 years of age). Mutations in the tumour suppressor gene WT1 (found on chromosome 11) are thought to be important in tumorigenesis. Prognosis (and treatment) depends on the degree of spread (stage) of the tumour and whether or not it contains high grade areas ('anaplasia').

10.4 The ureters

Learning objectives

You should:

- Know the normal histology and function of the ureters

- Have a basic knowledge of congenital and acquired abnormalities of the ureter

Table 28 Benign tumours of the kidney*

Structure	Possible benign tumours
Renal capsule/perinephric fat	Fibroma, leiomyoma, lipoma
Renal parenchyma	Adenoma (often defined as a very small renal cell carcinoma < 0.5 cm in diameter; these tiny lesions very rarely metastasise)
	Oncocytoma (some authorities believe that these tumours virtually never metastasise)
	Angiomyolipoma (may be seen in tuberose sclerosis; considered by some authorities to be a hamartoma)
Renal vessels	Haemangioma

*As in all organs, benign tumours can arise from any of the anatomical structures of the kidney

These epithelium-lined, muscular tubes convey the urine form the kidney to the bladder.

Congenital abnormalities

There are many congenital abnormalities of the ureters from reduplication to stenosis and atresia. Congenital pelviureteric junction obstruction may be picked up in utero as hydronephrosis.

Acquired abnormalities

Many of the acquired abnormalities of the ureters lead to obstruction (see Table 29).

10.5 The bladder

Learning objectives

You should:

- Have a sound knowledge of the normal anatomical relations and histology of the bladder

- Have a working knowledge of the important congenital abnormaltites of the bladder

- Be acquainted with the important acquired bladder diseases (particularly inflammation-related and tumours)

The mature urinary bladder is essentially a distensible, muscular bag found in the pelvis. Urine is conveyed to the bladder by the ureters. The lining of the urinary bladder (and that of the ureters, renal pelvis and proximal urethra) is transitional cell epithelium (urothelium). Irrespective of its site, the urothelium is a watertight, multilayered epithelium covered by large specialised cells called 'umbrella cells'. The urothelium rests on a basal lamina and subjacent to this is the lamina propria (in which is found loose connective tissue, thin-walled blood vessels, twigs of smooth muscle and scattered inflammatory cells). There is a thick muscular coat to the human bladder (detrusor muscle), which consists of interwoven bundles. This allows complete emptying of the bladder. The bladder is innervated by both sympathetic and parasympathetic fibres originating from T11 to S4.

Congenital abnormalities

There are numerous congenital abnormalities of the bladder, including diverticula and fistulas (an important example is a fistula between the bladder and umbilicus, persistent urachus). Exstrophy is a rare, but important, abnormality in which there is absence of part of the anterior abdominal wall and anterior (ventral) bladder wall with eversion and exteriorisation of the rest of the urinary bladder. Other urinary tract and non-urinary tract abnormalities are often associated with exstrophy.

Vesicoureteric reflux (VUR) is also an important congenital abnormality. This may be caused by abnormal positioning (altered angle of entry) of one or both ureters as they course into the bladder wall (to open into the trigone of the bladder). Severe VUR can lead to UTI, reflux-type CPN and advanced renal scarring in children (see section on pyelonephritis above).

Acquired abnormalities

The most important acquired pathologies of the bladder are inflammation (cystitis) and neoplasms (transitional cell carcinoma, TCC). As in other sites along the urinary tract, stones can also cause problems.

Table 29 Abnormalities of the ureters

Congenital		Acquired	
Mega ureter	Large, dilated ureters	Ureteric obstruction due to abnormalities:	
Ureteral stricture or valves	Congenital narrowing of the ureter or 'flaps' obstructing lumen	in lumen of ureter	Stones, fragments of renal papillae (sickle cell disease)
Diverticula	Outpouchings made up of all layers of the ureteral wall	of ureteric wall	Inflammation/scarring tumours (benign or malignant)
Duplication	Double ureters on either one or both sides	from outside ureter	Inflammation/scarring/tumour (can cause dilatation above blockage)

Cystitis

Inflammation of the bladder is common. Usually it is bacterial in origin. Bacterial colonisation of the urine may be asymptomatic (e.g. as has been found when screening the urine of normal schoolgirls) or symptomatic (features include pain on micturition and increased frequency of passing urine). The diagnosis is, not surprisingly, made on examination of a urine sample, which will show large numbers of bacteria. These bacteria are usually intestinal in origin with *E. coli* being the commonest. Cystitis/UTI is more common in women (presumed to be because of the shorter female urethra), but becomes more frequent in older males (presumed to be secondary to bladder outflow obstruction, which occurs with an enlarging prostate). Any trauma to, or congenital/acquired abnormalities of, the bladder often increases the risk of cystitis/UTI.

Bladder biopsies taken during an 'attack' of cystitis often show rather non-specific features such as congestion or acute or chronic inflammation.

Infection/inflammation of the bladder can also be caused by *Mycobacterium tuberculosis* (usually by way of infected urine from a tuberculous kidney), *Candida* species (especially in neonates and the immunosuppressed) and schistosomes (in particular, *Schistosoma haematobium* causing Bilharzia). Adenovirus infection can also cause cystitis.

Cystitis may also be caused by non-infective agents such as radiation and drugs (e.g. cyclophosphamide causing haemorrhagic cystitis).

Two 'special' forms of cystitis are important to know:

1. **Interstitial cystitis (sometimes called Hunner's ulcer)**—usually occurs in middle-aged women and often causes pain. Histologically there may be ulceration of the urothelium and mast cells are very numerous, particularly in the muscular layer.
2. **Malacoplakia**—this appears to be a reaction to bacterial infection. The bladder shows yellow patches on the urothelium and down the microscope numerous foamy and granular macrophages are seen containing intracellular structures (partially digested bacterial debris) called Michaelis–Guttmann bodies. Malacoplakia is not confined to the kidney, but may be found widely in the urinary tract, lungs or bones.

Tumours of the bladder

Benign tumours of the bladder
These are rare, but include haemangiomas, neurofibromas and paragangliomas.

Malignant tumours of the bladder
By far the commonest malignant tumour of the bladder in adults is the urothelial-derived transitional cell carcinoma (TCC).

However, in the paediatric age group a common malignant tumour of the bladder is the rhabdomyosarcoma (see Box 21).

Transitional cell carcinoma-in-situ (TCCis)—believed by many authorities to precede the development of TCC in some patients (as evidenced by the presence of TCCis in the majority of cases of TCC), TCCis is characterised by flat and thickened or gently undulating full-thickness dysplastic urothelium (nuclear pleomorphism, abnormal mitoses and apoptotic figures are seen). Often appearing as a red patch, the disease may be multifocal within the bladder.

Transitional cell carcinoma (TCC)—overall, TCC accounts for about 5% of all malignancies in adults in the UK. Most patients are over 50 years of age and there are definite risk factors for development of TCC, the most important of which are shown in Box 22. The tumour may present with haematuria, frequency or urgency. TCC may be multifocal either within the bladder or the urinary tract.

As in other parts of the urothelium-lined urinary tract, the tumour can have a very varied appearance, both macroscopically (fronded and seaweed-like to solid) and microscopically (well differentiated and papillary to poorly differentiated and widely muscle-invasive). The grading and staging system for bladder TCC is shown in Box 23, together with prognosis.

Numerous cytogenetic and molecular alterations have been found in TCC, including monosomy or deletions of the short (p) or long (q) arm of chromosome 9 and deletions of 17p (which involves the *p53* gene).

Squamous metaplasia of the urothelium can occur in a variety of circumstances, for example as a response to

Box 21 Bladder rhabdomyosarcoma	
Definition	Malignant mesenchymal tumour, showing evidence of skeletal muscle differentiation
Age group	Usually ≤ 5 years old
	Male > female
Naked-eye appearance	May look like a 'polyp' or 'bunch of grapes' protruding into the bladder lumen
Microscopic appearance	May have very cellular areas and acellular areas
	Malignant cells may be small and nondescript or 'strap like', or even look like mature skeletal muscle
Prognosis	Generally good but depends on subtype and stage

Box 22 Confirmed or suspected risk factors for transitional cell carcinoma of the bladder

Smoking	Increases risk up to five times
Analgesics	Mainly associated with renal pelvis transitional cell carcinoma, but also bladder tumours
Occupation	Workers in aniline dye, rubber and chemical industries due to exposure to β-naphthylanine (which in the liver is converted to a carcinogen that must be activated in the bladder) These workers need regular bladder checks
Cyclophosphamide	Can cause bladder cancer in the long term (although used for cancer treatment)
Schistosomiasis	Causes chronic inflammation and metaplasia (squamous) of the bladder mucosa (leading to squamous cell carcinoma)
Chronic infections/ inflammation	Some authorities believe that any chronic inflammatory process may predispose to cancer

Box 23 Grading and staging of bladder transitional cell carcinoma (TNM)

Grade	Definition
G1	Well differentiated
G2	Moderately differentiated
G3	Poorly differentiated/undifferentiated

Stage	Definition
Tis	In situ carcinoma
Ta	Non-invasive, papillary tumour
T1	Tumour invades subepithelial connective tissue
T2	Tumour invades muscularis propria
T3	Tumour invades beyond muscularis propria
T4	Tumour invades prostate, uterus, vagina or pelvic wall/abdominal wall
N1	Single lymph node metastasis ($\leq$ 2 cm)
N2	Single metastasis (> 2 cm) or multiple metastases ($\leq$ 5 cm)
N3	Multiple metastases (> 5 cm)

Prognosis
- About half (or more) of all newly diagnosed bladder TCCs are G1 or G2, Ta or T1 (good prognosis)
- Most patients who have had a G1/G2 Ta/T1 tumour and have a recurrence will have another similar tumour
- 10% of patients with these tumours eventually develop invasive or metastatic tumours (poor prognosis)
- About 25% of newly diagnosed bladder TCCs will be muscle invasive (and G2/G3), and about half will have metastases
- Most patients with metastatic bladder TCC die within five years

bladder stones, indwelling catheters and infection by *Schistosoma* (schistosomiasis is endemic in countries such as Egypt). Under these circumstances, squamous cell carcinoma of the bladder can develop. Often this tumour has invaded the bladder wall at presentation.

10.6 The urethra

Learning objectives

You should:

- Know the normal anatomy and histology of the urethra
- Know the principal diseases that affect this structure

The mature male urethra is lined predominantly by transitional epithelium and has a spindle-shaped expansion in its prostatic portion (the verumontanum) into which the ejaculatory ducts drain. The distal end of the penile urethra is lined by squamous epithelium. The female urethra is much shorter than in the male and is lined mainly by squamous epithelium.

Inflammation of the urethra is relatively common (but rarely biopsied) and is caused by gonococci (gonorrhoea, *Neisseria*) and non-gonococcal organisms (such as *E. coli*, *Chlamydia* and *Mycoplasma*).

A urethral caruncle is essentially a painful, red, polypoid nodule found in females at the urethral meatus (it may represent inflamed, prolapsed tissue). The lesion is usually about 1 cm in diameter and excision is curative.

Urethral malignancies are rare. Squamous cell carcinoma of the distal urethra is the commonest.

Self-assessment: questions

Multiple choice questions

1. Concerning the kidney:
   a. There are approximately 1000 nephrons in each kidney
   b. The glomerular basement membrane is a positively charged filtration unit
   c. The tubular compartment is the largest, by volume, in the kidney
   d. Acute renal failure may be caused by drugs
   e. Chronic renal failure inevitably leads to dialysis or transplantation.

2. The following statements are correct:
   a. Membranous glomerulonephritis is the commonest cause of the adult nephrotic syndrome
   b. Minimal change disease is immune complex-mediated
   c. The glomerular basement membrane is full of cationic macromolecules
   d. Post-infectious glomerulonephritis is usually triggered by viruses
   e. IgA disease is a rare form of glomerulonephritis.

3. Acute pyelonephritis:
   a. Is commonly due to blood spread of organisms to the kidney
   b. Is commoner in men than women
   c. Is often caused by *E. coli*
   d. Even if promptly treated results in scarring of the kidney
   e. Classically results in two small, but symmetrical, kidneys.

4. Concerning the renal tubules and interstitium:
   a. Tubular diseases are usually immune complex-mediated
   b. Interstitial nephritis may be caused by non-steroidal anti-inflammatory drugs (NSAIDs)
   c. The amount of inflammation and scarring in the interstitium is important in the progression of renal disease
   d. Acute tubular necrosis (ATN) is usually irreversible and leads to permanent kidney damage
   e. Granulomas may be seen in the interstitium in renal sarcoidosis.

5. The following are correctly paired:
   a. Renal cell carcinoma—schistosomal infestation
   b. Renal angiomyolipoma—massive haemorrhage
   c. Transitional cell carcinoma of the bladder—cigarette smoking
   d. Wilms' tumour—nephroblastoma
   e. Malacoplakia—malignant tumour of B lymphocytes

6. The following statements are correct:
   a. Diabetes mellitus is a cause of hyaline arteriolosclerosis
   b. Haemodialysis is the only method of long-term renal replacement therapy
   c. Renal amyloidosis is seen in patients with multiple myeloma
   d. Vesicoureteric reflux may lead to kidney scarring in children
   e. Acute renal failure is commonly caused by IgA disease.

Case histories

Case history 1

A 75-year-old man presents to his GP with a three-month history of feeling generally unwell. He has noted that both his legs are puffy and he thinks his urine seems rather frothy. Blood tests show that his albumin is 9 g/L (normal about 40) and his urine contains about 10 g/L of protein.

1. What is the syndrome that this patient is suffering from called?
   His renal function (i.e. creatinine clearance) is normal and he has a renal biopsy.
2. What is the likeliest cause of his syndrome?
   He is treated appropriately, but three months later is found to have lung cancer.
3. What is the relationship between the tumour and his renal disease?

Case history 2

Whilst having a routine life assurance medical, a 52-year-old man is found to present with haematuria.

1. List the common causes of haematuria in this man.
   Further tests show that he has a 10 cm mass replacing one pole of his right kidney.
2. What could this mass be?
   A biopsy of the mass is performed and it is found to be a renal cell carcinoma. At operation, it appears to have invaded into the right renal vein.

3. How do renal cell carcinomas spread?
4. What is understood by the 'stage' of a tumour?

Short note questions

1. Briefly describe the possible mechanisms of pathogenesis of immune-mediated glomerulonephritis.
2. Write short notes an pyelonephritis.
3. Write short notes an bladder cancer.

Viva questions

Discuss:
1. Grading and staging of urinary tract tumours.
2. UTIs and common organisms/complications.
3. The immune system and glomerular disease.

Self-assessment: answers

Multiple choice answers

1. a. **False.** The quoted figure is 1 000 000.
   b. **False.** The glomerular basement membrane is certainly a charge-selective filtration barrier. However, it is full of *negatively* charged macromolecules such as collagen and heparan sulphate.
   c. **True.**
   d. **True.** Drugs (often widely used drugs such as non-steroidal anti-inflammatories, NSAIDs) can cause acute renal failure (often by provoking an interstitial nephritis). It is important to remember that ARF can be classified as:
   - pre-renal, i.e. caused by poor perfusion of the kidney as seen in severe heart failure or patients with extensive burns
   - renal, i.e. the abnormality causing renal dysfunction is in the kidney itself, e.g. glomerulonephritis
   - post-renal, i.e. usually caused by relatively sudden blockage to urine flow, e.g. prostatic enlargement with urine retention.
       In any of these instances, there may be dramatic, life-threatening alterations in electrolyte, water and acid–base balance. Acute renal failure is a medical emergency.
   e. **False.** There are many patients with renal disease who have impaired renal function, but it is not severe enough to require dialysis or transplantation. Chronic renal failure will often be characterised by a slow, predictable decline in renal function, which can be monitored by urea and creatinine levels in the blood. There will be wide-ranging changes in salt and water, acid–base and calcium and phosphate homeostasis (to name but a few). Chronic renal failure is also a cause of (normocytic normochromic) anaemia.

2. a. **True.** The nephrotic syndrome is defined as heavy proteinuria (the cut off point is often quoted as 3.5 g/day) combined with hypoalbuminaemia and peripheral oedema. In addition, nephrotic patients often have hypercholesterolaemia and a tendency to thrombosis.
   b. **False.** No immune complexes can be demonstrated.
   c. **False.** Cationic molecules are *positively* charged.
   d. **False.** PIG is usually triggered by bacteria (especially Group A β-haemolytic streptococci).
   e. **False.** Many authorities believe it is the commonest glomerulopathy in the world.

3. a. **False.** Ascending infection is far more common.
   b. **False.** Females are far more likely to suffer urinary tract infections (UTIs) than men and acute pyelonephritis is a sequel to this. This is probably due, at least in part, to the shorter urethra in females.
   c. **True.**
   d. **False.** Early treatment should lead to complete resolution of the inflammatory process.
   e. **False.** Interestingly, recurrent attacks of acute pyelonephritis may lead to chronic pyelonephritis and scarred kidneys, but there is usually asymmetrical, coarse scarring. Thus, one kidney may be very shrivelled and shrunken (perhaps because there was severe bladder-to-ureter-to-kidney reflux on this side) while the other is relatively normal or shows only one or two small scars. In chronic glomerular diseases and hypertension the kidneys become symmetrically reduced in size with a finely granular surface (due to loss of nephrons).

4. a. **False.** They are usually caused by ischaemia, toxins and infections.
   b. **True.**
   c. **True.**
   d. **False.** Many cases of acute renal failure due to acute tubular necrosis will, with supportive measures, completely resolve.
   e. **True.** Sarcoidosis is a multisystem granulomatous disease of unknown aetiology that usually targets lymph nodes, the lung and liver. The kidney can be involved. The two 'oids', amyloid and sarcoid often crop up in multiple choice or short answer questions and it is worth knowing a few facts about each.

5. a. **False.** Schistosomiasis is endemic in countries such as Egypt and causes squamous metaplasia of the bladder urothelium. Thus, there is an unusually high number of cases of squamous cell carcinoma of the bladder in these countries.
   b. **True.** Angiomyolipoma is a rare (benign) kidney tumour (some authorities think that it is a hamartoma rather than a tumour—i.e. a haphazard collection of tissue normally found in and around the kidney). The 'tumour' is made up of adipose tissue with thick-walled blood vessels. This tumour has an association with tuberose sclerosis, an autosomal dominant disease in which patients can also have rhabdomyomas of

the heart and skin lesions (called adenoma sebaceum). Angiomyolipomas can be very vascular and may present as a massive bleed into the retroperitoneum.

c. **True.** Cigarette smokers have a significantly increased risk of bladder transitional cell carcinoma. Other 'smoking-related' tumours are found in the mouth, oesophagus, lung and cervix.

d. **True.** Wilms' tumour is also known as nephroblastoma. There are several important childhood 'solid tumours' that you should be aware of (remember than haematological malignancy is common in children, e.g. acute leukaemia). Many of the childhood solid malignancies look similar down the microscope and are often called 'small blue cell tumours'. Among these are neuroblastomas, rhabdomyosarcomas, nephroblastomas, and some lymphomas. Many of these tumours contain primitive or precursor cells normally found in the developing tissue/organ. Deciding which tumour is which can be difficult, but is helped by immunocytochemistry and molecular biology.

e. **False.** Malacoplakia is a rare disease. In the bladder (it can also occur in the bowel and respiratory tract), yellowy mucosal plaques are seen and histologically these are collections of macrophages with cytoplasmic and extruded, dark-coloured, Michaelis–Guttmann bodies (which are probably bacterial-derived).

6. a. **True.** Hyaline arteriolosclerosis, thick, bright pink arteriolar walls on staining with haematoxylin and eosin, is seen in conditions such as diabetes, amyloidosis and hypertension.

b. **False.** Peritoneal dialysis and transplantation are two others.

c. **True.** In multiple myeloma, the amyloid is light chain derived (AL amyloid).

d. **True.** See 3e above.

e. **False.** IgA disease could theoretically cause acute renal failure, but usually presents as haematuria +/– proteinuria.

Case histories

Case history 1

1. This man has the nephrotic syndrome.

2. The commonest cause of the nephrotic syndrome in adults is membranous glomerulopathy.

3. Interestingly, although in the vast majority of cases this is idiopathic it can be rarely associated

with/caused by tumours (possibly by tumour-containing immune complexes becoming lodged in the glomerulus). There have been cases where removal of the tumour has lead to resolution of the glomerular disease.

Case history 2

This is quite a common exam question. Essentially, whether in an essay, short answer or viva format, this type of question tests how well you can logically approach a clinical problem (and mimics how, for instance, casualty officers or GPs have to think with the patient in front of them). The best way to tackle this type of question is to mentally (or physically, on a piece of exam paper) jot down the components of the urinary tract (kidney-to-ureter-to-bladder, etc.) and then use a set of general headings to describe the possible pathologies (usable for any organ), e.g. congenital vs. acquired, inflammatory (bacterial, viral, etc.), neoplastic (benign vs. malignant, primary vs. secondary), metabolic, etc. The list you make should, of course, be modified to the age of the patient (it is less likely that a congenital abnormality will present in a man of 52 than an acquired, inflammatory or neoplastic condition).

1. The commoner causes of haematuria in a 52-year-old man include:
   Kidney
   - tumours (renal cell carcinoma, transitional cell carcinoma)
   - stones with inflammation/ulceration
   - trauma.

   Ureter
   - tumours (transitional cell carcinoma)
   - stones +/– inflammation.

   Bladder
   - tumours (transitional cell carcinoma)
   - acquired diverticula with inflammation/stones
   - infection (less likely than in females but instrumentation, diabetes, etc.).

   Prostate
   - benign prostatic enlargement/tumours.

2. The mass is a renal cell carcinoma.

3. Renal cell carcinomas may spread locally or to distant sites. Classically, the tumour may permeate the renal vein and may grow up this structure as far as the right atrium. Distant metastases can occur in any organ but particularly the bones.

4. Remember that *stage* is a reflection of the degree of spread of a tumour (*grade* is how malignant the tumour looks down the microscope).

Short note answers

1. Include circulating and in situ immune complex formation and the possibility of T cell/macrophage products as a cause of glomerular dysfunction.

2. Set out your answer logically. Tackle acute and chronic pyelonephritis (have your memory-jogger headings ready: definition; incidence; age of patient; sex distribution; aetiology/pathogenesis; naked eye, i.e. macroscopic, appearances; microscopic appearances; spread; complications; treatment; etc.).

3. Set out your response in a logical fashion (remember bladder cancer implies a malignant process, so spend most of your time on transitional cell carcinoma).

Viva answers

1–3. All three questions should be approached logically, remember to define the terms you use, this shows the examiner that you understand the nomenclature that you are using.

11 Lymphoreticular system

Overview

The lymphoreticular system consists of organs (lymph nodes, spleen, thymus) and ill-defined tissues (mucosa-associated lymphoid tissue) that are concerned with the growth, development, and deployment of white blood cells. White blood cells are crucial for immune responses. The lymph nodes lie along the course of the lymphatics, receiving lymph from the tissues and destroying or mounting immune responses to foreign agents before they reach the bloodstream. Both benign and malignant disorders of the lymph nodes often manifest as lymph node enlargement (lymphadenopathy), and lymph node biopsy is sometimes necessary to determine the diagnosis and indicate further management. The spleen receives blood from the arterial system. It functions as a filter by removing obsolescent red blood cells and particulate matter from the blood, and mounts immunological responses against foreign agents. Most benign and malignant disorders of the spleen manifest as splenic enlargement (splenomegaly). Rupture of the spleen is a potentially life-threatening condition that requires prompt management. The thymus is an important component of the lymphoreticular system in fetal life, but probably has no significant role in adults. Failure of normal development of the thymus causes deficient immune responses and, in adults, thymic hyperplasia and thymic tumours may develop.

Basic principles

The cells which circulate in the peripheral blood can be classified simply into those that are non-nucleated (erythrocytes and platelets) and those that are nucleated (leukocytes or white blood cells). White blood cells can be further subclassified into three main cell types:

- granulocytes
- monocytes
- lymphocytes.

The main function of these cells is to protect against infection. Lymphocytes and monocytes circulate around the body in blood vessels and lymphatic vessels, but they also accumulate in organised masses called lymphoid tissues. These organised masses together are known as the lymphoreticular system and the main components of this system are the lymph nodes, thymus, spleen, tonsils, adenoids, and the Peyer's patches. The latter three tissues are known as mucosa-associated lymphoid tissue (MALT).

11.1 Lymph nodes

Learning objectives

You should:

- Understand the structure and function of lymph nodes

- Know the causes of lymphadenopathy

- Have a basic understanding of the lymphoid neoplasms

Structure and function

Lymph nodes are ovoid, encapsulated structures, which range in size from a few millimetres to a few centimetres. They are situated along the course of lymphatic vessels and tend to occur in groups where these vessels converge (e.g. the axilla, groin, neck and mediastinum). Lymph is essentially interstitial fluid containing proteins that need to return to the bloodstream, but which are prevented from doing so within the tissues because of overwhelming hydrostatic pressure. Lymph is therefore carried away from the tissues in small peripheral lymphatic vessels, which converge to form larger vessels, until eventually a single large lymphatic vessel called the thoracic duct ultimately drains the lymph into the bloodstream at the root of the neck. Before the lymph enters the blood-stream, it must pass through one or more lymph nodes. Within the lymph nodes, foreign agents and unwanted materials, which have gained access to the tissues, are entrapped and an immune response is mounted.

Each lymph node is divided into three main regions: the cortex; the paracortex; and the medulla (Fig. 36).

The cortex

This is the area just beneath the capsule, and it contains spherical aggregations of B lymphocytes (B cells). These aggregations are called primary follicles. B cells are involved in humoral immunity and the primary follicle is the principle site of B-cell activation in response to antigenic stimulation. Antigens that enter the lymph node are presented to the B cells in the primary follicle. Activated B cells enlarge and undergo a series of changes, resulting ultimately in the production of immunoglobulin-secreting plasma cells. Hence, after antigenic stimulation, the primary follicle enlarges and develops a pale-staining germinal centre that contains large, activated B cells. The germinal centre is surrounded by a rim of small unchallenged B cells called the mantle zone.

The paracortex

The paracortex is the area between the follicles and is rich in T lymphocytes (T cells). T cells are involved in cell-mediated immunity. Scattered histiocytic cells are also present.

The medulla

This region contains the medullary cords and sinuses. The sinuses are lined by macrophages, which phago-cytose particulate material within the lymph. The medullary cords contain numerous plasma cells, which secrete immunoglobulins (antibodies).

Lymph enters the lymph node via multiple afferent lymphatic vessels, which perforate the fibrous capsule and empty into a slit-like space just beneath the capsule called the subcapsular sinus. From there, the lymph enters the cortex via multiple, small cortical sinuses, which penetrate into the node. In the medulla, these sinuses begin to converge into larger sinuses (the medullary sinuses) and, in turn, the medullary sinuses join to form a single efferent lymphatic vessel.

Lymphadenopathy

When there is a pathological process affecting a lymph node, it usually becomes enlarged. Lymphadenopathy is a term used to denote lymph-node enlargement. Lymphadenopathy may be localised or widespread. There are two main causes:

1. Non-neoplastic (reactive) lymphadenopathy
2. Neoplastic lymphadenopathy.

Neoplasms of the lymph nodes can be divided into primary (lymphoma) or secondary (metastases).

Non-neoplastic (reactive) lymphadenopathy

Lymph node enlargement is a common response to antigenic stimuli. These may be:

- infecting organisms
- non-infectious agents such as foreign material, cell debris, metabolites, or drugs
- unknown agents.

Reactive lymph nodes enlarge because there is proliferation of one or more cell types within them. The various antigenic stimuli evoke the reactive proliferation of particular cell types within the lymph node, and may induce other changes. In many cases, the morphological changes induced by these aetiological agents are non-specific, such that precise diagnosis of the causal agent is not possible on histological grounds alone (blood tests may be needed). In other cases, the reactive changes are entity specific, such that the pathologist is able to make an exact diagnosis.

Non-specific reactive changes
Lymph nodes may react in one of five different ways to antigenic stimulation. Often, a combination of one or more of these patterns is seen.

Acute non-specific lymphadenitis—occurs when there is direct drainage of pyogenic infectious microbes into a lymph node, causing a localised acute inflammatory response. Affected lymph nodes become enlarged

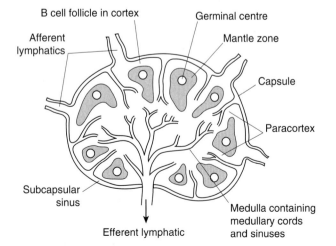

B cell follicle in cortex

Germinal centre

Afferent lymphatics

Mantle zone

Capsule

Paracortex

Subcapsular sinus

Medulla containing medullary cords and sinuses

Efferent lymphatic

Fig. 36 Diagram of a lymph node.

and tender. Microscopically, there is lymph node oedema and hyperaemia, and neutrophil polymorphs migrate from the vasculature into the nodal parenchyma. There may be progression to abscess formation.

Follicular hyperplasia—occurs when there is a B-cell response, and is characterised by marked enlargement and prominence of the germinal centres.

Paracortical hyperplasia—is the result of a T-cell response. The paracortex expands and encroaches on the follicles. This pattern is often encountered in reactions induced by drugs and acute viral infections.

Sinus histiocytosis—is seen if there is a marked proliferation of histiocytic cells, which normally occupy the sinuses. The sinuses become dilated and engorged with numerous histiocytes.

Granulomatous lymphadenitis—refers to the formation of granulomas within a lymph node. A granuloma is a collection of macrophages. Causes include:

- tuberculosis
- sarcoidosis
- cat scratch disease
- Crohn's disease
- toxoplasmosis
- reaction to foreign material.

Entity-specific reactive changes

A number of reactive conditions affecting lymph nodes induce morphological appearances which, although often complex, may be distinctive enough to enable the pathologist to make an exact diagnosis. Such conditions include certain infections (e.g. toxoplasmosis, HIV, Epstein–Barr virus), some connective tissue diseases (e.g. systemic lupus erythematosus), reactions to types of foreign material (e.g. silicone), certain drug reactions (e.g. some anticonvulsants), and conditions of uncertain aetiology (e.g. Castleman's disease).

Lymphoma

Lymphomas are primary neoplasms of the cells native to the lymphoid tissues. The term 'lymphoma' is a misnomer, because all lymphomas are potentially malignant.

Lymphomas are classified into subtypes according to histological appearance and immunophenotype (i.e. the staining patterns on immunohistochemistry). Different subtypes behave differently, have different prognoses, and require different treatments. Hence, classification of lymphoma is the means by which pathologists convey meaningful information to the clinicians. There have been a number of classification systems in the past (e.g. Keil classification, Working Formulation for Clinical Usage), all of which have had their merits. However, many entities went by different names in the different classification systems, and this was a source of confusion for both pathologists and clinicians. In addition, there have been major advances in our knowledge and understanding of lymphoid neoplasms since the 1980s, and many new entities have now been recognised. To overcome these problems, a new unifying lymphoma classification system was devised and published by the International Lymphoma Study Group in 1994, and it was called the 'Revised European–American Classification of Lymphoid Neoplasms' (REAL). A few years later, when the World Health Organization (WHO) were developing a new classification system for neoplastic diseases of the haematopoietic and lymphoid tissues, they adopted the REAL classification, making only a few modifications. It is the 2001 WHO Lymphoma Classification System that is currently used in clinical practise.

There are two main types of lymphoma—Hodgkin's lymphoma and non-Hodgkin's lymphoma. They are separated for two main reasons:

1. Hodgkin's lymphoma is characterised morphologically by the presence of unique neoplastic cells called Reed–Sternberg cells.
2. Hodgkin's lymphoma may be associated with certain clinical symptoms.

Hodgkin's lymphoma

Hodgkin's lymphoma is differentiated from the other types of lymphoma by the presence of distinctive and diagnostic tumour cells called Reed–Sternberg cells (RS cells), although for the diagnosis of Hodgkin's lymphoma to be made, the RS cells must be associated with the appropriate cellular background. Classically, the RS cell is large with a pale, bilobed nucleus and large, prominent, eosinophilic nucleoli. The nucleoli are bounded by a clear zone, giving the cell a characteristic 'owl-eye' appearance. The various subtypes of Hodgkin's lymphoma are shown in Table 30.

Clinical features

Typical patients are young adults, the peak incidence being in the third and fourth decades of life. Patients usually present with painless lymphadenopathy, which typically affects the upper half of the body. The enlarged lymph nodes are discrete, mobile, and rubbery in consistency. Patients may also present with systemic symptoms (unexplained pyrexia, drenching night sweats, unexplained weight loss).

Staging

Staging is an important determinant of treatment and prognosis. The staging system used is the Ann Arbor system:

Stage I—involvement of a single lymph node region (I) or single extranodal organ or site (Ie).

Table 30 The WHO lymphoma classification system

Hodgkin's lymphoma	Nodular lymphocyte-predominant Hodgkin's lymphoma		
	Classical Hodgkin's lymphoma		Nodular sclerosing Hodgkin's lymphoma Lymphocyte-rich classical Hodgkin's lymphoma Mixed-cellularity Hodgkin's lymphoma Lymphocyte-depleted Hodgkin's lymphoma
Non-Hodgkin's lymphoma[*]	B-cell neoplasms	Precursor B-cell neoplasms	Precursor B-lymphocytic leukaemia/lymphoma[§]
		Mature B-cell neoplasms	B-cell chronic lymphocytic leukaemia/small lymphocytic lymphoma[†] Plasma cell myeloma[†] Extranodal marginal zone B-cell lymphoma of MALT type Follicular lymphoma[†] Mantle cell lymphoma Diffuse large B-cell lymphoma[†] Burkitt's lymphoma[§]
	T/NK-cell neoplasms	Precursor T-cell neoplasms	Precursor T-lymphoblastic lymphoma[§]
		Mature T-cell neoplasms	Mycosis fungoides/Sezary syndrome Peripheral T-cell lymphoma Angioimmunoblastic T-cell lymphoma Anaplastic large-cell lymphoma

[*]Within the non-Hodgkin's group, only the most common subtypes are shown.
[†]The subtypes which constitute the majority of lymphoid neoplasms in adults.
[§]The subtypes most common in children.

Stage II—involvement of two or more lymph node regions on the same side of the diaphragm (II), or one extranodal organ plus one or more lymph node regions on the same side of the diaphragm (IIe).

Stage III—involvement of lymph regions on both sides of the diaphragm (III), which may be associated with splenic involvement (IIIs), or localised involvement of an extranodal site (IIIe), or both (IIIse).

Stage IV—diffuse or disseminated involvement of one or more extralymphatic sites, such as the liver, lung, or bone marrow, with or without lymph-node involvement.

Any of these stages may be followed by the suffix A or B, depending on whether the systemic symptoms are absent (A) or present (B). The presence of systemic symptoms is associated with a poorer prognosis.

Treatment and prognosis

Factors associated with a poorer prognosis are:

- advancing age
- systemic symptoms
- advanced stage
- aggressive histological subtype (e.g. lymphocyte-depleted Hodgkin's lymphoma)
- abnormal blood markers.

With advances in treatment during the late 1990s, the prognosis of Hodgkin's lymphoma has generally improved, so that even with advanced disease, the five-year disease-free survival is 60–70%.

Non-Hodgkin's lymphoma

Within this category, there is a much wider spectrum of lymphoid neoplasms, showing a marked diversity in their histological appearance, immunophenotype, biological behaviour, response to therapy, prognosis, and clinical settings, including typical age at onset. Because of the extremely complex nature of this group of lymphoid neoplasms, only a framework for the basic understanding of non-Hodgkin's lymphoma will be presented here as detailed descriptions of the various subtypes are not necessary in this text. The most frequently encountered subtypes are shown in Table 28. In basic terms, non-Hodgkin's lymphoma can be subdivided according to the type of lymphoid cell of origin into B-cell non-Hodgkin's lymphoma and T-cell/NK-cell non-Hodgkin's lymphoma. These B- and T-cell neoplasms can be further subdivided into precursor (lymphoblastic) neoplasms or mature (peripheral) neoplasms. Within these categories, the various distinct entities are then listed.

In the past, grading of lymphomas has sometimes been used, but the current convention is to grade only follicular lymphomas, because only for this particular lymphoma subtype does grading add any further information. Low-grade follicular lymphomas have an indolent clinical course but respond poorly to therapy, and high-grade follicular lymphomas behave more aggressively but respond well to therapy. With all other subtypes of lymphoma, the behaviour and expected response to therapy is implied by the diagnosis. For example, Burkitt's lymphoma is always a high-grade tumour, and therefore behaves aggressively but responds quite well to very aggressive therapy.

Diagnosis of lymphoma

In order to make a definitive diagnosis of lymphoma, a lymph node biopsy is often performed and the node examined histologically. In some cases, cytogenetic analysis is used in conjunction with histological assessment in order to make the correct diagnosis. Lymphnode biopsy may be preceded by fine-needle aspiration cytology.

Secondary tumours

The tumours most often encountered in the lymph nodes are metastatic rather than primary. Most carcinomas, melanomas, and some sarcomas have the capacity to metastasise via the lymphatic system.

11.2 The thymus

Learning objectives

You should:

- Understand the structure and function of the thymus
- Know the common disorders of the thymus

Structure and function

The thymus is an encapsulated bilobed structure, which is situated in the anterior superior mediastinum.

It is embryologically derived from the third and, occasionally, fourth pharyngeal pouches. The gland grows in size until puberty (weighing up to 50 g), thereafter undergoing progressive atrophy and gradual replacement by fibrofatty tissue.

The thymus has a central role in cell-mediated immunity. During fetal development, bone-marrow derived stem cells migrate to the thymus where they differentiate and mature into T cells. A small population of B cells is also present. The thymus has a lymphoid component and an epithelial component.

Disorders of the thymus

Agenesis and aplasia

These conditions are the result of failure of development of either the epithelial or lymphoid component of the thymus. In di George syndrome, there is failure of development of the third and fourth pharyngeal pouches that normally give rise to the thymus and parathyroid glands. Affected infants have grossly reduced cell-mediated immunity due to absence of the thymus, and hypocalcaemia leading to tetany due to absence of the parathyroids. Cardiac defects and abnormal facies may also be a feature. In Nezelof syndrome, which is an inherited condition, only the thymus is affected.

Thymic hyperplasia (thymic follicular hyperplasia)

This condition is characterised by the presence of lymphoid follicles with germinal centres within the thymus. Thymic hyperplasia is seen in ~70% of patients with the autoimmune condition myasthenia gravis. In these patients, the thymus appears to be the main source of the autoantibody, and thymectomy may therefore be of benefit. A degree of thymic hyperplasia may also be seen in other autoimmune disorders such as Graves' disease, SLE, systemic sclerosis, and rheumatoid arthritis.

Neoplasms of the thymus

The main types of neoplasms that can arise within the thymus are:

- thymoma
- thymic carcinoma
- lymphoma
- germ cell tumours (rare)
- neuroendocrine tumours (rare).

Thymomas—are tumours of thymic epithelial cells. Many are asymptomatic and are only detected on chest X-ray performed for other reasons. Others become manifest clinically through local pressure symptoms, e.g. stridor, cough, or dyspnoea, or through their association with myasthenia gravis. The majority of thymomas are completely benign.

Thymic carcinomas—are usually highly aggressive.

Lymphoma—can occur in the thymus. The thymus is not an uncommon site for Hodgkin's lymphoma and thymic involvement by non-Hodgkin's lymphoma, mostly T-cell neoplasms or large B-cell lymphomas, is frequently encountered.

Germ cell tumours—such as seminomas and teratomas, may be encountered. They are derived from germ cells that have failed to migrate to the gonads during fetal life.

Neuroendocrine tumours—such as thymic carcinoids, may arise from neuroendocrine cells that are scattered throughout the gland.

11.3 The spleen

Learning objectives

You should:

- Understand the structure and function of the spleen
- Know the major causes of splenomegaly
- Understand the importance of splenic rupture

Structure and function

The spleen is an encapsulated organ, which is situated in the left upper quadrant of the abdomen. The spleen receives blood from the splenic artery and, in general, it is to the circulatory system what the lymph nodes are to the lymphatic system. The adult organ has two main functions:

1. Filtration and phagocytosis of obsolescent red blood cells and bacteria
2. Mounting immunological responses.

Reflecting these functions, the spleen has two main components: the white pulp, which is lymphoid tissue and is where immunological responses are mounted; and the red pulp, which is the site of blood filtration and phagocytosis.

The white pulp

The splenic artery enters the spleen at the hilum and then divides to give rise to numerous central arteries, which ramify through the organ. Each central artery becomes ensheathed in lymphoid cells, which constitute the white pulp. The white pulp consists of periarteriolar lymphoid sheaths (PALS) of T cells, which are intermittently expanded by B-cell follicles. The unstimulated B-cell follicle consists of a nodule of small B lymphocytes surrounded by a rim of larger, marginal zone B cells. If the B-cell follicle is stimulated, a germinal centre forms in the centre, surrounded by a mantle zone of small unchallenged B cells, which are surrounded by the marginal zone (Fig. 37).

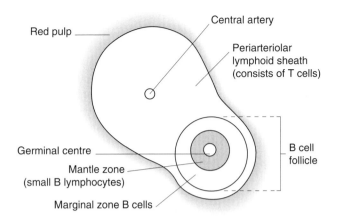

Fig. 37 Diagrammatic representation of splenic white pulp.

The red pulp

The red pulp consists of sinusoids separated by splenic cords (Fig. 38). The splenic cords contain numerous macrophages. Once blood has left the central artery of the white pulp, it passes into capillaries. Blood within the capillaries can either drain directly into the sinusoids and then into the splenic veins ('closed' circulation), or it can first enter the splenic cords and then pass into the sinusoids through fenestrations in the sinusoid epithelium ('open' circulation). In the open circulation, red blood cells must undergo extreme deformation to pass from the cords into the sinusoids. Obsolescent, damaged or abnormal red blood cells have reduced deformability and, therefore, become trapped within the splenic cords where they are phagocytosed.

Macroscopically, the cut surface of the spleen is red (red pulp) dotted with grey specks (white pulp).

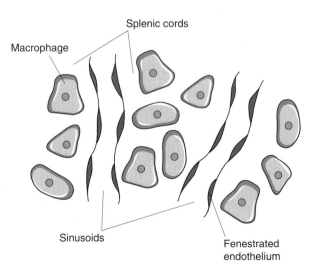

Fig. 38 Diagrammatic representation of splenic red pulp.

Disorders of the spleen

Congenital abnormalities

An accessory (supernumerary) spleen is not uncommon, the most usual location being the hilum of the spleen. Congenital absence of the spleen (asplenia) and polysplenia are rare and are often associated with other congenital defects.

Splenomegaly

This term refers to enlargement of the spleen. With very few exceptions, pathological states in the spleen are manifest as splenomegaly, and there are numerous causes. However, apart from being an indicator of an underlying disorder, splenomegaly may itself cause problems by inducing portal hypertension (because of increased blood flow though the organ) and hypersplenism. Hypersplenism is characterised by splenomegaly, a deficiency in one or more of the cellular elements in the blood, and correction of the cytopenia(s) by splenectomy.

Causes of splenomegaly include:

- infections (e.g. acute non-specific splenitis, infectious mononucleosis, malaria, miliary TB)
- congestion (e.g. cardiac failure, cirrhosis, portal hypertension)
- lymphohaematogenous disorders and neoplasms (e.g. lymphoma, leukaemia, haemolytic anaemia)
- immune inflammatory disorders (e.g. rheumatoid arthritis, SLE)
- storage diseases (e.g. Gaucher's disease)
- amyloidosis and sarcoidosis.

Infection
The morphological changes which occur in the spleen during infection often vary depending on the particular infecting organism. In acute non-specific splenitis due to sepsis, the spleen becomes very soft and, when sliced, the substance of the spleen typically flows out from the cut surface. In infectious mononucleosis the splenic capsule is particularly vulnerable to rupture. In malaria, the spleen can reach a massive size and is markedly congested.

Congestive splenomegaly
Persistent elevation of the splenic or portal venous blood pressure can cause splenomegaly. The pressure may be raised due to prehepatic, hepatic, or posthepatic causes. Prehepatic causes include thrombosis of the splenic or portal veins. The most important hepatic cause is cirrhosis. Posthepatic causes include thrombosis of the hepatic veins (Budd–Chiari syndrome), and raised inferior vena cava pressure associated with right heart failure.

The spleen may be considerably enlarged and the capsule is often thickened and fibrotic. The cut surface is dark red with inconspicuous white pulp. Microscopically, the increased venous pressure is reflected by distension of the sinusoids by red blood cells. Collagen may be laid down in the basement membranes of distended sinusoids, resulting in impairment of blood flow from the cords to the sinusoids. The red blood cells are therefore exposed to the cord macrophages for much longer, and hypersplenism may result. The elevated venous pressure can lead to sinusoid rupture and intraparenchymal haemorrhage. Organisation of these areas gives rise to small brown nodules called Gamna–Gandy bodies, which are visible with the naked eye.

Lymphohaematogenous neoplasms
The spleen is not infrequently involved in a number of lymphoid and haematological neoplasms. Each type of neoplasm is associated with a different pattern of splenic involvement. For example, in chronic myeloid leukaemia, the red pulp is filled with mature myeloid precursors, and in Hodgkin's lymphoma, the white pulp is preferentially involved with the formation of expansile nodules.

Non-lymphohaematogenous tumours of the spleen are rare, but include hamartomas, lymphangiomas and haemangiomas.

Splenic infarction

Splenic infarcts are due to occlusion of the splenic artery or one of its branches, and are usually secondary to emboli that arise in the heart. Occasionally, infarction is due to localised thrombosis (e.g. in sickle cell disease). Infarcts are characteristically pale and wedge-shaped. They may be single or multiple, and healing leads to the formation of scars, which depress the surface.

Splenic rupture

Rupture of the spleen is most commonly the result of blunt trauma, such as can occur during a car accident when the steering wheel may inflict a severe blow to the upper abdomen. Spontaneous splenic rupture may occur if the organ is enlarged and abnormally soft, as in infectious mononucleosis. Rupture is followed by extensive intraperitoneal haemorrhage. Prompt splenectomy is necessary to prevent death from hypovolaemic shock.

Self-assessment: questions

Multiple choice questions

1. The following statements are correct:
   a. Lymph nodes are only found in the neck
   b. After passing through lymph nodes, lymph enters the bloodstream via the thoracic duct
   c. Lymph node enlargement always indicates a malignant process
   d. Acute viral infections cause paracortical expansion
   e. The primary follicles within a lymph node are composed of T cells.

2. The following statements are correct:
   a. Lymphomas may affect the gastrointestinal tract
   b. Hodgkin's lymphoma is one of the most common forms of malignancy in young adults
   c. Lymph nodes involved by Hodgkin's lymphoma may become painful on consumption of alcohol
   d. Non-Hodgkin's lymphomas are characterised by the presence of Reed–Sternberg cells
   e. The definitive diagnosis of lymphoma requires histological assessment of a lymph-node biopsy.

3. The following statements regarding the thymus are correct:
   a. The thymus is situated in the anterior superior mediastinum
   b. Thymomas are tumours of thymic T cells
   c. Thymic hyperplasia may be associated with myasthenia gravis
   d. di George syndrome is associated with thymic enlargement
   e. The thymus is most active in late adult life.

4. The following statements regarding the spleen are correct:
   a. The spleen is composed of white pulp and red pulp
   b. Malaria is associated with development of massive splenomegaly
   c. Splenomegaly may be associated with leucopenia
   d. Spontaneous rupture of the spleen refers to splenic rupture when there is no underlying pathology
   e. Splenectomy should be supplemented by vaccination against pneumococcus.

Case histories

Case history 1

A 32-year-old female presented to her GP with unexplained weight loss and drenching night sweats for the last six months. On examination she has right-sided cervical lymphadenopathy.

1. What diagnoses would you consider?
2. What further information would you seek from the history and examination to help determine the diagnosis?
3. What tests might you perform to establish the diagnosis?

Viva questions

1. How are lymphomas classified?
2. How might thymic tumours present clinically?
3. What are the main causes of congestive splenomegaly?

Self-assessment: answers

Multiple choice questions

1. a. **False.**
   b. **True.**
   c. **False.**
   d. **True.**
   e. **False.** Primary follicles are composed predominantly of B cells.

2. a. **True.** The gastrointestinal tract contains mucosa-associated lymphoid tissue within its wall, which may be involved by lymphoma.
   b. **True.**
   c. **True.**
   d. **False.** Reed–Sternberg cells are seen in Hodgkin's lymphoma.
   e. **True.**

3. a. **True.**
   b. **False.** Thymomas are tumours of thymic epithelial cells.
   c. **True.**
   d. **False.**
   e. **False.** The thymus undergoes progressive atrophy after puberty.

4. a. **True.**
   b. **True.**
   c. **True.** Splenomegaly may induce hypersplenism.
   d. **False.** Spontaneous splenic rupture refers to non-traumatic rupture. If rupture is spontaneous, an underlying pathology predisposing to rupture must be considered.
   e. **True.** Patients who have had a splenectomy have a life-long increased risk of infection by pneumococcus and other encapsulated bacteria. Hence they should be considered for vaccination.

Case histories

Case history 1

1. There are two main causes of lymph node enlargement—a reactive process and a neoplastic process. In this case the lymphadenopathy is associated with a six-month history of unexplained weight loss and drenching night sweats. This should raise the possibility of Hodgkin's lymphoma, and the age of the patient and apparent involvement of only one group of nodes in the upper part of the body is supportive of this diagnosis. However, this combination of symptoms and findings is also seen during the course some infections. Although an acute infection is unlikely with this long history, a chronic infection should be considered. For example, TB could cause pyrexia with night sweats, weight loss and cervical lymphadenopathy. Secondary involvement of the lymph nodes by a malignant tumour is unlikely in this age group.

2. Ask questions to determine if an infective process could be causing the symptoms, e.g. chronic cough, pharyngitis, laryngitis, etc. You should also ask if there has been any recent travel abroad where an unusual infection, such as TB, could have been contracted. Remember that lymph nodes affected by Hodgkin's lymphoma may be painful on consumption of alcohol, so you should enquire about this. All systems should be examined in the physical examination to exclude an infective aetiology. Remember that a low-grade pyrexia may be present in Hodgkin's lymphoma. Lymph nodes involved by an infective process may be tender on palpation. Lymph nodes affected by Hodgkin's lymphoma are said to be discrete, mobile and rubbery in consistency. You would also need to examine for lymphadenopathy elsewhere on the body, and see if there is any associated splenomegaly or hepatomegaly. Remember that the spleen may be enlarged in some infective processes, most notably infectious mononucleosis.

3. If the possibility of lymphoma is not excluded on history or examination, the next step is either to remove part, or all, of an affected lymph node for formal histological assessment or to perform a fine-needle aspiration (FNA) and examine the extracted cells for any signs of a neoplastic process. If signs of neoplasia are present on FNA, the lymph node must then be removed for formal histological assessment and diagnosis. Other tests may aid the diagnosis of infections. To diagnose TB, a chest X-ray should be the performed but ultimately the bacillus must be isolated in a tissue specimen, usually either sputum or a biopsy. Serology may be helpful in the diagnosis of some infections, e.g. infectious mononucleosis.

Viva answers

1. Lymphoma classification has been a hot topic lately. The classification system now employed by most clinicians is the WHO classification, which is based on the REAL classification. Lymphomas are divided

into two main types—Hodgkin's lymphoma and non-Hodgkin's lymphoma. Within these two groups there are a number of separate entities that differ in their histological appearance, immunophenotype, clinical behaviour and prognosis.

2. Many thymic tumours are discovered incidentally during the course of thoracic surgery or imaging studies. Thymic abnormalities are actively sought in patients with myasthenia gravis. When they reach a certain size they produce local pressure symptoms relating to their location in the anterior mediastinum, e.g. stridor, cough or dyspnoea.

3. Congestive splenomegaly arises when there is persistent or chronic venous congestion. The venous congestion may be systemic (such as in right-sided cardiac failure) or localised, but traditionally the causes of congestive splenomegaly are divided into three categories:

- prehepatic causes
- hepatic causes
- posthepatic causes.

Prehepatic causes include obstruction of the extrahepatic portal vein or splenic vein by thrombus or an inflammatory process. By far the most common hepatic cause is cirrhosis. Posthepatic causes include right-sided cardiac failure and thrombosis of the hepatic veins (Budd–Chiari syndrome).

12 Bones and soft tissue

Overview

Within the osteoarticular system, the bones provide structural support for the body and have an important role in mineral homeostasis and haematopoiesis, and the joints permit movement. Disorders of the osteoarticular system can, therefore, cause significant disability and deformity. Most of the more common disorders such as osteoarthritis, osteoporosis and rheumatoid arthritis are chronic and progressive causing significant morbidity among the general population, especially the elderly. Bone tumours affect all age groups, show marked diversity in their behaviour and different types target particular age groups and anatomic sites. Connective tissue diseases form an important group of multisystem disorders, and they are presented here because a feature common to most of them is their propensity to involve the joints and soft tissues. 'Soft tissue tumours' form a highly heterogeneous group of neoplasms that are important because benign tumours are relatively frequent and sarcomas are often highly aggressive.

12.1 Bone

Learning objectives

You should:

- Know the structure and function of bones

- Know the major bone diseases, their pathogenesis and clinicopathological features

- Know the major types of bone tumour

Structure and function

The skeletal system is composed of 206 bones, and has a number of functions:

1. Provides structural support.
2. Protective. The skull and the vertebral column protect the brain and spinal cord respectively. The ribs protect the thoracic and upper abdominal organs to a lesser degree.
3. Mineral homeostasis. Bone is a reservoir for the body's calcium, phosphorus, and magnesium.
4. Haematopoiesis. Under normal conditions in the adult, bone is the sole site of haematopoietic marrow.

Bone is a special type of connective tissue, which is mineralised, and therefore has an organic and inorganic component. The organic component is the connective tissue matrix composed predominantly of Type I collagen. The organic matrix undergoes mineralisation by the deposition of the mineral calcium hydroxyapatite. This mineral is the inorganic component of bone. Mineralisation gives bone its strength and hardness. Unmineralised bone is called osteoid. Bone formation, maintenance and remodelling is performed by the bone cells, of which there are three main types:

1. **Osteoblasts**—these cells are responsible for bone formation. They synthesise the Type I collagen that forms osteoid, and also initiate the process of mineralisation.
2. **Osteoclasts**—these are multinucleate cells responsible for bone resorption.
3. **Osteocytes**—evidence suggests that these cells play an important role in the control of the daily fluctuations in serum calcium and phosphorus levels and the maintenance of bone.

Bone can be formed quickly or slowly. When bone is formed quickly, such as in fracture repair or fetal development, the osteoblasts deposit the collagen in a random weave arrangement. This type of bone is called woven bone. Woven bone is replaced by lamellar bone, which is formed much more slowly.

In lamellar bone, the collagen is arranged in parallel sheets. Lamellar bone can also form without a woven bone framework. There are two types of mature lamellar bone:

1. **Cortical (compact) bone**—is composed of numerous units called Haversian systems. In each Haversian system the lamellar bone is arranged concentrically around a central canal called the Haversian canal, through which arteries and veins run.
2. **Cancellous (spongy) bone**—consists of lamellar bone arranged in a meshwork of bone trabeculae.

Most bones are tubular, hollow structures that consist of a shaft, called the diaphysis, expanded end regions, called the epiphyses, and a region between the diaphysis and each epiphysis, called the metaphysis (Fig. 39). The sleeve-like tube (or cortex) of each bone is composed of compact sheets of cortical bone. The inner portion of bone is not quite hollow and is called the medulla. The medulla contains cancellous bone, connective tissue, nerves, blood vessels, fat, and haematopoietic tissue. All bones are covered by a connective-tissue periosteum.

Development and growth of the skeleton

During fetal development, bone can be formed either directly in mesenchyme, as in the case of the skull and clavicles (intramembranous ossification), or on pre-existing cartilage (endochondral ossification). In intramembranous ossification, bone is laid down as woven bone that eventually matures into lamellar bone. In endochondral ossification, the cartilaginous template undergoes ossification at particular sites along the bone known as ossification centres. In long bones, the cartilage at the epiphysis persists until after puberty, allowing growth. This area of persisting cartilage is called the growth plate. Once the bones are fully formed, further growth occurs by the laying down of further bone onto the pre-existing bone. The coordinated actions of the osteoblasts and osteoclasts are paramount in bone development and maintenance. In bone development, the action of osteoblasts predominates. When the skeleton has reached maturity, the bones are continually renewed and remodelled, which requires the actions of the osteoblasts and osteoclasts to be in equilibrium. By the third decade, osteoclastic resorption begins to predominate, with a resultant steady decrease in skeletal mass.

Developmental disorders

Achondroplasia

Achondroplasia is a major cause of dwarfism, and is due to mutation of a single gene. The condition can be familial, with autosomal dominant inheritance, or sporadic. The defective gene leads to abnormal ossification at the growth plates of bones formed by endochondral ossification. Intramembranous ossification is unaffected. Affected individuals have a characteristic appearance, with shortening of the proximal extremities, a relatively normal-sized trunk, and a disproportionately large head with typical bulging of the forehead and depression of the nasal bridge.

Osteogenesis imperfecta ('brittle bone' disease)

This is a rare group of genetic disorders that have in common the abnormal synthesis of Type I collagen. In addition to bone, the other tissues rich in Type I collagen are tendons, ligaments, skin, dentin, and sclera. Affected individuals have brittle bones and spontaneous fractures may occur. The sclera appears blue because it is so thin that the underlying uveal pigment becomes visible. Some variants of osteogenesis imperfecta are fatal early in life while others are associated with survival.

Osteoporosis

Osteoporosis is characterised by reduced bone mass, making bone vulnerable to fracture. Trabecular bone is affected before cortical bone. Trabecular bone is found in the greatest amounts in the vertebral bodies and pelvis,

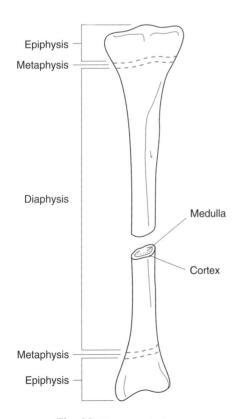

Epiphysis
Metaphysis
Diaphysis
Medulla
Cortex
Metaphysis
Epiphysis

Fig. 39 Diagram of a bone.

and cortical bone is found in the greatest amounts in the long bones.

Aetiology and pathogenesis

Osteoporosis may be primary or secondary. Primary osteoporosis refers to senile osteoporosis and post-menopausal osteoporosis. Secondary osteoporosis is due to conditions other than age or menopause, such as reduced mobility (e.g. after fracture or associated with rheumatoid arthritis), smoking and alcohol consumption, endocrine disorders (e.g. Cushing's syndrome, hyperthyroidism, diabetes) and corticosteroid therapy. Obesity and exercise appear to be protective against osteoporosis.

Senile osteoporosis—there is a normal progressive loss of bone mass after around the age of 30 years, and so all elderly people will have some degree of osteoporosis. Bone loss rarely exceeds 1% per year. The higher the initial bone density, the lower the risk of significant osteoporosis. Women are at higher risk than men, and whites are at higher risk than blacks.

Postmenopausal osteoporosis—this type of osteoporosis is characterised by hormone-dependent acceleration of bone loss. Postmenopausal women may lose up to 2% of cortical bone per year and up to 9% of trabecular bone per year for 8–10 years, declining to the normal rate of bone loss after that. Oestrogen deficiency is thought to play a major role, and oestrogen replacement at the beginning of the menopause reduces the rate of bone loss.

Clinical features

The major complication of osteoporosis is bone fracture. The sites most commonly affected are the vertebral bodies, the distal radius (Colles' fracture) and the hips. Fractures of the vertebral bodies can be of the 'crush' variety leading to progressive loss of height and considerable pain, or of the 'wedge' variety causing deformity of the spine (kyphosis). Hip fractures are important because they cause major disability and lead to hospital admission. Secondary complications such as pneumonia and pulmonary thromboembolism are common, and account for the high mortality rate associated with hip fractures.

Treatment

Women who take hormone replacement therapy have a reduced risk of developing postmenopausal osteoporosis. Also, oral bisphosphonates and vitamin D may be effective.

Metabolic bone disease

Rickets and osteomalacia

Osteomalacia is characterised by defective mineralisation of the osteoid matrix, and is associated with lack of vitamin D. When the condition occurs in the growing skeleton (children) it is called rickets. Vitamin D is important in the maintenance of adequate serum calcium and phosphorus levels, and deficiency impairs normal mineralisation of osteoid laid down in the remodelling of bone. The result is osteomalacia. In children, lack of vitamin D leads to inadequate mineralisation of the epiphyseal cartilage as well as the osteoid, resulting in rickets.

Aetiology

There are two main sources of vitamin D—dietary and endogenous. Consequently, there are four main causes of osteomalacia:

1. **Dietary deficiency of vitamin D**—this used to be a common cause of rickets and osteomalacia. Improvements in diet and the addition of vitamin D to foodstuffs has drastically reduced the incidence of osteomalacia due to nutritional deficiency.
2. **Intestinal malabsorption**—this is now the commonest cause of osteomalacia. Vitamin D is fat soluble. Any condition that causes malabsorption or poor absorption of fat (steatorrhoea) can cause osteomalacia. Causes include coeliac disease and Crohn's disease.
3. **Deficiency of endogenous vitamin D due to defective synthesis in the skin**—more than 90% of circulating vitamin D is photochemically synthesised in the skin. A steroid molecule precursor found in the epidermis is converted to vitamin D by UV light from the sun. Decreased exposure to sunlight or increased skin pigmentation hinders synthesis of vitamin D.
4. **Renal or liver disease**—newly synthesised vitamin D is biologically inactive. A number of metabolic steps are required to convert vitamin D into its active form. The first of these steps is carried out by hepatocytes. The resulting compound is converted to the active form of vitamin D (1,25-dihydroxycalciferol) in the kidney. Hence, renal disease and, to a lesser extent, liver disease can lead to a deficiency in the active form of vitamin D.

Clinicopathological features

The basic abnormality is deficient mineralisation of the organic matrix of the skeleton. In children, the skeleton becomes deformed because there is reduced structural rigidity and inadequate ossification at the growth plates. In preambulatory infants, there is flattening of the occipital bones, and in ambulatory children, bowing of the legs and lumbar lordosis are characteristic. A pigeon breast deformity may develop due to the forces incurred on the weakened bones of the chest during normal respiration. Excess osteoid may cause frontal bossing of the head. Inadequate calcification of the epiphyseal cartilage in long bones leads to cartilaginous overgrowth at the growth plates, resulting in localised enlargement, which is seen especially at the wrists, knees, and ankles. Overgrowth of the cartilage at the costochondral junctions of the chest results in an appearance that is referred to as a 'rachitic rosary'.

In adults, the osteoid that is laid down in the remodelling of bone is inadequately mineralised. The shape of the bone is usually not affected, but the bone becomes vulnerable to spontaneous fractures. Looser zones (pseudofractures) are the hallmark of osteomalacia, and they appear on X-rays as transverse linear lucencies perpendicular to the bone surface. Persistent inadequate mineralisation may eventually lead to generalised osteopenia.

Hyperparathyroidism and renal osteodystrophy

These are discussed in Chapter 6 (the endocrine system).

Paget's disease (osteitis deformans)

In this condition, which is of uncertain aetiology, there is an initial phase of osteoclastic resorption of bone followed by a 'reparative phase' in which there is intense osteoblastic activity and overproduction of disordered and architecturally abnormal bone. Bones may become larger than normal, and are composed of structurally unsound cortical bone and thickened trabeculae with numerous prominent cement lines, which give the bone its characteristic 'mosaic pattern' on microscopy. Later, bone may become ivory hard ('sclerosis'). The abnormal bone is vulnerable to fracture.

Clinical features and complications
The clinical features and complications of Paget's disease are:

- bone pain
- fractures
- neuropathies
- deformities
- deafness
- high-output heart failure
- osteosarcoma and other bone tumours.

The usual presenting features are bone pain, deformities, and fractures. The axial skeleton, skull and proximal femur are involved in the vast majority of cases. Pain is a common problem, and is localised to the affected bone. Deformities are most common when the skull is involved resulting in enlargement of the head with protuberance of the frontal lobes and lion-like (leo-

nine) facies. When the long bones of the lower extremities are involved, weight-bearing leads to anterior bowing of the legs. Fractures occur most commonly in the long bones of the legs, and 'crush' fractures of the spine may lead to spinal cord injury and kyphosis. The spinal cord and nerve roots are also at risk of compression due to enlargement of the vertebral bodies. Distortion of the middle ear cavity and VIIIth nerve compression may lead to deafness. Other cranial nerves may be affected by compression. The bones in Paget's disease are extremely vascular, and the subsequent increased blood flow can (rarely) lead to high-output heart failure. Paget's disease may be complicated by the development of bone tumours, the most sinister being osteosarcoma.

Diagnosis and treatment
Paget's disease may be detected incidentally on X-ray or become manifest through the development of typical clinical features. Intense osteoblastic activity means that affected individuals have raised serum alkaline phosphatase levels. Treatment is by medical therapy with calcitonin and bisphosphonates.

Osteomyelitis

Osteomyelitis refers to inflammation of the bone and marrow, and is usually the result of infection.

Aetiology
Organisms may gain access to the bone by bloodstream spread from a distant infected site, by contiguous spread from neighbouring tissues, or by direct access via a penetrating injury. Almost any organism can cause osteomyelitis, but those most frequently implicated are bacteria. *Staphylococcus aureus* is responsible for many cases. Patients with sickle cell disease are predisposed to *Salmonella* osteomyelitis. *Mycobacterium tuberculosis* is sometimes implicated.

Pathogenesis
The location of the lesions within a particular bone depends on the intraosseous vascular circulation, which varies with age. In infants less than one year old the epiphysis is usually affected. In children the metaphysis is usually affected, and in adults the diaphysis is most commonly affected. In acute osteomyelitis, once the infection has become localised in bone, an intense acute inflammatory process begins. The release of numerous mediators into the Haversian canals leads to compression of the arteries and veins, resulting in localised bone death (osteonecrosis). The bacteria and inflammation spread via the Haversian systems to reach the periosteum. Subperiosteal abscess formation and lifting of the periosteum further impairs the blood supply to the bone, resulting in further necrosis. The dead piece of

bone is called the sequestrum. Rupture of the periosteum leads to formation of drainage sinuses, which drain pus onto the skin. If osteomyelitis becomes chronic, a rind of viable new bone is formed around the sequestrum and below the periosteum. This new bone is called an involucrum. An intraosseous abscess, called a Brodie abscess, may form.

Clinical features and treatment

Acute osteomyelitis presents with localised bone pain and soft tissue swelling. If there is systemic infection, patients may present with an acute systemic illness. Presentation may be extremely subtle in children and infants, who may present only with a pyrexia (pyrexia of unknown origin, PUO). Characteristic X-ray changes consist of a lytic focus of bone surrounded by a zone of sclerosis. Treatment requires aggressive antibiotic therapy. Inadequate treatment of acute osteomyelitis may lead to chronic osteomyelitis, which is notoriously difficult to manage. Surgical removal of bony tissue may be required.

Avascular necrosis

This is necrosis of bone due to ischaemia. Ischaemia may result if the blood supply to a bone is interrupted, which may occur if there is a fracture particularly in areas where blood supply is suboptimal (e.g. the scaphoid and the femoral neck). Most other cases of avascular necrosis are either idiopathic or follow corticosteroid administration.

Bone tumours

Primary bone tumours are uncommon. They can generally be classified according to whether they are cartilage-forming or bone-forming.

Benign cartilage-forming tumours

Osteochondroma (exostosis)—these tumours are cartilage-capped bony outgrowths, which most frequently occur near the metaphysis of long bones. Affected individuals are usually less than 20 years of age. Exostoses are usually solitary. Malignant change is very rare.

Chondroma (enchondroma)—these cartilaginous tumours usually arise within the medullary cavity of the bones of the hands and feet. They occur most frequently in the third to fifth decades of life. The lesions can sometimes cause localised pain, swelling, tenderness or pathological fracture. X-rays show the characteristic 'O-ring' sign—oval-shaped radiolucent cartilage surrounded by a dense rim of bone. Most chondromas are solitary. Malignant change is extremely rare.

Other rare benign cartilage-forming tumours include chondroblastomas and chondromyxoid fibromas.

Malignant cartilage-forming tumours

Chondrosarcoma—this is the second most common primary tumour of bone, being half as frequent as osteosarcoma. Chondrosarcomas occur most frequently in the trunk bones (ribs, spine and pelvis). A few develop within pre-existing osteochondromas, chondroblastomas, or bones affected by Paget's disease. They present as painful enlarging masses, and their nodular growth pattern gives them a scalloped appearance on X-ray. Most chondrosarcomas are low-grade, and therefore pursue a relatively indolent course. However, high-grade tumours metastasise in 70% of cases, usually to other parts of the skeleton or the lungs.

Benign bone-forming tumours

Osteoma—these are bosselated tumours of bone, which most frequently occur in the skull and facial bones. Symptoms depend on the site at which they occur, e.g. symptoms due to obstruction of paranasal sinuses, symptoms related to impingement on the brain.

Osteoid osteoma—these round tumours consist of a small central area (called the 'nidus') surrounded by dense sclerotic bone. Affected individuals are usually less than 25 years old. The lesions are characteristically painful.

Malignant bone-forming tumours

Osteosarcomas—these are the commonest primary malignant tumour of bone, and they usually affect young adults. The metaphysis of long bones are the most frequently affected sites, particularly the distal femur. They present as painful enlarging masses. The tumours usually penetrate the bone cortex, causing elevation of the periosteum. This produces the characteristic triangular shadow (Codman's triangle) seen on X-ray, formed by the bone cortex and the elevated ends of the periosteum. Patients with hereditary retinoblastoma are at significantly increased risk of developing osteosarcomas. Mutations in the p53 gene have also been implicated in some cases. A few cases are secondary to Paget's disease or previous radiation. These aggressive tumours can metastasise widely, especially to the lungs, but due to advances in treatment, the five-year survival has improved to around 50%.

Miscellaneous bone tumours

Ewing's sarcoma—this tumour is composed of small, round, darkly staining cells, which are now believed to be neuroectodermal in origin. The tumour affects children and adolescents, the average age at presentation being 10–15 years. The pelvis and the diaphysis of long bones are the most frequently affected sites. The tumour presents as a painful enlarging mass, and some patients may have systemic features such as a fever, raised white-cell count, or raised erythrocyte sedimentation rate (ESR). Treatment with radiotherapy and chemotherapy has drastically improved survival rates.

Fibroblastic tumours—although fibroblastic tumours such as malignant fibrous histiocytomas and fibrosarcomas more frequently arise within soft tissues, they can also occur in bones. One-quarter of cases are secondary to pre-existing conditions such as Paget's disease, radiation, or bone infarct. The prognosis for high-grade tumours is poor.

Secondary bone tumours

The commonest malignant tumours of bone are secondary deposits from other sites. Most skeletal secondary deposits originate from malignancies at the following sites:

- lung
- breast
- thyroid
- kidney
- prostate.

These deposits cause osteolytic lesions to the bone, with the exception of secondaries originating from prostate tumours, which cause osteosclerotic lesions.

12.2 Joints

Learning objectives

You should:

- Know the structure and function of joints

- Know the major joint diseases, their pathogenesis and clinicopathological features

Structure and function

Joints can be of two main types:

1. **Solid joints**—these joints are fixed and rigid, and allow only minimal movement. Examples of solid joints include the skull sutures (where the skull bones are bridged by fibrous tissue) and the symphysis pubis (where the bones are joined by cartilage).

2. **Synovial joints**—these joints have a joint space, which allows a wide range of movement. The articular cartilage in synovial joints is a specialised hyaline cartilage, which is an excellent shock absorber. The synovial membrane secretes synovial fluid into the joint space. Synovial fluid acts as a lubricant and provides nutrients for the articular hyaline cartilage (Fig. 40).

Osteoarthritis (degenerative joint disease)

This is the most common type of joint disease, and is characterised by the progressive erosion of articular cartilage in weight-bearing joints. The incidence increases with age. Osteoarthritis can be primary or secondary to other bone or joint diseases, systemic diseases such as diabetes, a congenital or developmental deformity of a joint, or previous trauma including repetitive trauma.

Pathology and pathogenesis
In the early stages of osteoarthritis, the articular cartilage becomes eroded and fragmented (fibrillated), and portions of the cartilage flake off. In contrast to joints affected by simple wear and tear, these changes occur well away from the articular margins, and there is eventual full thickness loss of cartilage with the underlying bone becoming exposed and developing a polished ivory appearance (eburnation). Loss of articular cartilage stimulates thickening of the subchondral plate and the adjacent cancellous bone, which impairs the ability of the joint to act as a shock absorber and results in increased damage to the residual cartilage. Small fractures develop

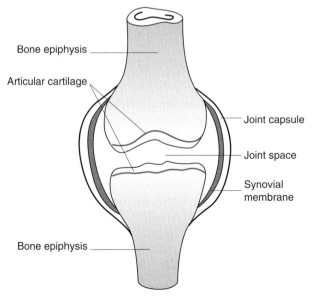

Fig. 40 Diagram of a synovial joint.

in the now articulating bone, allowing synovial fluid to enter the subchondral regions, with resultant formation of subchondral pseudocysts. Fragments of cartilage and bone fall into the joint space forming loose bodies (joint mice). Bony outgrowths, known as osteophytes, form at the margin of the articular cartilage. The articular surfaces become increasingly deformed.

The reason why the articular cartilage becomes predisposed to this damage appears to be related to biochemical alterations in the hyaline. In hyaline cartilage affected by osteoarthritis, the water content is increased and the proteoglycan content is decreased. The elasticity and compliance of the cartilage is, therefore, reduced. The very first change seen in osteoarthritis is proliferation of chondroblasts, and it has been proposed that these cells produce enzymes that induce these biochemical changes in the hyaline cartilage.

Clinical features

The most frequently affected joints are the hips, the knees, the cervical and lumbar vertebrae, the proximal and distal interphalangeal joints of the hands (PIP and DIP joints), the first metacarpophalangeal joint, and the first metatarsophalangeal joint. In affected women, osteophytes at the DIP joints produce nodular swellings called Heberden's nodes. With increasing deformity of the joint the typical symptoms develop, which are pain (which is worse with use), morning stiffness, and limitation in joint movement. With involvement of the cervical and lumbar spine, osteophytes may impinge on the nerve roots causing symptoms such as pain and pins and needles in the arms or legs. The overall result is disability. The process cannot be halted.

Rheumatoid arthritis

Rheumatoid arthritis is a chronic inflammatory multisystem disorder, but the joints are invariably involved. The condition can affect all age groups. When children are affected, the condition is designated Still's disease. Females are affected more often than males. The pathogenesis is not well understood, but it is thought that an initiating agent, possibly an organism, triggers immunological dysfunction resulting in persistent chronic inflammation in genetically susceptible individuals. In the joints, the ongoing inflammation causes destruction of the articular cartilage. Circulating autoantibodies (rheumatoid factors), which are directed against autologous IgG immunoglobulins, can be detected in the serum of around 80% of affected individuals. The exact role of these autoantibodies is uncertain.

Pathological features

Joints—the most severe morphological changes of rheumatoid arthritis are manifest in the joints. In the early stages the synovium becomes thickened, oedematous and hyperplastic. With ongoing inflammation, a pannus is formed. A pannus is a chronically inflamed fibrocellular mass of synovium and synovial stroma, which develops over the articular cartilage. As the pannus slowly spreads, it degrades the underlying cartilage, and erosions and subchondral cysts develop in the underlying bone. Small detached fragments fall into the joint space and are called rice bodies. Localised osteoporosis may also occur. The fibrous pannus eventually bridges the opposing bones causing limitation of movement, and ossification of this fibrous tissue leads to bony ankylosis. The inflammation also affects the joint capsule, tendons and ligaments causing characteristic deformities.

Skin—the most common cutaneous lesions are rheumatoid nodules, which arise in areas exposed to pressure, e.g. the extensor surfaces of the arms and the elbows. They are seen in ~30% of patients. They arise in the subcutaneous tissue and manifest as firm, nontender skin nodules. Microscopically, they consist of a central area of fibrinoid necrosis surrounded by a palisade of histiocytes and fibroblasts.

Blood vessels—patients with severe disease may develop a rheumatoid vasculitis. Peripheral neuropathy, skin ulceration, gangrene and nail-bed infarcts may develop. Impairment of blood supply to vital organs can be fatal.

Lungs—parenchymal rheumatoid nodules (usually asymptomatic), chronic interstitial fibrosis and pleurisy can occur.

Eyes—scleritis and uveitis can develop.

Heart—the development of rheumatoid nodules in the conduction system may occur, and coronary artery vasculitis may result in myocardial ischaemia. Pericarditis can also be a feature.

Bones—patients are at increased risk of localised and generalised osteoporosis.

Lymphoreticular—patients may develop lymphadenopathy, with or without splenomegaly. The combination of rheumatoid arthritis, splenomegaly, and neutropenia is called Felty's syndrome. Approximately 50% of patients with Felty's syndrome develop secondary Sjögren's syndrome. Patients may have a normocytic normochromic anaemia.

Miscellaneous—patients are at an increased risk of developing amyloidosis.

Clinical features

The clinical course of rheumatoid arthritis is very variable. Some patients have mild disease, whereas others have severe progressive disease quickly leading to disability. Initially patients may suffer constitutional symptoms and only after a few weeks or months do the joints become involved. Generally, the small joints (especially those in the hands) are affected before the large joints. The affected joints are swollen, painful and stiff following a period of inactivity. Symptoms may improve with the administration of anti-inflammatory drugs or immunosuppressants. As a result of the pathological processes within the articular and periarticular tissues, characteristic deformities develop, and these include:

- radial deviation at the wrists
- ulnar deviation at the fingers
- flexion and hyperextension deformities of the fingers (swan neck and boutonnière deformities).

Typical X-ray changes include:

- loss of articular cartilage leading to narrowing of the joint space
- joint effusions
- localised osteoporosis
- erosions.

Fatalities are usually the result of complications such as amyloidosis, vasculitis or the iatrogenic effects of therapy (e.g. gastrointestinal bleed secondary to NSAIDs, infections secondary to steroids).

Seronegative spondyloarthropathies

The spondyloarthropathies are a group of disorders characterised by arthropathy associated with disease in other systems. Many are associated with human lymphocyte antigen (HLA)-B27 positivity. The term 'seronegative' is used because affected individuals are seronegative for rheumatoid factors.

Ankylosing spondylitis

This condition typically affects young men and ~90% of patients are HLA-B27 positive. The changes are first seen in the sacroiliac joints and the spine. In the early stages there is inflammation of the tendoligamentous insertion sites, which is followed by reactive bone formation in the adjacent ligaments and tendons. This is compounded by a chronic synovitis causing destruction of the articular cartilage. With attempts at healing, the overall result is bony ankylosis and severe spinal immobility. Patients present with chronic progressive lower back pain. Further progression of the disease leads to spinal kyphosis and neck hyperextension (question mark posture). Characteristic X-ray changes include a 'bamboo spine' and squaring of the vertebral bodies. Extra-articular manifestations include the following:

- uveitis
- apical lung fibrosis
- aortic incompetence
- amyloidosis.

Reiter's syndrome

This condition is defined as a triad of:

- arthritis
- urethritis (non-gonococcal)
- conjunctivitis.

Typical patients are young men, and ~80% of patients are HLA-B27 positive. The condition usually follows infection of the gastrointestinal or genitourinary tract. Several weeks after the diarrhoea or urethritis, an arthritis develops, which may persist for many months. The joints of the leg are the most commonly affected sites.

Enteropathic arthropathy

Salmonella, *Shigella*, *Yersinia* and *Campylobacter* gastroenteritis may be complicated by arthritis, with HLA-B27 positive individuals being at an increased risk of developing this complication. Arthritis is also seen in 20% of patients with Crohn's disease or ulcerative colitis.

Psoriatic arthritis

An arthritis is developed by ~5% of patients with psoriasis, and these individuals are usually HLA-B27 positive.

Infective arthritis

Organisms can gain access to the joint by three main routes:

1. Haematogenous spread from a distant infected site (most common)
2. Direct access via a penetrating injury
3. Direct spread from a neighbouring infected site, e.g. osteomyelitis, soft-tissue abscess.

Infective arthritis, particularly bacterial and tuberculous arthritis, is potentially serious because it can cause rapid destruction of the joint.

Bacterial arthritis

Most cases of infective arthritis are caused by bacteria. The most common organisms are gonococcus (*Neisseria*), *Staphylococcus*, *Streptococcus*, *Haemophilus influenzae*, and gram negative bacilli. In general, children are affected more commonly than adults. Gonococcal arthritis is seen mainly in late adolescence and adulthood, and patients with sickle-cell diseases tend to develop *Salmonella* arthritis. Affected patients develop pain and swelling of the affected joint, and there may be systemic indicators of infection, e.g. fever. Aspiration and culture of the joint fluid gives the diagnosis. Prompt treatment with antibiotics is paramount.

Viral arthritis

Infections such as viral hepatitis, rubella and Parvovirus B19 may be complicated by an arthritis. Symptoms are of a mild arthralgia (aching joints). It is not certain whether the virus directly infects the joint, or whether the arthritis is simply a reactive process due to systemic viral infection.

Rare forms of infective arthritis

Lyme disease—this condition is caused by joint infection with the spirochete *Borrelia burgdorferi*, which is transmitted to humans via tick bites. Infection of the skin is followed by dissemination of the organism to many other sites, particularly the joints. Firstly, the patient usually develops a macular rash known as erythema migrans and there may be constitutional symptoms. This is followed by the development of an arthritis, which may affect more than one joint.

Tuberculous arthritis—this is due to haematogenous spread from an established focus of infection elsewhere, usually the lungs. Tuberculous arthritis usually presents with insidious development of joint pain associated with limitation of movement. The vertebral column is commonly involved, and when there is an associated osteomyelitis vertebral collapse may result (Pott's disease of the spine).

Crystal arthropathies

These are a group of disorders caused by the deposition of crystals within the joint resulting in an acute and chronic arthritis. Such crystals may be endogenous or exogenous. The most common crystal arthropathies, gout and calcium pyrophosphate arthropathy, are due to endogenous crystal deposition.

Gout

This condition is due to the crystallisation of mono-sodium urate within a joint, resulting in an acute (gouty) arthritis, which is characterised by extreme localised pain, erythema, and exquisite tenderness of the affected joint. The most commonly affected joint is the metatar-sophalangeal joint of the great toe, followed in decreasing frequency by the ankle, and then the knee. The disorder is due primarily to raised serum uric acid levels, but only around 3% of people with hyperuricaemia will develop gout. Uric acid is the end product of purine metabolism, and is excreted by the kidneys. Purines can either be derived from the breakdown of nucleic acids or

synthesised de novo. Hyperuricaemia has several main causes:

- idiopathic (80% of cases)
- overproduction of uric acid due to increased purine turnover (e.g. leukaemia) or an enzyme defect
- decreased excretion of uric acid (e.g. chronic renal failure, thiazide diuretics)
- high dietary purine intake.

The events which lead to the deposition of urate crystals in the joint are uncertain, but possible triggers include alcohol, trauma, surgery and infection. The presence of urate crystals within the joint causes the accumulation of numerous inflammatory cells. The resulting arthritis remits after a few days or weeks, even without treatment. The diagnosis can be confirmed by aspirating the joint fluid and using polarising microscopy to detect the needle-shaped crystals, which exhibit negative birefringence with a red filter.

Repeated attacks of acute gouty arthritis eventually lead to chronic tophaceous gouty arthritis, where the affected joint is damaged and function is impaired. Tophi are large aggregates of urate crystals, which are visible with the naked eye. They occur in the joints and soft tissues of people with persistent hyperuricaemia. A common site for tophi is the pinna of the ear.

Urate crystals can also become deposited in the kidney, resulting in acute uric acid nephropathy, chronic renal disease, or uric acid stones causing renal colic.

Calcium pyrophosphate arthropathy (pseudogout, chondrocalcinosis)

This condition is due to the deposition of calcium pyrophosphate crystals in the synovium (pseudogout) and articular cartilage (chondrocalcinosis). It can occur in three main settings:

1. Sporadic (more common in the elderly)
2. Hereditary
3. Secondary to other conditions, such as previous joint damage, hyperparathyroidism, hypothyroidism, haemochromatosis, and diabetes.

The crystals first develop in the articular cartilage (chondrocalcinosis), which is usually asymptomatic. From here the crystals may shed into the joint cavity resulting in an acute arthritis, which mimics gout and is therefore called pseudogout. Pseudogout can be differentiated from gout in three ways:

1. The knee is most commonly involved
2. X-rays show the characteristic line of calcification of the articular cartilage
3. The crystals look different under polarising microscopy—they are rhomboid in shape and exhibit positive birefringence with a red filter.

12.3 Connective tissue diseases

Basic principles

'Connective tissue diseases' is a convenient general term which covers a wide variety of disorders which have certain features in common, those being:

1. They are multisystem disorders and the joints, skin, and subcutaneous tissue are often affected
2. Females are more commonly affected than males
3. Immunological abnormalities are often present
4. A chronic clinical course is usual
5. They usually respond to anti-inflammatory drugs.

The conditions included in this group of disorders are:

- rheumatoid arthritis (presented above)
- systemic lupus erythematosus (SLE)
- polyarteritis nodosa (PAN)
- dermatomyositis and polymyositis
- polymyalgia rheumatica
- cranial arteritis
- scleroderma (systemic sclerosis).

Systemic lupus erythematosus (SLE)

This is a multisystem disorder of autoimmune origin. Females are affected more commonly than males (the female to male ratio is 9 : 1), and the disease usually arises in the second or third decade.

Aetiology and pathogenesis

The cause of SLE is unknown but most patients have circulating autoantibodies directed against nuclear antigens (antinuclear antibodies, or ANAs) and these autoantibodies are the mediators of the tissue damage. Hence B-cell hyper-reactivity is implicated in the pathogenesis and evidence suggests that it is excess T-cell help that drives self-reactive B cells to produce these autoantibodies. Genetic factors may also be important, since there is a strong familial tendency to develop SLE. Some cases of SLE are drug induced, hydralazine and procainamide being among those implicated.

Clinicopathological features

Most visceral lesions are mediated by Type III hypersensitivity (immune complex hypersensitivity reaction). The haematological effects are mediated by Type II hypersensitivity. The organs and tissues affected and the various pathological manifestations are shown in Table 31.

Table 31 Common clinicopathological features of SLE

Organ affected	Clinicopathological features
Skin (involved in most patients)	Symmetrical erythematous facial 'butterfly' rash, often precipitated by sun exposure Discoid lupus erythematosus (DLE)
Joints	Arthralgia
Kidneys	Glomerulonephritis, which may progress to renal failure
Central nervous system	Psychiatric symptoms Focal neurological symptoms due to non-inflammatory occlusion of small blood vessels
Cardiovascular system	Pericarditis Myocarditis Libman–Sacks endocarditis (rare) Necrotising vasculitis
Lungs	Pleuritis Pleural effusions
Lymphoreticular	Mild lymphadenopathy and splenomegaly
Haematological	Anaemia Leucopenia Thrombophilia (antiphospholipid antibody syndrome)

The typical presentation of SLE is of a young women with a butterfly rash on her face associated with a fever and arthralgia. Alternatively, fever or arthralgia may be the only symptoms, making diagnosis difficult. Some patients who have autoantibodies directed against cardiolipin develop the anti-phospholipid antibody syndrome, characterised by thrombophilia. Affected females may suffer recurrent miscarriages.

The clinical course of the condition is variable. That most frequently seen is a relapsing remitting course spanning years. Exacerbations are treated with steroids or other immunosuppressants. Death is usually due to renal disease, diffuse CNS disease or intercurrent infection.

Polyarteritis nodosa (PAN)

This disorder is characterised by inflammation and fibrinoid necrosis of small- or medium-sized arteries. The aetiology is unknown. Segmental artery wall damage may lead to aneurysm formation. The primary targets of PAN are the main visceral vessels, with the kidneys being affected most frequently, followed by the heart, liver and gastrointestinal tract. Joints, muscles, nerves, the skin, and the lungs may also be involved.

Clinical features

Patients usually present with non-specific features such as pyrexia and myalgia, with or without organ-specific symptoms. Renal vessel involvement may cause hypertension, haematuria, or proteinuria. Involvement of the mesenteric vessels causes abdominal pain, melaena, vomiting and diarrhoea. Involvement of the arteries supplying nerves is a cause of mononeuritis multiplex. Joint involvement causes arthralgia, skin involvement causes a rash, and lung involvement causes cough and dyspnoea.

The diagnosis depends on finding a necrotising vasculitis in a biopsy specimen. The serum of affected patients often contains pANCA (perinuclear antineutrophil cytoplasmic autoantibody).

Therapy with corticosteroids or cyclophosphamide causes remission in most cases. If left untreated, PAN is often fatal.

Dermatomyositis and polymyositis

Both of these conditions are inflammatory disorders of muscle, and they present with gradual onset of muscular weakness. More than one muscle is usually affected and the distribution is commonly bilateral, symmetrical, and proximal. The oesophagus, diaphragm and heart are not infrequently involved. In dermatomyositis, a distinctive skin rash precedes the muscular weakness.

The rash is a lilac discolouration of the upper eyelids associated with periorbital oedema. A more generalised dermatitis is often present. Ten per cent of patients with dermatomyositis have an underlying malignancy, most commonly carcinoma of the lung, breast or gastrointestinal tract. Polymyositis differs from dermatomyositis because it lacks the skin changes, and is seen only in adults. There is a slight increased risk of an underlying malignancy.

Diagnosis of these disorders depends on clinical symptoms, elevated muscle enzymes (e.g. creatinine phosphokinase) and muscle biopsy.

Polymyalgia rheumatica

This condition is seen in elderly individuals, and presents with pain and stiffness in the shoulder and pelvic girdles. Muscle weakness is not a feature. There may be non-specific features such as lethargy, raised ESR, and mild normochromic normocytic anaemia. The condition responds well to corticosteroid therapy.

Cranial arteritis (temporal or giant cell arteritis)

Cranial arteritis is a granulomatous inflammation of small- and medium-sized arteries, and is the commonest of the vasculitides. The inflammatory process principally affects the cranial vessels, especially the temporal arteries and the terminal branches of the ophthalmic artery. In such cases, prompt diagnosis is paramount because of the risk of blindness. Typical symptoms are headache, scalp tenderness in the region of the temporal artery, and jaw claudication. The condition may also be associated with polymyalgia rheumatica. An elevated serum ESR should raise the possibility of cranial arteritis.

Diagnosis depends on temporal artery biopsy, which should be performed immediately if the diagnosis is suspected. Histologically, the wall of the artery is infiltrated by inflammatory cells, with or without multinucleate giant cells, and the internal elastic lamina becomes fragmented. These changes may only be focal ('skip' lesions) and may be missed on biopsy. The treatment of choice is steroids.

Scleroderma (systemic sclerosis)

This condition is characterised by excessive fibrosis of organs and tissues. The skin is almost always affected with variable involvement of the gastrointestinal tract, heart, kidneys, lungs, arteries, and musculoskeletal system. The condition is more common in women than men. In a subset of patients where the skin is the main target organ and visceral involvement is uncommon, the condition is often associated with CREST syndrome. CREST is an acronym of:

Calcinosis

Raynaud's syndrome

Oesophageal dysfunction

Sclerodactyly

Telangiectasia.

Aetiology

The principle underlying abnormality is excessive production and deposition of collagen. The mechanism by which this occurs is uncertain, but disordered immune activation appears to be involved with excess T-cell help driving the production of fibrogenic mediators by inflammatory cells.

Clinicopathological features

Most patients present with Raynaud's phenomenon and the characteristic skin changes, but some patients also develop symptoms related to involvement of other organs.

Skin—becomes tight and tethered and joint mobility becomes impaired. The hands and fingers are usually affected first, the fingers become tapered and the hand takes on a claw-like configuration. Involvement of the face causes taut facial skin and the mouth appears small. At a microscopic level, there is skin oedema followed by progressive fibrosis of the dermis and epidermal atrophy. Impaired blood supply due to arterial involvement may lead to skin ulceration and autoamputation of digits.

Gastrointestinal tract—there is fibrous replacement of the muscularis. This change can affect any part of the GI tract, but the oesophagus is frequently involved resulting in dysphagia. When other parts of the GI tract are affected, malabsorption may result.

Kidneys—the renal abnormalities are due to changes in the vasculature. Vascular lesions are confined to the medium-sized arteries and are similar to those seen in hypertension. Ten to thirty per cent of patients with scleroderma develop hypertension, and in a proportion of these cases there is malignant hypertension, which may prove fatal.

Lungs—patients may develop interstitial fibrosis causing dyspnoea.

Heart—pericarditis with effusions and myocardial fibrosis are seen rarely.

Musculoskeletal—there may be a polyarthritis and a myositis.

Progression of the disease is usually slow, unless superseded by malignant hypertension. Death may occur from:

- renal failure secondary to malignant hypertension
- severe respiratory compromise
- cor pulmonale
- cardiac failure or arrhythmias secondary to myocardial fibrosis.

12.4 Soft tissue tumours

Soft tissue can be defined as non-epithelial, extra-skeletal tissue of the body, exclusive of the reticulo-endothelial system, glia, meninges, and the visceral

Learning objectives

You should:

- Understand what defines soft tissue tumours
- Understand the classification of soft tissue tumours
- Know how benign and malignant soft tissue tumours behave
- Know some common types of soft tissue tumour

parenchyma. Soft tissue tumours are a highly heterogeneous and complex group of neoplasms, which are classified according to the mature tissues that they most closely resemble. For example, lipomas and liposarcomas resemble to a varying degree normal fatty tissue. Benign soft tissue tumours are extremely common among the general population, and many never need medial attention. Malignant soft tissue tumours (sarcomas) on the other hand are relatively rare, accounting for less than 1% of all cancers. However, sarcomas often behave extremely aggressively and are capable of metastasising widely. This, together with the fact that most sarcomas tend to arise within deep soft tissues and have often grown to a large size before they become clinically apparent, means that the prognosis is generally quite poor.

Because of the complex nature of this group of tumours, we present only a framework for the basic understanding of the various types of soft tissue tumours that exist (see Table 32). For the purposes of this book, it is not necessary to detail each specific entity, but some of the more common soft tissue tumours (e.g. leiomyoma of the uterus) are presented in other chapters.

Table 32 Examples of benign and malignant soft tissue tumours

Mature tissue resembled	Benign	Malignant
Fat	Lipoma	Liposarcoma
Smooth muscle	Leiomyoma	Leiomyosarcoma
Skeletal muscle	Rhabdomyoma	Rhabdomyosarcoma
Blood vessels	Haemangioma	Angiosarcoma
Perivascular tissue	Glomus tumour	Malignant glomus tumour
Fibrous tissue	Fibroma	Fibrosarcoma
Fibrohistiocytic tumours	Fibrous histiocytoma	Malignant fibrous histiocytoma
Nerves	Schwannoma, neurofibroma	Malignant peripheral nerve sheath tumour

Self-assessment: questions

Multiple choice questions

1. The following statements are correct:
   a. Osteogenesis imperfecta is caused by dietary insufficiency
   b. Osteoporosis rarely occurs in men
   c. Osteomalacia and rickets are caused by a lack of vitamin K
   d. Bowing of the legs is a feature of osteomalacia
   e. In Paget's disease, affected bones become enlarged and are therefore not vulnerable to fracture.

2. The following statements are correct:
   a. *Staphylococcus aureus* is responsible for the majority of cases of pyogenic osteomyelitis
   b. Osteomyelitis may complicate compound fractures
   c. Following its fracture, the scaphoid bone is particularly vulnerable to avascular necrosis
   d. Osteosarcomas are the most common bone tumours
   e. Bone tumours may form cartilage.

3. Osteoarthritis:
   a. Is caused by bacterial infection of the articular cartilage
   b. Is a multisystem disorder
   c. Is characterised by pannus formation
   d. Usually affects the weight-bearing joints
   e. Is associated with Heberden's nodes, which represent prominent osteophytes at the distal interphalangeal joints.

4. The following statements are correct:
   a. Rheumatoid arthritis is a multisystem disorder
   b. Rheumatoid factor is an autoantibody that is directed against articular cartilage
   c. In rheumatoid arthritis, joint deformities may develop in the hands
   d. The majority of patients with ankylosing spondylitis are HLA-B27 positive
   e. In ankylosing spondylitis, the most frequently affected joints are those of the lower limbs.

5. The following statements are correct:
   a. Bacterial infective arthritis may cause joint destruction
   b. Gout is due to deposition of calcium pyrophosphate crystals within the joint
   c. The joint most frequently affected by gout is the knee joint
   d. Use of diuretics may predispose to the development of gout
   e. The crystal seen in joints affected by pseudogout are rhomboid in shape and exhibit positive birefringence on polarising microscopy.

6. Systemic lupus erythematosus:
   a. Is more common in females than males
   b. In most cases is characterised by circulating antinuclear antibodies, which mediate the tissue damage
   c. May be drug-induced
   d. Causes renal abnormalities in almost all patients
   e. May be associated with a skin rash that is limited to the trunk.

7. The following statements are correct:
   a. Patients with dermatomyositis have an increased risk of developing visceral malignancies
   b. cANCA is often detected in the serum of patients with polyarteritis nodosa
   c. Cranial (temporal) arteritis may lead to blindness if untreated
   d. Systemic sclerosis is characterised by excess deposition of collagen
   e. Skin involvement, which is characteristic of systemic sclerosis, is not seen in patients with CREST syndrome.

Case histories

Case history 1

A 60-year-old woman attends the accident and emergency department complaining of pain in her left hip following a trivial fall. A history reveals that she has been getting backache for some time. She is otherwise well but has been on steroids for Crohn's disease for some time. An X-ray demonstrates a fractured femoral neck.

1. What underlying diagnoses would you consider?
2. How would this patient be managed?

Case history 2

A 71-year-old man with a 20-year history of rheumatoid disease regularly attends an outpatient rheumatology clinic for investigation, physiotherapy and adjustment of his drug treatment. He is presently on non-steroidal anti-inflammatory drugs and cyclo-phosphamide. At his last clinic appointment he complained of increasing shortness of breath on exertion. Auscultation of the chest revealed late inspiratory crepitations. A chest X-ray shows a finely reticulated appearance. Serum haematology showed a normocytic normochromic anaemia.

1. What deformities might you expect to see in the hands of this patient?
2. What might be the cause of his increasing shortness of breath?
3. What are the possible causes of his anaemia?

Short note questions

Write short notes on:
1. The aetiology of osteomalacia.
2. The pathogenesis of osteomyelitis.
3. CREST syndrome.
4. Autoantibodies.

Viva questions

1. What functions does bone perform?
2. How are bone tumours classified?
3. What features do the seronegative spondyloarthropathies have in common as a group of disorders?

Self-assessment: answers

Multiple choice answers

1. a. **False.**
   b. **False.** Osteoporosis occurs in both males and females.
   c. **False.**
   d. **False.** In osteomalacia the shape of the bone is not affected.
   e. **False.** Affected bones are more vulnerable to fracture because the enlarged bone is structurally unsound.

2. a. **True.**
   b. **True.**
   c. **True.**
   d. **False.** Metastases are the most common tumours of bone. Osteosarcomas are the most common primary bone cancers.
   e. **True.**

3. a. **False.**
   b. **False.**
   c. **False.** Pannus formation is seen in rheumatoid arthritis.
   d. **True.**
   e. **True.**

4. a. **True.**
   b. **False.**
   c. **True.**
   d. **True.**
   e. **False.**

5. a. **True.**
   b. **False.**
   c. **False.**
   d. **True.**
   e. **True.**

6. a. **True.**
   b. **True.**
   c. **True.**
   d. **True.**
   e. **False.** The skin rash is not limited to the trunk.

7. a. **True.**
   b. **False.** pANCA (not cANCA) is often detected in PAN.
   c. **True.**
   d. **True.**
   e. **False.**

Case histories

Case history 1

1. In this situation, a number of underlying pathologies should be considered. Most cases of fractured neck of femur are due to underlying osteoporosis. The recent history of backache and the fact that this woman is taking steroids would support this diagnosis. The other main diagnosis to consider is a pathological fracture secondary to bony metastases. The recent history of backache may be due to the presence of metastatic deposits in the spine. It is also important to realise that bones affected by Paget's disease and osteomalacia are prone to fracture. The appearance of the bone adjacent to the fracture on X-ray may help establish the diagnosis.

2. The patient would need to have surgery to remove the head of the femur and replace it with a prosthesis. It is unlikely that the fracture would have healed by itself since fractures through the neck of the femur interrupt the blood supply to the head, which makes fracture healing difficult. Surgery is performed as soon as possible so that the patients can be mobilised quickly. Patients immobilised after hip fractures are prone to developing pneumonia, which can be rapidly fatal.

Case history 2

1. This man has had rheumatoid arthritis for some time now and so many deformities may be present in the hands including swelling of the interphalangeal joints, flexion and hyperextension deformities of the fingers, radial deviation at the wrists and ulnar deviation at the metacarpophalangeal joints. In elderly individuals, you may also see changes related to osteoarthritis.

2. Increasing shortness of breath associated with coarse crackles on auscultation of the lung fields and a ground-glass appearance on chest X-ray would raise the suspicion of interstitial lung disease, which patients with rheumatoid arthritis are at increased risk of developing. Lung function tests could be performed to confirm this.

3. A normocytic normochromic anaemia is seen in anaemia of chronic disease, which is the most likely cause of the anaemia in this case. However, when

you discover anaemia in a patient on long-term non-steroidal anti-inflammatory drug treatment, you should consider the possibility of chronic blood loss owing to drug-induced peptic ulceration, but this would characteristically induce a microcytic anaemia.

Short note answers

1. Osteomalacia is caused by vitamin D deficiency. To give a full account of the aetiology, you must understand how vitamin D deficiency may arise. There are two main sources of vitamin D—diet and endogenous synthesis in the skin. Hence, poor diet, intestinal malabsorption and reduced exposure to sunlight may all lead to osteomalacia. Newly synthesised vitamin D is biologically inactive and conversion to its active form occurs in the liver and kidneys. Hence renal disease and liver disease may also lead to osteomalacia.

2. Remember that the term 'pathogenesis' refers to the process of production and development of a lesion, i.e. the mechanism through which the aetiology operates to produce the pathological and clinical manifestation. Hence, a sequence of events linking the aetiological agent to the end lesion is what is wanted here. The aetiological agent in osteomyelitis is a microorganism, which may gain access to bone via several routes. When the infection has been localised in bone, the ensuing inflammation causes a sequence of events culminating in bone necrosis.

3. CREST syndrome is associated with systemic sclerosis. There are two main forms of systemic sclerosis: diffuse and localised. The diffuse form is characterised by widespread skin involvement and early visceral involvement. The localised form is characterised by usually localised skin involvement and late visceral involvement. Calcinosis, Raynaud's phenomenon, oesophageal dysmotility, sclerodactyly and telangiectasia are features often seen in the localised form, and affected patients are then

sometimes said to have CREST syndrome (CREST being an acronym of these five features).

4. Start by giving a definition of what an autoantibody is: an antibody directed against self-antigens (or autoantigens). Interactions between autoantibodies and autoantigens evoke an immune response against the individual's own tissues, a process known as autoimmunity. The immune reaction is self-perpetuating, causing chronic inflammatory disorders, which are known as autoimmune diseases. At this point, it would be a good idea to list the main autoimmune diseases, such as SLE and rheumatoid arthritis, remembering also to include some 'organ-specific' autoimmune diseases such as Grave's disease, Hashimoto's thyroiditis and myasthenia gravis.

Viva answers

1. Remember that bone performs a number of functions other than just providing structural support. It is protective to certain organs, and it is involved in mineral homeostasis and haematopoiesis.

2. You should devise a system that enables you to classify all tumours. A simple one is to divide them into primary tumours and secondary tumours. Primary tumours are then subdivided into benign and malignant. Further classification is usually according to the cell of origin or histological appearance, and for bone tumours this means dividing them into those that are bone-forming, those that are cartilage-forming, and miscellaneous tumours such as Ewing's sarcoma and fibroblastic tumours.

3. The seronegative spondyloarthropathies are a group of disorders characterised by an inflammatory arthritis associated with disorders (usually infectious) in other systems. They include ankylosing spondylitis, Reiter's syndrome, enteropathic arthropathy and psoriatic arthritis. Patients are seronegative for rheumatoid factors, and many are HLA-B27 positive.

13 Skin

Overview

The skin is a multifunctional organ involved in structural support, protection from injury and infection and temperature regulation. When these functions are dramatically disturbed—in extensive burn injuries, for example—patients are at risk of fatal metabolic and fluid homeostasis disruption or overwhelming bacterial infection. Skin neoplasms are very common in white skinned races, with malignant melanoma rising rapidly in incidence. There are many inflammatory diseases of the skin that cause significant morbidity and cosmetic problems.

13.1 Inflammation and infection

Learning objectives

You should:

- Understand the terminology used to described skin lesions macroscopically

- Know how inflammatory skin diseases can be classified according to the pattern of microscopic changes; this will help your understanding of clinical dermatology

- Understand the classification and complications of burns

One of the common difficulties students encounter when learning about skin diseases is the large number of specific terms used to describe both macroscopic and microscopic appearances. The following list includes the naked-eye descriptive terms used later in this chapter:

Macule—flat area of altered colour
Papule—small raised lesion
Plaque—slightly raised, flat-topped lesion
Erythema—reddening of the skin
Vesicle—small fluid filled lesion
Bulla—larger fluid filled lesion
Blister—non-specific term that includes vesicle and bulla

The following terms are microscopic descriptions:

Hyperkeratosis—increased thickness of the superficial keratin
Parakeratosis—presence of residual nuclear material within the superficial keratin (implies abnormal maturation)
Spongiosis—intercellular oedema in the epidermis, characteristically seen in eczematous lesions
Acanthosis—thickening of the epidermis
Acantholysis—discohesion, 'falling apart', of epidermal cells

Inflammatory skin diseases can be classified according to the pattern of histological changes (Table 33).

Eczema—is a common inflammatory skin disease presenting clinically with red papules or plaques containing small vesicles, which may itch, ooze and crust. There are several clinical subtypes. The characteristic histological feature is intercellular oedema in the epidermis (spongiosis), which separates the keratinocytes and can cause vesicle formation. Chronic inflammation with lymphocytic infiltration of the epidermis and dermis is often seen. Pathogenesis is variable and includes:

- direct toxic effects (irritant contact dermatitis)
- delayed hypersensitivity reaction (allergic contact dermatitis)
- combination of IgE-mediated and T-cell mediated reaction (atopic eczema).

Psoriasis—is a common chronic relapsing dermatitis that classically manifests as circumscribed red skin plaques often several centimetres in diameter, with silvery surface scale. Extensor surfaces of knees and elbows, the sacral region and the scalp are common sites. Nail changes are common and arthritis develops in a small percentage of patients. Onset is usually in early adult life. The pathogenesis is unclear but there is

Table 33 Major skin inflammatory disease patterns

Spongiotic	Spongiosis—intraepidermal oedema	Eczema
Psoriasiform	Regular epidermal hyperplasia (thickening)	Psoriasis
Lichenoid	Damage to basal epidermis, often with chronic inflammatory infiltrate along dermo–epidermal junction	Lichen planus Lupus erythematosus Erythema multiforme Graft versus host disease
Vesico-bullous	Vesicle or blister (bulla) formation	Pemphigoid Dermatitis herpetiformis Pemphigus
Granulomatous	Chronic inflammation with aggregates of enlarged (epithelioid) histiocytes	Sarcoidosis Infection (tuberculosis, fungal) Reaction to foreign material
Vasculitis	Inflammation of vessel walls (see Chapter 1, Section 1.6)	Primary cutaneous vasculitis Skin involvement by systemic vasculitis
Panniculitis	Inflammation of the subcutaneous fat	Erythema nodosum

hyperproliferation of keratinocytes, with the epidermal turnover time reduced from the normal 13 days to 3–4 days. The histological features of classical psoriasis are:

- regular epidermal hyperplasia (thickening)
- parakeratosis (retained nuclei within the surface keratin layer)
- thinning of the granular layer
- neutrophil microabscesses
- increased mitotic activity (cell turnover).

Lichen planus—presents clinically as multiple small itchy violet papules, around the wrist and elbows. Oral and genital lesions also occur. Skin lesions often resolve after several months or years. Histological features include:

- irregular epidermal hyperplasia
- damage to the basal epidermis with vacuolation and apoptotic epidermal cells
- band-like ('lichenoid') chronic inflammatory infiltrate at the dermo-epidermal junction.

Erythema multiforme (EM)—is an uncommon but potentially serious hypersensitivity response to certain infections (herpes simplex and *Mycoplasma*) and drugs (including sulphonamides, penicillin and aspirin). Clinical lesions include red macules, papules

and vesicles. The characteristic 'target' lesion has a pale, raised or eroded centre and erythematous (red) rim. Symmetrical involvement of the limbs is most commonly seen. Stevens–Johnson syndrome is severe erythema multiforme with oral mucosal lesions. Toxic epidermal necrosis is the most serious manifestation of EM, with a high risk of systemic sepsis and fluid imbalance due to extensive loss of skin and mucosal epithelium; mortality is 35%. Histology shows a lichenoid inflammatory infiltrate with epidermal cell apoptosis.

Vesico-bullous diseases—are classified according to the site of the vesicle formation, which may be within the epidermis or at the dermo-epidermal junction. The pathogenesis in many cases involves immune complex formation with autoantibodies. Examples are shown in Table 34. Many of these diseases are described further in the text of this chapter.

Burns

Burns can be caused by hot liquids (scalds), gases or solids, as well as fire. Burn injuries are classified as:

- partial thickness (1st and 2nd degree burns)
- full thickness (3rd degree burns).

Table 34 Vesico-bullous skin diseases

Site of blistering	Disease example	Pathogenesis
Within epidermis	Impetigo Staphylococcal scalded skin syndrome	Bacterial infection
	Pemphigus	Autoantibody formation
	Spongiotic dermatitis	Extreme intercellular oedema
At dermo-epidermal junction	Epidermolysis bullosa	Hereditary defect in proteins that anchor basal epidermis cells to basement membrane
	Porphyria	Enzyme deficiency causing skin fragility
	Dermatitis herpetiformis	IgA antibody deposition
	Pemphigoid	Autoantibody formation

In 1st degree burns there is endothelial injury and leakage of intravascular fluid into the surrounding tissue. There is vascular congestion with pain and erythema, but no skin necrosis. Second degree burns show epidermal necrosis with blistering as the epidermis separates from the dermis. Regeneration of the skin surface cells can occur from adjacent viable epidermis or from surviving skin adnexal structures. More severe damage occurs in 3rd degree burns, with necrosis of the epidermis and dermis. As the extent of severe burn injuries increases, so does the risk of serious or fatal complications, including:

- septic shock
- renal failure
- adult respiratory distress syndrome (ARDS)
- scarring and contractures in survivors.

Skin grafting is often required for healing of 3rd degree burns.

Infectious disease

Skin infections are common, with a wide variety of potential pathogens, including:

- **Bacteria**
  impetigo (staphylococcal or streptococcal infection, particularly in children)
  staphylococcal scalded skin syndrome (infants and children)
  furuncles ('boils')
  cellulitis
  cutaneous tuberculosis.
- **Viruses**
  varicella-zoster (chicken pox and shingles)
  verrucae (common warts—HPV infection)
  molluscum contagiosum (poxvirus).
- **Fungi**
  Candida
  tinea (ringworm, athlete's foot).
- **Arthropods**
  scabies
  lice

13.2 Immunological disorders

Learning objective

You should:

- Appreciate that certain skin diseases are immunologically mediated (specialist immunofluorescence tests may be needed for precise diagnosis in these lesions)

Lupus erythematosus (LE)—lichenoid inflammatory pattern skin lesions may be part of systemic lupus erythematosus or more commonly isolated cutaneous disease, called discoid LE. Immunoglobulins and complement are deposited along the dermo-epidermal junction.

Graft-versus-host disease (GvHD)—recipients of immunocompetent bone marrow transplants often develop lesions in the skin, gastrointestinal tract and liver, when grafted lymphocytes attack host tissue. Cutaneous GvHD has a lichenoid pattern.

Bullous pemphigoid—is a blistering skin disease that occurs in the elderly. Up to 90% have IgG autoantibodies against the bullous pemphigoid major antigen located in the epidermal basement membrane. The vesicles and bullae usually contain eosinophils.

Pemphigus—is an intraepidermal blistering disease with autoantibodies to various structural proteins involved in intercellular adhesion.

Dermatitis herpetiformis—is a subepidermal blistering disease characterised by IgA antibody deposition, although the exact pathogenesis is unclear. There is a strong association with coeliac disease.

13.3 Genetic disorders

Learning objective

You should:

- Understand that inherited skin disease can manifest as inflammatory disease or neoplastic disease

Epidermolysis bullosa—is a rare, blistering, skin disease with several subtypes that have dominant or recessive inheritance. Some variants are lethal in early life, others cause disfiguring scars with increased risk of developing squamous cell carcinoma. Blisters develop at sites of skin trauma or rubbing.

Xeroderma pigmentosum—is a rare, autosomal-recessive disease with defective DNA repair. There is extremely high incidence of epidermal and melanocytic malignancies.

Porphyria—describes a group of rare diseases with deficiencies of enzymes involved in haem production. Porphyrins are pigments present in haemoglobin, myoglobin and cytochrome enzymes. In the skin, vesicle formation and scarring occurs, and symptoms may be precipitated by exposure to sunlight.

13.4 Neoplasia

Learning objectives

You should:

- Know the pathology of the common skin cancers—basal cell carcinoma, squamous cell carcinoma and malignant melanoma

- Understand the spectrum of benign and malignant melanocytic lesions in the skin and be able to recognise clinically suspicious 'moles'

- Be able to interpret the prognostic information provided in a histopathology report of a malignant melanoma

Neoplasms of the skin can arise from many of the component cells and tissues. The most common tumours arise from the epidermal cells and from melanocytes. The adnexal structures—eccrine sweat glands, sebaceous glands, hair follicles, and apocrine glands—can give rise to a huge range of different tumours, both benign and malignant (see Box 24).

Basal cell papilloma—also known as seborrhoeic keratosis or seborrhoeic wart. These are very common benign warty tumours arising in adults. They occur almost anywhere on the body and are often pigmented. Microscopically the tumour consists of papillary projections of uniform cells resembling normal basal epidermal keratinocytes. There is hyperkeratosis and frequent formation of keratin nodules (horn cysts).

Basal cell carcinoma—is the commonest human malignant neoplasm. Basal cell carcinoma typically arises in chronically sun-exposed skin of older adults;

80% develop on the head or neck. Metastasis is very rare occurs in less than 0.05% of patients but, if untreated, basal cell carcinoma may cause extensive local tissue erosion, hence the historical name of 'rodent ulcer'. Basal cell carcinoma has several microscopic growth patterns:

- nodular—commonest (70%)
- superficial multifocal
- infiltrative (morphoeic)—highest risk of recurrence.

The tumour cells resemble those of the normal basal epidermis and are recognised histologically by their small hyperchromatic nuclei, mitotic figures and palisading (regular arrangement) of cells at the periphery of the tumour nests.

Squamous cell carcinoma—is also a common tumour arising on sun-exposed skin of older adults. The tumour cells resemble those of the suprabasal epidermis in normal skin. Well-differentiated squamous cell carcinomas produce keratin and microscopically show thin cytoplasmic extensions or 'prickles', which represent desmosomal cell junctions, between the tumour cells. Squamous cell carcinomas have a low incidence of metastasis to local lymph nodes and distant sites (approximately 1%).

Squamous cell carcinoma often develops within a pre-existing dysplastic epidermal lesion, such as actinic keratosis or Bowen's disease (carcinoma in situ). Rarely, squamous cell carcinoma can arise in a chronic ulcer (Marjolin's ulcer), burn or scar. Immunosuppressed patients (e.g. following renal transplantation) have an increased incidence of squamous cell carcinoma.

Keratoacanthoma—is a rapidly growing keratotic nodule that resembles well-differentiated squamous cell carcinoma, both clinically and microscopically, and the distinction between the two lesions can be very difficult. Keratoacanthomas tend to involute spontaneously, but can leave marked scarring.

Box 24 Skin tumours—a simple classification

	Benign	Malignant
Epidermal	Basal cell papilloma Squamous cell papilloma	Basal cell carcinoma Squamous cell carcinoma
Melanocytic	Naevus (junctional, compound, intradermal, Spitz)	Malignant melanoma
Adnexal	Syringoma Pilomatrixoma Cylindroma	Adnexal carcinomas (rare)
Lymphoid		Cutaneous T-cell lymphoma Cutaneous B-cell lymphoma
Connective tissue	Dermatofibroma Lipoma Haemangioma	Dermatofibrosarcoma protruberans Liposarcoma Kaposi's sarcoma Angiosarcoma
	Neurofibroma Leiomyoma	Malignant nerve sheath tumours Leiomyosarcoma

Melanocytic lesions—pigmented skin lesions can be due to:

- increased melanin pigmentation of the epidermis without melanocytic proliferation (pigmented basal cell papillomas, lentigo simplex)
- benign proliferation of melanocytes (naevi)
- malignant melanoma.

Clinical features that raise suspicion of melanoma in a pigmented lesion include:

- itching, crusting or bleeding
- change in size
- change in colour
- change in shape (irregularity of lesion border)
- size > 7 mm—although malignant melanomas can be smaller than this.

Benign naevi (singular = naevus)—are extremely common and may be congenital or acquired. Most arise in childhood or adolescence. Naevi are classified according to the distribution of the melanocytic cells:

- junctional (naevus cells confined to epidermis)
- compound (naevus cells in epidermis and dermis)
- intradermal (naevus cells found only in dermis)
- blue naevi (intradermal, composed of spindle cells with marked melanin pigmentation).

Malignant change in acquired naevi is rare. However, large numbers of moles (> 50 per individual) do appear to confer an increased risk of melanoma. Up to 10% of giant congenital naevi (> 20 mm diameter) will develop melanoma within them.

The incidence of melanoma in the UK is rising more rapidly than that of any other malignancy. The pathogenesis is clearly linked to UV-induced cell damage. Individuals with fair skin and hair, a history of sunburn and repeated high-intensity sun exposure are at particular risk. A strong family history is also significant.

Traditionally, classification of melanoma has been by architectural type (Fig. 41):

- lentigo maligna melanoma
- superficial spreading melanoma (commonest, > 50%)
- acral lentiginous melanoma (palm and soles—rare)
- nodular melanoma.

Lentigo maligna—arises mainly on the chronically sun-exposed skin of the head and neck in the elderly. Atypical melanocytes replace the normal basal epidermis. The tumour may be present as an irregular pigmented macule for several years before invasive dermal malignancy with metastatic potential develops.

Superficial spreading melanoma—is characterised by atypical melanocytes scattered irregularly at all levels of the epidermis; this pattern is also known as 'pagetoid spread'. It can develop at any age, and is commonest on the back in males and lower leg in females.

More recently, melanomas have been classified according to their growth pattern into **radial growth phase** or **vertical growth phase**. It is proposed that only tumours showing evidence of proliferation in the

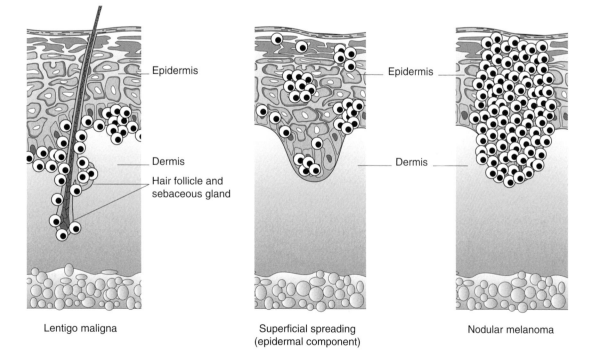

Epidermis

Dermis

Hair follicle and sebaceous gland

Epidermis

Dermis

Lentigo maligna

Superficial spreading (epidermal component)

Nodular melanoma

Fig. 41 Common growth patterns of melanoma.

dermis (vertical growth phase) have the capacity to metastasise (Table 35).

Classical melanoma cells are 'epithelioid'—large polygonal or cuboidal cells with copious cytoplasm and a large single eosinophilic nucleolus. Pigmentation is often found in a percentage of cells, but amelanotic lesions do occur and may be misdiagnosed clinically. Melanoma cells can also be spindle shaped. The histological diagnosis can be confirmed with immunocytochemistry with antibodies to S100 (a marker of neural crest origin) and HMB45 (see Box 25).

The most important prognostic factor in melanoma is the depth of invasion (Breslow thickness), measured from the top of the granular epidermal layer to the deepest dermal melanoma cell. The anatomical depth of invasion is also expressed as Clark's level (Fig. 42). Other adverse prognostic factors include:

- ulceration
- vascular invasion
- lack of a host inflammatory response
- male gender
- anatomical site (lesions on the back have worse prognosis than those on the extremities)
- high mitotic rate
- the presence of satellite lesions (cutaneous metastases) in adjacent skin.

Survival in malignant melanoma is improving as a result of greater public and medical awareness with earlier clinical presentation. Radial growth phase lesions have virtually 100% five-year survival. When the Breslow thickness exceeds 1.5 mm, five-year survival drops to 34%.

Metastatic tumours—deposits in the skin most frequently arise from:

- melanoma
- carcinoma (particularly breast, bronchus and large-intestine adenocarcinomas).

Cutaneous infiltration by lymphoma and leukaemia can also occur.

Box 25 Immunohistochemistry

What is it?
Immunohistochemistry is a histological technique in which labelled antibodies to specific proteins are applied to tissue sections. If the protein antigen is present in the cells they will bind the antibody, which can be detected on microscopy by the attached coloured label.

When is it used?
- to confirm the nature of a cell or tumour when the morphological appearances alone are not diagnostic
- for prognosis and treatment, e.g. oestrogen receptor status in breast carcinoma.

Examples of commonly used immunohistochemical antibodies

Epithelial markers	Cam 5.2 (low-molecular-weight cytokeratin) AE1/AE3 (a 'cocktail' of cytokeratins)
Lymphocyte markers	LCA (leucocyte common antigen) CD3 (T cells) CD20 (B cells)
Melanocytic markers	S100 (also stains neural tissue) HMB-45 (a marker of melanosomes)
Connective tissues	
Muscle	Desmin, myoglobin, anti-smooth muscle actin
Vascular endothelium	Factor-8-related antigen
Nerve	S100
Others	Prostatic specific antigen (PSA) α-Fetoprotein (hepatocellular carcinoma and certain germ-cell tumours) Oestrogen receptor (ER)—breast cancer prognosis

---

Table 35 Melanoma growth-phase classification

Radial growth phase melanoma	Vertical growth phase melanoma
Tumour grows within epidermis, with only single cells or small nests of melanocytes in the papillary dermis	Tumour usually involves the reticular dermis
Melanocyte cell groups in the epidermis larger than those in the dermis	Melanocyte cell groups in the dermis larger than those in the epidermis
No dermal mitoses are present	Dermal mitoses are often present

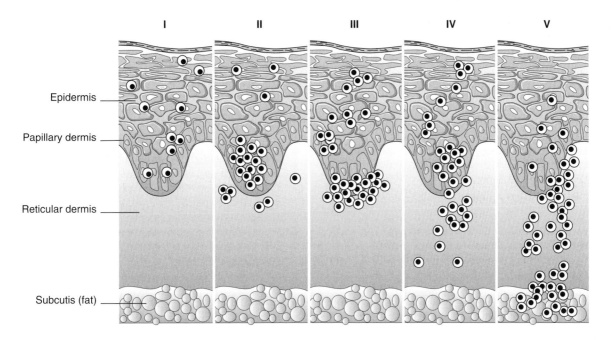

Fig. 42 Clark's levels (I–V) for staging of malignant melanomas: I, confined to epidermis; II, papillary dermal invasion; III, papillary-reticular dermis junction invasion; IV, reticular dermis invasion; V, subcutis invasion.

Self-assessment: questions

Multiple choice questions

1. Granulomatous inflammation is typically seen in:
   a. Tuberculosis
   b. Ulcerative colitis
   c. Erythema multiforme
   d. Foreign body reaction
   e. Sarcoidosis.

2. In psoriasis:
   a. The flexor surfaces are mainly affected
   b. The epidermis shows regular thickening
   c. Epidermal turnover time is increased
   d. Nail changes are common
   e. Skin lesions consist of red plaques with silvery scale.

3. The following are correctly paired:
   a. Spongiosis—dermal oedema
   b. Erythema multiforme—lichenoid inflammation
   c. Xeroderma pigmentosum—squamous cell carcinoma
   d. Pemphigoid—bullae formation
   e. Dermatitis herpetiformis—granulomatous inflammation.

4. In a pigmented lesion, the following clinical features are suggestive of malignant melanoma:
   a. Irregular border
   b. Uniform pigmentation
   c. Itching
   d. Changing size
   e. Bleeding.

5. The following are risk factors for squamous cell carcinoma:
   a. Bowen's disease
   b. Chronic skin ulceration
   c. Psoriasis
   d. Actinic keratosis
   e. Irradiation.

6. Regarding basal cell carcinoma:
   a. 5% of tumours metastasise
   b. It is commonest on the lower limbs
   c. The microscopic growth pattern influences the risk of local recurrence
   d. If left untreated, it can erode into underlying bone
   e. It occurs exclusively in patients aged over 50.

Case histories

Case history 1

A 34-year-old male presents to his GP with an enlarging lesion on his back which has recently bled. On examination there is a 7 mm papule with variable pigmentation and an irregular border. The GP decides to perform an incisional biopsy for diagnosis. Histopathology shows an ulcerated vertical growth phase superficial spreading malignant melanoma, Breslow thickness 2.1 mm, Clark's level IV.

1. Is incisional biopsy appropriate for the initial diagnosis in this situation?
2. What do Breslow thickness and Clark's level mean?
3. What does the histopathology report tell you about the likely behaviour of this tumour?

Case history 2

A 43-year-old female presents to her GP with a linear vesicular rash around the left flank and back, which is painful. On examination, the GP also notes several warty growths on the hands, arms and neck. The patient underwent renal transplantation two years earlier and is taking immunosuppressive drugs to prevent rejection of the transplanted kidney.

1. What is the likely cause of the rash?
2. Give a differential diagnosis for the warty growths.

Viva questions

1. What advice would you give to a group of healthy school children about skin cancer prevention?
2. Discuss the classification and complications of burns.

Self-assessment: answers

Multiple choice answers

1. a. **True.** Often with central caseous necrosis.
   b. **False.** Granulomas are a feature of Crohn's disease.
   c. **False.**
   d. **True.** Common foreign bodies may be exogenous, such as surgical sutures, or endogenous (liberated keratin from inflamed hair follicles or sebaceous cysts).
   e. **True.** Sarcoid granulomas do not show central necrosis.

2. a. **False.** Extensor surfaces are typically involved.
   b. **True.**
   c. **False.** Cell turnover time is decreased.
   d. **True.**
   e. **True.**

3. a. **False.** Spongiosis is intraepidermal oedema.
   b. **True.**
   c. **True.** Xeroderma pigmentosum confers a greatly increased risk of all forms of skin cancer.
   d. **True.**
   e. **False.** Dermatitis herpetiformis is a vesico-bullous disease, which microscopically shows neutrophilic inflammation.

4. a. **True.**
   b. **False.** Uniform pigmentation can be seen in benign and malignant lesions.
   c. **True.**
   d. **True.**
   e. **True.**

5. a. **True.**
   b. **True.**
   c. **False.**
   d. **True.**
   e. **True.**

6. a. **False.** The rate of metastasis is less than 1 in 1000.
   b. **False.**
   c. **True.**
   d. **True.**
   e. **False.** Although commonest in the elderly, basal cell carcinoma does occasionally occur in young adults, particularly white adults with a history of high sun exposure. Rare inherited skin disease syndromes can give rise to basal cell carcinoma in childhood.

Case histories

Case history 1

1. As the clinical features here are very suspicious of melanoma, the lesion should initially be excised complete with a narrow margin rather than biopsied, to allow accurate histological diagnosis. If this confirms melanoma, a further wider excision of the surrounding skin will be required.

2. These are described in the text and Figure 42.

3. The tumour is in the vertical growth phase, and therefore there is a risk of lymph node and distant metastasis. The Breslow thickness of over 2 mm is a poor prognostic factor as is ulceration. Statistically, male gender and lesion location on the back are also adverse features. This patient's chance of being alive five years from diagnosis is probably less than 50%.

Case history 2

1. This description of a painful, linear, vesicular rash arising in an immunosuppressed patient is virtually diagnostic of herpes zoster ('shingles'). The patient may recall a previous episode of chicken pox, representing initial infection with varicella-zoster virus. The virus persists as a latent infection in dorsal root ganglia and may become reactivated at any time, but particularly with increasing age and in periods of 'stress' or reduced immune-system functioning. The virus travels via sensory nerves to the skin, where it replicates, causing the characteristic lesions.

2. Many skin lesions can manifest as warty growths—including true viral warts and hyperkeratotic lesions. The latter include benign tumours (seborrhoeic warts/basal cell papillomas), dysplastic epithelial growths (actinic keratoses) and squamous cell carcinoma. Many of these lesions occur with increased frequency in immunosuppressed patients, reflecting the role of HPV infection in their pathogenesis.

Viva answers

1. Points to discuss would include:

   - The danger of episodic high sun exposure throughout life but particularly in childhood and young adulthood

- The rapidly increasing incidence of malignant melanoma, which is clearly linked to the increasing popularity of foreign holidays in hot places
- The need to apply appropriate sun protection products to exposed skin, and to reapply these regularly, especially before and after swimming, even on hazy days
- Covering exposed skin with hats, sleeves, skirts, long trousers, etc.

- Avoiding sun beds and tanning salons, the long-term reward of a manufactured 'healthy' tan is skin damage and tumour formation
- You could also discuss the features of a changing mole that should prompt the patient to seek medical help; these are discussed in the text.

2. Burns are discussed in the text under Section 13.1.

14 Nervous system

Overview

Diseases of the central nervous system—particularly strokes, head injuries and dementia—are major causes of morbidity and mortality. Neurons do not divide in postnatal life (they are 'permanent' cells), and neuronal cell death is repaired by proliferation of supporting cells and 'gliosis' (the CNS equivalent of scarring). Children and young adults are not immune to serious CNS pathology—meningitis, congenital malformations, birth injuries, multiple sclerosis and certain neoplasms can particularly affect this population group.

The fixed available volume within the rigid skull means that an expanding mass lesion often results in raised intracranial pressure, which is frequently fatal without prompt medical intervention. Primary and secondary tumours are not uncommon in the CNS, and again the anatomical confines of the skull and vertebral column are important factors in prognosis, due to the effects of raised intracranial pressure and the physical limitation imposed on surgical resection.

14.1 Infection and inflammation

Learning objectives

You should:

- Know the spectrum of organisms that can cause meningitis and encephalitis
- Understand the pathology of acute bacterial meningitis and the information that can be obtained from investigation of cerebrospinal fluid in suspected meningitis
- Be aware of how HIV infection can manifest in the CNS
- Understand the basic pathology of spongiform encephalopathies

Intracranial infection—can affect the arachnoid and pial membranes (meningitis) or the underlying brain itself (encephalitis). Viral, bacterial, protozoal, fungal and protein (prion) agents all contribute. Routes of entry into the CNS include:

- blood-borne spread from distant site of infection
- direct inoculation of organisms (traumatic or iatrogenic)
- local extension of sepsis (e.g. dental or sinus infection)
- via the peripheral nervous system (viral agents including herpes simplex and rabies).

Meningitis can be:

- pyogenic (bacterial)
- aseptic (viral)
- chronic (bacterial or fungal).

The microorganisms likely to be responsible vary with age and immunocompetence. Clinical symptoms include headache, neck stiffness, photophobia, irritability and altered consciousness. A skin rash may only be present with certain strains of meningococcal bacteria causing systemic sepsis. Biochemical analysis and microscopic examination of cerebrospinal fluid (CSF) obtained at lumbar puncture is helpful in discriminating the causative agent (Box 26). Bacteria and protozoa may be directly identified by microscopy.

Acute bacterial meningitis—can be fatal if not treated at an early stage. Complications include:

- extension of infection into brain tissue with abscess formation
- venous thrombosis with cerebral infarction
- meningeal fibrosis with hydrocephalus.

The infective organisms vary with the age of patients and immunisation status but include: *E. coli*, group B streptococci and *Haemophilus influenzae* in infants; *Neisseria meningitidis* and *Streptococcus pneumoniae* in older children and young adults; and *Listeria monocytogenes* in the elderly.

Viral meningitis—is clinically less important and usually self-limiting.

Tuberculous meningitis—is rare, but is increasing in frequency among AIDS patients. The onset is clinically more insidious with non-specific symptoms such as headache, confusion and vomiting. Chronic meningeal inflammation with granuloma formation and fibrosis can cause hydrocephalus and cranial nerve damage. Syphilis is a rare cause of neurological disease in the UK today, but a small percentage of those with tertiary syphilis develop chronic meningitis, sensory spinal cord damage (tabes dorsalis) or brain infection (dementia, Argyll Robertson pupils). The risk of developing neurosyphilis is increased in AIDS.

Viral infections can cause encephalitis, with lymphocytic inflammation of the brain parenchyma and proliferation of glial cells. Intraneuronal inclusions may be seen in herpes simplex Type 1 (HSV-1), cytomegalovirus (CMV) and rabies encephalopathy. Viral infections can be particularly damaging if acquired in fetal life (e.g. rubella, CMV-related congenital malformations) or during delivery (e.g. HSV-2-related neonatal sepsis).

Specific areas of the brain may be damaged; for example HSV-1 encephalitis particularly affects the temporal lobe.

Human immunodeficiency virus (HIV)—infects CNS macrophages and microglial cells. HIV infection and AIDS can cause numerous neurological lesions including:

- mild meningitis at seroconversion
- dementia-like illness
- spinal cord damage

- neuropathies
- congenital AIDS (microcephaly, motor delay and mental retardation)
- opportunistic infections
    —toxoplasmosis
    —CMV
    —cryptococcal meningitis
    —progressive multifocal leucoencephalopathy (PML)—a papovavirus infection, which affects oligodendrocytes, causing demyelination and multifocal white-matter damage.

Rabies virus—gains entry to the brain by ascending along peripheral nerves. Symptoms arise weeks after initial infection and include abnormal CNS excitability (excessive pain on light touch, convulsions), paralysis, mania, stupor and coma. Local paraesthesia around the entry wound is a diagnostic pointer.

Poliomyelitis—now very rare in industrialised countries, initially infects the gut but in a small number of cases there is spread to lower motor neurons in the spinal cord, leading to muscle wasting and paralysis. Death can occur acutely due to a myocarditis or chronically due to respiratory muscle involvement.

Fungal infections of the CNS—mainly occur in immunocompromised patients. Organisms include *Candida*, *Mucor*, *Aspergillus* and *Cryptococcus*.

Spongiform encephalopathies—are characterised by spongiform change (vacuolation) in the cerebral white matter. They are transmitted by prion protein, an abnormal form of a cellular protein that has undergone a conformational change and is able to induce a further conformational change in native protein when inoculated into previously normal cells. The prion protein gene is located on chromosome 20. It is highly conserved across species, and infectious particles in one species can corrupt the normal protein in other species. Spongiform encephalopathies include:

- scrapie in sheep
- bovine spongiform encephalopathy (BSE) in cattle
- transmissible encephalopathy in mink
- Creutzfeldt–Jakob disease (CJD), new variant CJD, and kuru in humans.

Prions are neither destroyed by most normal disinfectants nor by formalin fixation.

Box 26 CSF analysis in meningitis

Infectious agent	Predominant cell content	Protein	Glucose
Pyogenic bacteria	Neutrophil polymorphs	Increased	Marked decrease
Viral	Lymphocytes	Mild increase	Normal, occasionally decreased
Tuberculosis	Lymphocytes	Marked increase	Decreased or normal

Until the last decade, the incidence of CJD was approximately 1 per million, occurring sporadically in older adults. Iatrogenic transmission via corneal grafts, cadaveric growth hormone extracts or implanted electrodes has been documented. Recently there has been extensive debate about new variant (nv) CJD, which is thought to represent human infection by BSE transmitted by ingestion of contaminated meat products. Both CJD and new variant disease are characterised by rapidly progressive dementia with movement disorder (myoclonic jerks) and death is usual within two years of symptom onset. The eventual number of individuals likely to be affected by nv CJD remains unknown.

Brain abscesses—can occur secondary to:

- acute bacterial meningitis
- direct extension of sepsis from outside brain
- penetrating injury
- blood-borne infection (infective endocarditis, cyanotic congenital heart disease, pulmonary sepsis).

The bacteria responsible are usually streptococcal or staphylococcal. Clinical symptoms include progressive focal neurological deficit and raised intracranial pressure.

14.2 CNS trauma and raised intracranial pressure

Learning objectives

You should:

- Know the patterns of tissue damage and intracranial haemorrhage that can follow head injury
- Understand the causes and consequences of raised intracranial pressure

Mechanisms of traumatic brain injury

Contusion

Brain tissue is bruised on impact with the bony skull surface. A 'coup' injury occurs to the brain tissue underlying the point of external injury. A 'contre-coup' injury affects an area of brain directly opposite the impact. For example, a fall backwards onto the occiput causes contre-coup injury to inferior frontal lobes and inferior poles of temporal lobes (which is often more severe and clinically significant than the coup injury to the occipital lobe directly underlying the point of impact).

Laceration

Brain substance is torn, usually as a result of penetrating injury.

Diffuse axonal injury (DAI)—deceleration and rotational forces to the brain cause shearing injury to neurons and axonal processes. If extensive, this can cause coma and death. DAI is graded according to the extent of damage and the presence of grossly visible brain haemorrhage. Severe DAI can occur in the absence of any externally evident head trauma.

Tissue displacement following head injury damages blood vessels, causing haemorrhage and oedema with consequent mass effect (see *raised intracranial pressure*, below). Vascular injury and subsequent haemorrhage can be extradural, subdural, subarachnoid or intra-parenchymal.

Extradural haemorrhage—is classically seen in association with a skull fracture involving the temporal bone with laceration of the middle meningeal artery. The typical clinical history includes a 'lucid interval' of several hours between the injury and neurological deterioration.

Subdural haemorrhage—usually originates from tearing of bridging veins that pass through the subdural space between the brain and the dural sinuses. The elderly are at increased risk, as brain atrophy increases stretching of the bridging veins and allows greater movement of the smaller brain within the skull following trauma. The precipitating head injury may be so trivial as to have gone unnoticed. Subdural haemorrhage usually becomes clinically evident within hours, with non-specific signs (diminishing consciousness, headache) but may present chronically. Rebleeding is common, and may occur from vascular granulation tissue within the organising haematoma.

Subarachnoid haemorrhage (SAH)—occurring after trauma is usually secondary to brain tissue disruption. Non-traumatic SAH is more common and is discussed later in Section 14.3.

Raised intracranial pressure—the fixed skull volume allows very little room for the intracranial contents to expand in the presence of haemorrhage, tumour, abscess or oedema. Therefore a mild increase in intracranial mass can lead to increased intracranial pressure with serious consequences. Brain tissue becomes displaced (herniation). The site of herniation partly depends on whether mass increase is focal or diffuse (Fig. 43):

- cingulate gyrus (inferior frontal lobe) can herniate across the midline under the dural fold of the falx cerebri, compressing the anterior cerebral artery
- uncal gyrus (inferior temporal lobe) can herniate under the tentorium cerebelli and compress the midbrain (leading to altered consciousness),

oculomotor nerve, contralateral cerebral peduncle, aqueduct and posterior cerebral artery

- cerebellar tonsils can herniate through the foramen magnum, compressing the brainstem ('coning').

Compression of blood vessels supplying the midbrain causes venous stagnation with haemorrhage, necrosis and irreversible neuronal injury in this vital area.

Cerebral oedema—can be focal or diffuse. Oedema often makes a significant contribution to the mass effect of tumours and abscesses. The development of cerebral oedema indicates impaired function of blood–brain barrier, which normally tightly controls fluid movement within the brain. Mechanisms of cerebral oedema include:

- increased vascular permeability (vasogenic oedema)
- altered cell regulation of fluid (cytotoxic oedema)
- movement of fluid from the ventricular system into the brain.

Hydrocephalus—describes an increased volume of cerebrospinal fluid, usually due to a blockage in the CSF pathway. If occurring prior to the fusion of skull bone sutures in young children, hydrocephalus will result in head enlargement. The development of hydrocephalus may result from blood, postinflammatory fibrosis or tumour blocking CSF flow. Apparent hydrocephalus in older adults due to atrophy of brain tissue and expansion of the ventricular system is sometimes called 'hydrocephalus ex vacuo'.

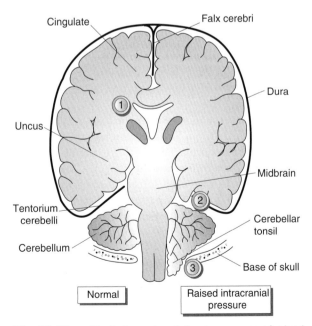

Fig. 43 Sites of brain tissue herniation in presence of raised intracranial pressure.

14.3 Cerebrovascular disease

Learning objectives

You should:

- Understand the pathogenesis of thrombotic and embolic stroke, and be able to identify clinical risk factors
- Know the causes and consequences of subarachnoid and intracerebral haemorrhage

Cerebral infarction

Normal brain function ceases within a few seconds of loss of oxygen supply; irreversible neuronal damage occurs after 6–8 minutes of anoxia. Most cerebrovascular disease results from focal impairment of blood supply causing cerebral infarction. This manifests clinically as a 'stroke'—a neurological deficit of sudden onset but lasting more than 24 hours, caused by vascular insufficiency (neurological symptoms caused by lack of blood flow but resolving within 24 hours are known as transient ischaemic attacks or 'TIA'). Stroke can be due to thrombosis or embolus.

Thrombotic stroke—usually complicates atherosclerosis in the basilar artery, proximal middle cerebral artery or at the carotid bifurcation.

As thrombotic stroke arises on a background of atheroma, risk factors include hypercholesterolaemia, hypertension, diabetes mellitus and ischaemic heart disease.

Embolic stroke—when stroke occurs secondary to embolism, the source of the embolus is usually the heart. Cardiac mural thrombus can complicate myocardial infarction and atrial fibrillation. Thrombus may also embolise from abnormal heart valves, arterial walls (especially atherosclerotic carotid arteries) or from sites of cardiac surgery. Less commonly the embolus may consist of fat, air or tumour. Cerebral fat embolus should be suspected when neurological signs develop following non-head trauma with multiple bone fractures. Most embolic strokes affect the middle cerebral artery territory. Identification of the embolus at post mortem is often not possible, as a high percentage will have lysed.

Cerebral infarction can be haemorrhagic or non-haemorrhagic, as demonstrated by CT or MRI scanning. The distinction is of therapeutic importance, as anticoagulation therapy is contraindicated in the presence of intracerebral bleeding. Thrombotic strokes are not usually complicated by bleeding. Haemorrhage can be secondary to reperfusion following an embolic stroke, but is more commonly seen in spontaneous intracerebral haemorrhage (ICH) associated with hypertension. ICH usually arises in:

- deep white matter of cerebral hemispheres/basal ganglia (> 50%)
- pons (10%)
- cerebellum (10%).

Microscopically, the small arterial branches that rupture may show fibrinoid necrosis of the vessel wall and formation of microaneurysms known as Charcot–Bouchard aneurysms. Severe bleeding can cause rapid mass effect with an acute fatal rise in intracranial pressure. Haemorrhage may rupture internally into the ventricular system or externally into the subarachnoid space.

Hypertension can also result in small, often multiple lacunar infarctions (< 15 mm in diameter) in the basal ganglia, deep white matter and pons. In accelerated or malignant hypertension, an encephalopathy may develop with headaches, vomiting, convulsions and altered conscious level.

The sequelae of stroke depend on the area of the brain involved and the extent of the infarction. Anterior circulation infarcts (internal carotid supply) affect cerebral hemispheres and can cause hemiparesis, sensory loss, dysphasia, incontinence and hemianopia. Posterior circulation infarcts (vertebrobasilar circulation) affect the brainstem and cerebellum. Neurological deficits may include ataxia and gaze abnormalities. Even small posterior circulation infarcts can cause coma and death due to involvement of vital regulatory centres in the brainstem.

Multiple small strokes can cause vascular (multi-infarct) dementia, with a stepwise deterioration in cognitive function. Cerebrovascular disease is the second commonest cause of dementia in the UK.

Rarer causes of intracerebral haemorrhage include:

- arteriovenous malformations
- tumours
- bleeding diatheses or anticoagulation therapy
- amyloid angiopathy.

Cerebral amyloid angiopathy occurs in the elderly and is associated with Alzheimer's disease (see Section 14.4). Haemorrhage is usually peripheral (lobar) in distribution.

Diffuse cerebral ischaemia can result following profound systemic hypertension. Clinically this may manifest as transient confusion with no permanent damage, or may result in widespread cerebral infarction with coma and death. The watershed areas of the brain—at the margins of perfusion by the major circle of Willis arterial branches—are particularly susceptible to such global ischaemia. Other brain regions particularly sensitive to hypoxia include:

- cerebellar Purkinje cells
- pyramidal neurones of hippocampus
- deeper neuronal layers of the cerebral cortex.

Subarachnoid haemorrhage—is a relatively frequent natural cause of sudden unexpected death in young and middle-aged adults. The pathogenesis involves a congenital defect in the muscle wall of the cerebral arteries, which becomes manifest in later life as saccular dilatations known as 'berry aneurysms'. There is an association with adult polycystic renal disease (see Chapter 10) and hypertension. The aneurysms develop mainly in the anterior part of the circle of Willis (Fig. 44), around the origin and proximal branches of the anterior and middle cerebral arteries. In 25% of cases there are multiple aneurysms. Rupture causes subarachnoid haemorrhage and clinically manifests with a sudden very severe headache. Bleeding may be precipitated by an acute rise in blood pressure (e.g.

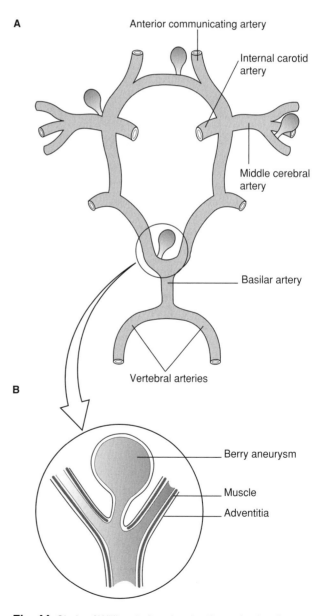

Fig. 44 Circle of Willis arteries showing the main sites for berry aneurysms.

during sexual intercourse). Females are more frequently affected than males. As with aneurysms elsewhere in the vascular system, the risk of rupture increases in proportion with the aneurysm size. Rebleeding is common in those who survive the initial insult. As the haemorrhage resolves, fibrosis of the meninges at the base of the brain can lead to subsequent hydrocephalus.

14.4 Degenerative and demyelinating diseases

Learning objective

You should:

● Understand the pathology of Alzheimer's disease, Huntington's disease and multiple sclerosis

Dementia

Alzheimer's disease

Dementia is the progressive loss of cognitive function, manifest by memory loss and global intellectual impairment without diminished consciousness. The commonest cause of dementia in the UK is Alzheimer's disease (AD). AD is uncommon in people under 75 but thereafter its incidence increases dramatically. Up to 10% of cases are familial. Down's syndrome patients can develop AD changes at an earlier age but appear to progress at a slower rate. CT head scan and brain examination at autopsy show cortical atrophy with widened sulci and compensatory dilatation of the ventricular system ('hydrocephalus ex vacuo'). Microscopically, three lesions are seen:

● neurofibrillary tangles
● senile plaques
● amyloid angiopathy.

Neurofibrillary tangles are bundles of intracytoplasmic filaments present within neurons. The tangles are often rounded or flame shaped. They can be seen on routine histological staining (haematoxylin and eosin, 'H&E') but are better demonstrated with silver impregnation stains or by immunocytochemistry. Senile (neuritic) plaques are collections of neuronal processes surrounding an amyloid core. The main protein component of the core is β-amyloid protein, derived from amyloid precursor protein (APP). β-Amyloid protein is also present in the vascular amyloid deposits of amyloid angiopathy.

Plaques, tangles and amyloid angiopathy can all be seen to a certain extent in 'normal' brains and in individuals without clinical signs of AD. Amyloid angiopathy is a cause of peripheral intracerebral haemorrhage (see Section 14.3). It is the increased number and wide distribution of plaques and tangles that correlates with clinical dementia. In AD, cortical neurons, hippocampus and the amygdala are commonly involved sites.

Pick's disease

Pick's disease is a much less common form of dementia. There is severe atrophy of the frontal and temporal lobes, with basal ganglia involvement. Cytoplasmic Pick bodies (filamentous structures similar to those seen in AD) are present within neurons.

Huntington's disease

This is a progressive inherited dementia associated with uncontrolled movements (chorea). Onset is in middle age. Atrophy occurs in the caudate, putamen and frontal lobes. The involuntary movements result from loss of GABA-utilising inhibitory neurons, which regulate motor output in the basal ganglia. Huntington's is an autosomal dominant condition with full penetrance, and new mutations are very rare. The gene responsible lies on chromosome 4 and contains repeats of the trinucleotide base sequence CAG. The normal allele contains 11–34 CAG copies, but in Huntington's there is amplification of this base sequence, with up to several hundred copies. The age of onset of disease decreases with each successive generation as the number of CAG copies increases (this phenomenon is known as 'anticipation'). A similar mechanism of disease is seen in X-linked spinal muscular atrophy, which is linked to trinucleotide repeats in the androgen receptor gene.

Parkinson's disease

This is a movement disorder characterised by:

● abnormal gait and facial expression
● rigidity
● pill-rolling tremor
● difficulty in initiating movement
● dementia in a proportion of cases.

There is damage to dopamine-utilising neurones in the nigrostriatal tract. Loss of substantia nigra pigmentation can be identified at autopsy. Microscopically, Lewy bodies (cytoplasmic neuronal inclusions) can be seen in brain-stem nuclei, the cingulate gyrus and hippocampus.

Motor neuron disease

This is clinically manifest by progressive muscular atrophy, fasciculation and symmetrical weakness. There is atrophy of anterior motor roots of the spinal cord (lower motor neurons) and of corticospinal tracts (upper motor neurons). Patients are usually middle-aged males. Death is often due to respiratory complications.

Toxic and metabolic disorders

Toxic and metabolic disorders of the nervous system include thiamine (vitamin B_1) deficiency and B_{12} deficiency. The latter affects long tracts with lower-limb weakness, ataxia and sensory loss (known as subacute combined degeneration of the cord). Other uncommon but important causes of neurological damage include hypoglycaemia, hepatic encephalopathy and ethanol.

Fetal alcohol syndrome

Fetal alcohol syndrome, which is caused by excess maternal ethanol intake during pregnancy, comprises:

- growth restriction
- cardiac septal defects
- facial abnormalities
- mental retardation.

Demyelinating disorders

Demyelinating disorders affect oligodendrocytes in the CNS or the myelin sheath of peripheral nerves.

Multiple sclerosis (MS)

MS is characterised by repeated episodes of demyelination within the central nervous system. Neurological deficit is variable. It may be relatively mild, with relapses and remissions, or severe and chronically progressive. Unilateral optic neuropathy causing sudden visual deterioration is the commonest presentation, but the diagnosis is based on finding CNS lesions disseminated in time and space. The aetiology of MS is unknown. No specific infectious agent has been implicated, although there are increased serum and CSF antibody titres to common viruses. The pathogenesis may involve an immune reaction against myelin, possibly triggered by viral infection.

Epidemiology
- Incidence of MS increases with increasing distance from the equator, particularly in the northern hemisphere
- Peak onset age 20–35
- More common in females
- Increased risk for first degree relatives but no pattern of inheritance.

CSF analysis shows normal or increased protein and there is often an oligoclonal increase in IgG. Lymphocytes are usually increased in number.

The pathological lesions are plaques, a few millimetres in diameter, which can be seen on MRI scans and on examination of the brain and spinal cord at autopsy. Typical sites include:

- periventricular cerebral white matter
- optic nerves
- brainstem
- cervical cord.

Myelin is destroyed and oligodendrocytes lost but axons are preserved. There is a chronic inflammatory infiltrate. Older plaques become scarred ('gliotic').

14.5 Congenital malformations and genetic disease of the CNS

Learning objective

You should:

- Know the common types of congenital malformation in the CNS

CNS malformations

Neural tube defects
Neural tube defects (NTDs)—affect 2 per 1000 pregnancies in UK, although their frequency in live births is much lower (many such pregnancies are terminated). Many NTDs can be detected antenatally by serum α-fetoprotein measurement and ultrasound. Defects include anencephaly, encephalocoele and spinal fusion defects (Box 27). Recurrence rate in subsequent pregnancies is approximately 5%. The incidence of NTDs varies in different ethnic groups. Folate deficiency is a recognised aetiological factor. Spinal defects are commonest and usually involve the lumbosacral region, predisposing to infection and cord damage. Box 28 details other more common CNS malformations.

Cerebral palsy—is a non-progressive neurological defect arising in the perinatal period. The cause may not be apparent but intrauterine hypoxia, infection, birth trauma, kernicterus and hypoglycaemia may contribute. In premature babies, development of cerebral palsy is associated with cerebral haemorrhage and ischaemic damage to white matter (periventricular leucomalacia).

Inborn errors of metabolism in the CNS—include neuronal storage diseases and white-matter diseases (leucodystrophies) involving damage to myelin or oligodendrocytes. Storage diseases usually have an autosomal recessive pattern of inheritance. Enzyme deficiencies cause accumulation of substrate (e.g. mucopolysaccha-

Box 27 Neural tube defects

Anencephaly	Absence of brain and skull
Encephalocoele	Occipital bone defect with herniation of brain tissue
Meningomyelocoele	Spinal column bony defect with exposed CNS tissue
Meningocoele	Spinal column defect with herniation of meninges but no involvement of neural tissue
Spina bifida	Vertebral body bony defects but no involvement of spinal cord tissue

Box 28 CNS malformations

Microcephaly (small brain)	Fetal alcohol syndrome HIV CMV
Holoprosencephaly (incomplete separation of cerebral hemispheres)	Trisomy 13
Arnold–Chiari malformation	Multiple abnormalities involving cerebellum, medulla, aqueduct (stenosis) and lumbosacral spinal column (myelomeningocoele)
Dandy–Walker	Absent central cerebellum replaced by midline cyst

rides, sphingolipids) within neuronal lysosomes and ultimately cell death.

Friedreich's ataxia—is an inherited spinocerebellar degeneration with axonal loss in long tracts. Onset is usually in late childhood, with boys more commonly affected than girls. Symptoms include ataxia, dysarthria, sensory loss and progressive paralysis. There may be associated cardiomyopathy.

14.6 Neoplasms

Learning objectives

You should:

- Appreciate how the anatomy of the skull and spinal column influences the prognosis of both benign and malignant primary CNS tumours
- Know the types of tumours that can arise within the central and peripheral nervous systems

Primary nervous system tumours arise from:

- glial cells—astrocytes, oligodendrocytes and ependymal cells (60%)
- meningeal cells (20%)
- choroid plexus epithelium
- lymphoid cells
- nerve sheath (Schwann cells).

Central nervous system tumours

Intracranial tumours are ten times more frequent than spinal neoplasms. About 20% of childhood cancers arise in the CNS. Primary tumours of the CNS cannot be labelled as 'benign' or 'malignant' using the same criteria as for tumours arising elsewhere in the body. Cytologically benign tumours can show locally extensive growth patterns preventing surgical excision. Slow-growing lesions can prove fatal due to their location or mass effect (e.g. benign tumour of the brainstem). Even microscopically high-grade tumours rarely metastasise outside the CNS, although dissemination can occur via the subarachnoid space and CSF pathways. Up to half of all CNS neoplasms are primary. The rest are metastases arising largely from carcinoma of the lung, breast, kidney, gastrointestinal tract and from malignant melanoma.

Astrocytomas—are the most common adult primary brain tumours. High-grade tumours (glioblastoma multiforme) have a very poor prognosis. Low-grade astrocytomas often dedifferentiate to high-grade tumours over the course of several years.

Oligodendrocytomas—account for up to 15% of gliomas, and occur in middle-aged adults. Tumours arise in the cerebral hemispheres. Survival averages 5–10 years post-diagnosis.

Ependymomas—most commonly occur in the 4th ventricle in children, causing hydrocephalus. Their prognosis is poor as surgery is difficult and there is a tendency to dissemination via the cerebrospinal fluid.

Choroid plexus papillomas—mainly occur in the lateral ventricle during childhood. They cause hydrocephalus due to obstruction of CSF flow and increased CSF production.

Medulloblastoma—is a primitive neural tumour which accounts for 20% of childhood brain tumours. It is a rapidly growing lesion in the central cerebellum, which can cause hydrocephalus. Medulloblastoma spreads along CSF pathways, but is highly sensitive to radiotherapy.

Primary brain lymphoma—is increasing in incidence. The pathogenesis is linked to Epstein–Barr virus infection and immunosuppression, but the frequency of lymphoma is also rising in immunocompetent individuals. Tumour deposits are often multiple. Histologically,

Table 36 Cancer checklist: astrocytoma

Incidence	Commonest in middle-aged and elderly adults (cerebral hemispheres); cerebellar astrocytomas in children
Risk factors	Not established
Protective factors	Not established
Associated lesions	Occasional gliomas are part of neurofibromatosis or inherited cancer syndromes (e.g. Turcot's syndrome)
Common clinical presentation	Seizures, focal neurological signs Headache and vomiting if raised intracranial pressure
Location	Cerebral hemispheres most common, but can arise in brainstem, cerebellum and spinal cord
Macroscopic appearance	Poorly defined mass infiltrating adjacent brain
Histological features	Vary from low to high grade according to mitotic activity, nuclear pleomorphism and necrosis
Pattern of spread	Local brain infiltration
Prognosis (per cent 5-year survival)	Approximately 5–10 years' survival for low grade astrocytoma; 8–10 months' average survival in glioblastoma multiforme (high-grade tumour)

these are high-grade, B-lymphocyte, non-Hodgkin's lymphomas.

Meningiomas—are usually benign tumours of adulthood, arising from meningothelial cells of the arachnoid. Meningiomas are commoner in women and occur in young and middle-aged adults. Meningiomas can compress and invaginate into the brain substance but remain separate from it, which may permit surgical excision. Overlying bone can be eroded or infiltrated. There are many histological subtypes.

Metastatic tumours—frequently found in the CNS include lung and breast carcinomas and malignant melanomas.

Paraneoplastic symptoms

Paraneoplastic symptoms are defined as clinical phenomena associated with malignancy but not directly attributable to tumour infiltration. Paraneoplastic symptoms involving the CNS most commonly occur with small cell lung carcinoma. The pathogenesis is uncertain but may be immunologically mediated by antibodies against tumour expressed antigens cross-reacting against nervous system cells. CNS paraneoplastic syndromes include:

- cerebellar degeneration (antibody-mediated damage to Purkinje cells)
- spinal cord damage
- limbic encephalitis (a form of subacute dementia).

Peripheral nerve sheath tumours

Schwannoma is a benign tumour of cells that produce myelin in the peripheral nervous system. Schwannomas can involve cranial nerves, especially the VIIIth nerve, which gives rise to the name 'acoustic neuroma'. Schwannomas are encapsulated tumours attached to the nerve. Malignant change is very rare.

Neurofibroma—is a common tumour composed of Schwann cells, fibroblasts and perineural cells. Neurofibromas are unencapsulated, and cannot be separated from nerve in which they arise. Neurofibromas occur sporadically or in patients with neurofibromatosis (Box 29).

Malignant peripheral nerve sheath tumours—arise de novo or from transformation of neurofibromas in neurofibromatosis.

Box 29 Neurofibromatosis

Type 1
Mutation in tumour suppressor gene on chromosome 17
Autosomal dominantly inherited or spontaneous mutation
Characterised by:

- multiple neurofibromas (cutaneous and visceral)
- pigmented skin macules (café-au-lait patches)
- pigmented nodules on the iris (Lisch nodules)

There is an increased incidence of other tumours including acoustic neuromas, gliomas, meningiomas, phaeochromocytomas.

Mental retardation and skeletal abnormalities are common

Type 2
Bilateral acoustic schwannomas, with or without cutaneous neurofibromas.
No iris nodules.
Tumour suppressor gene involved is on chromosome 22

Self-assessment: questions

Multiple choice questions

1. Prion protein:
   a. Is degraded by formalin
   b. Is present in plaques of Alzheimer's disease
   c. Is highly conserved across species
   d. Causes cell damage by inducing a conformational change in normal protein
   e. Can be transmitted by corneal grafts.

2. Berry aneurysms:
   a. Are usually multiple
   b. Classically cause subdural haemorrhage
   c. Are associated with polycystic kidney disease
   d. Are present at birth
   e. Have a high risk of rebleeding following rupture.

3. In multiple sclerosis:
   a. There is loss of both myelin and axons
   b. Unilateral optic nerve involvement is a common presentation
   c. The incidence is highest in equatorial countries
   d. The cerebrospinal fluid often contains an oligoclonal increase in IgM antibodies
   e. Plaques are characteristically found in the periventricular white matter of the cerebral hemispheres.

4. Subdural haemorrhage:
   a. Is commonest in the elderly
   b. May not become clinically evident until several weeks after the event
   c. Is always preceded by a significant head injury
   d. Usually originates from the subdural sinuses
   e. Is rarely complicated by rebleeding.

5. The following are correctly paired:
   a. Huntington's disease—trinucleotide repeats
   b. Parkinson's disease—neurofibrillary tangles
   c. Pick's disease—frontal lobe atrophy
   d. Alzheimer's disease—amyloid angiopathy
   e. Fetal alcohol syndrome—cardiac septal defects.

6. The following are causes of non-traumatic intracranial haemorrhage:
   a. Hypertension
   b. Thrombocytopaenia
   c. Cerebral embolism
   d. Arteriovenous malformations
   e. Glioblastoma multiforme.

7. Concerning meningitis:
   a. Cerebrospinal fluid neutrophils are always increased
   b. Cerebral infarction is a complication
   c. *Neisseria meningitidis* is the commonest causative organism in infants
   d. Cryptococcal meningitis is increasing in incidence
   e. Viral meningitis is associated with markedly low CSF glucose.

8. Neural tube defects:
   a. Affect 2 per 1000 live births in the UK
   b. Can be detected by serum CEA measurement
   c. Of the spine are commonest in the cervical region
   d. Recur in 10% of subsequent pregnancies with the same parents
   e. Are associated with folate deficiency.

9. Concerning CNS tumours:
   a. The commonest primary glial tumours are astrocytomas
   b. Twenty per cent of childhood malignancy occurs in the CNS
   c. Glioblastoma multiforme metastasises widely outside the CNS
   d. Medulloblastoma is usually radiosensitive
   e. Primary brain lymphoma is associated with herpes simplex virus.

10. The following are risk factors for cerebral infarction:
    a. Myocardial infarction
    b. Infective endocarditis
    c. Fat embolism
    d. Diabetes insipidus
    e. Septic shock.

Case histories

Case history 1

A 56-year-old man presents with a nine-month history of worsening concentration and forgetfulness. He is anxious because his wife has noticed his behaviour has changed and he is worried that he has a brain tumour.

1. What clinical diagnosis do these symptoms suggest?
2. What further information would you seek from the history and clinical examination to help determine the underlying cause?

Case history 2

You are a consultant histopathologist, and have been asked by the Coroner to carry out a post-mortem examination on a 19-year-old male who died unexpectedly. The deceased had been out with friends the night before his death and had consumed several pints of lager. He had been involved in a fight and had briefly been knocked unconscious but appeared to recover within a few minutes and did not seek medical help. He had later felt tired and had been taken home to bed by his friends, where he was found dead the morning after.

1. What causes of death would you consider likely in this scenario?
2. On exposing the skull, you identify a fracture of the right temporal bone. What other abnormalities do you now expect to find inside the cranial cavity?

Case history 3

A 32-year-old female presents with a two-week history of headaches and recent onset of left-arm weakness. A CT head scan (with contrast) shows an intracerebral mass with rim enhancement and a low-density centre.

1. What is the differential diagnosis?
2. What further information would you seek from the history and clinical examination to help determine the underlying cause?

Viva questions

1. How can tumour involvement of the CNS present clinically?

Self-assessment: answers

Multiple choice answers

1. a. **False.**
   b. **False.**
   c. **True.**
   d. **True.**
   e. **True.**

2. a. **False.** Twenty-five per cent are multiple.
   b. **False.** Subarachnoid.
   c. **True.** In a proportion of cases.
   d. **False.** The weakness of the arterial wall is present at birth but the aneurysms develop in later life.
   e. **True.**

3. a. **False.** Axons are not damaged.
   b. **True.**
   c. **False.**
   d. **False.** There may be oligoclonal IgG antibody increase.
   e. **True.**

4. a. **True.** Alcoholics are another high risk group.
   b. **True.**
   c. **False.** The injury may be trivial and may have gone unnoticed or not be remembered.
   d. **False.** From bridging veins.
   e. **False.** Rebleeding from vascular granulation tissue in the organising thrombus is common.

5. a. **True.**
   b. **False.**
   c. **True.**
   d. **True.**
   e. **True.**

6. a. **True.**
   b. **True.**
   c. **True.**
   d. **True.**
   e. **True.**

7. a. **False.** Neutrophil polymorphs are inconsistently present in tuberculous meningitis and are absent in viral meningitis.
   b. **True.**
   c. **False.** *Haemophilus influenzae* in young children and *E. coli* in babies.
   d. **True.** Through its association with HIV infection.
   e. **False.** CSF glucose is usually normal in viral meningitis.

8. a. **False.** Many are detected antenatally and may be aborted spontaneously or by medical intervention.
   b. **False.** Maternal serum AFP may be raised.
   c. **False.** Spinal NTDs are most common in the lumbosacral region.
   d. **False.** Recurrence rate is less than 5%.
   e. **True.**

9. a. **True.**
   b. **True.**
   c. **False.**
   d. **True.**
   e. **False.** It is associated with Epstein–Barr virus infection in HIV-positive patients.

10. a. **True.** Cardiac mural thrombi are a source of cerebral emboli.
    b. **True.** Embolisation of valve vegetations.
    c. **True.**
    d. **False.**
    e. **True.** Profound hypotension can cause global cerebral ischaemia.

Case histories

Case history 1

1. The symptoms are those of a chronic decline in cognitive function, suggesting dementia. The commonest causes in the UK are Alzheimer's disease and multiple cerebral infarctions. The age of onset in this patient is unusually young for Alzheimer's but certainly does not exclude the diagnosis. A family history of dementia, especially with decreasing age of onset in successive generations, should raise the suspicion of Huntington's disease; a history of movement disorders should also be sought. CJD and nvCJD are very rare conditions (at least currently) and the typical history is of a more rapidly progressive dementia often with psychiatric symptoms and muscle disease (myoclonia or wasting).

2. The history and clinical examination must also include assessment of cerebrovascular and cardiovascular disease (previous strokes, hypertension, atrial fibrillation, etc.). Bear in mind other conditions in which dementia can arise, such as HIV infection.

Case history 2

1. The history raises the suspicion of traumatic injuries, either to the head or the viscera. Catastrophic haemorrhage could have occurred from a ruptured spleen. Acute alcohol intoxication certainly needs to be excluded (post-mortem blood samples for alcohol and drugs would be taken).

2. The history of brief loss of consciousness followed by a 'lucid interval' and the finding of a temporal bone fracture are highly suggestive of extradural haemorrhage. The bleeding is arterial in nature, with origin from a torn middle meningeal artery. At post mortem you would expect to see the extradural haematoma, and if this is the cause of death, there will almost certainly be signs of raised intracranial pressure.

Case history 3

1. The radiological appearances here suggest either an abscess or a tumour (primary or secondary).

2. You should specifically ask about and look for sepsis—either a local infection (middle ear or sinuses) or a distant source of septic embolism (infective endocarditis from congenital heart disease, IV drug abuse, etc.). You must establish whether the patient is immunosuppressed (diabetes, HIV, steroid therapy, organ transplant), which would increase the risk of brain abscess following infection with virulent and opportunistic organisms. Although metastatic tumour is rare in this age group, remember that breast cancer and melanoma in particular can affect young adults and are common tumours to metastasise to the CNS. Primary glial malignancies are most frequently seen in older adults but can present at any age.

Viva answers

Think logically:

- Localising neurological signs of gradual onset—focal weakness or sensory deficit, hearing loss (acoustic neuroma), spinal cord level of dysfunction for intravertebral tumours. Sudden severe neurological deficit may be caused by haemorrhage from the tumour.
- Focal or generalised epilepsy.
- Local mass of tumour +/− oedema causing raised intracranial pressure with headaches and vomiting.
- Remember that primary brain malignancies very rarely metastasise outside the CNS, but some will disseminate along the CSF pathway.
- Remember that some paraneoplastic syndromes occur in the CNS.

Index